Architecture and Health

T0172866

Architecture and Health recognizes the built environment and health as inextricable, encouraging a new mind-set for the profession. Over 40 international award-winning projects are included to explore innovative design principles linked to health outcomes. The book is organized into three interdependent health domains—individual, community, and global—in which each case study proposes context-specific architectural responses. Case studies include children's hospitals, rehabilitation facilities, elderly housing, mental health facilities, cancer support centers, clinics, healthy communities, healthcare campuses, wellness centers, healing gardens, commercial offices, infrastructure for developing countries, sustainable design, and more. Representing the United States, Africa, Asia, Europe, and Australia, each author brings a new perspective to health and its related architectural response.

This book brings a timely focus to a subject matter commonly constricted by normative building practices and transforms the dialogue into one of creativity and innovation. With over 200 color images, this book is an essential read for architects, designers, and students to explore and analyze designed environments that promote health and well-being.

Dina Battisto, BArch, MArch, MS, PhD, is an associate professor of architecture at Clemson University, where she teaches in the graduate Architecture + Health program. Her research and scholarship activities focus on studying relationships between health, healthcare, and the built environment.

Jacob J. Wilhelm works in architectural practice and publication, exploring hospitality, housing, and vernacular solutions for growing mountain and remote regions.

"One of the traps experienced healthcare architects fall into is replicating the status quo. The primary strengths of this book are, firstly, the diversity of ideas and approaches from all over the world force the reader to explore new ideas and approaches. Secondly, the use of case studies takes ideas beyond the conceptual and demonstrates their execution, thereby, helping the reader to understand the applicability to his or her situation. I would highly recommend this book to those who want to step back and reflect on the greater issue of health and environment."

Joyce Durham RN, AIA, EDAC, Director of Facilities
Strategic Planning; New York-Presbyterian

"*Architecture and Health* reflects the broadened identity of both the architecture and health professions: architects now recognize that their responsibilities include the global built environment, while health professionals have begun to embrace global health and well-being as central to their work. The essays in this book also help us understand why that change has happened: both our built environment and our health system are unsustainable, inequitable, and unaffordable in their current form."

Thomas Fisher Professor, School of Architecture; Director,
Minnesota Design Center, University of Minnesota

Architecture and Health

Guiding Principles for Practice

Edited by
Dina Battisto
and
Jacob J. Wilhelm

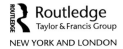

Routledge
Taylor & Francis Group

NEW YORK AND LONDON

First published 2020
by Routledge
52 Vanderbilt Avenue, New York, NY 10017

and by Routledge
2 Park Square, Milton Park, Abingdon, Oxon, OX14 4RN

Routledge is an imprint of the Taylor & Francis Group, an informa business

Library of Congress Cataloging-in-Publication Data
Names: Wilhelm, Jacob J., editor. | Battisto, Dina, editor.
Title: Architecture and health : guiding principles for practice / edited by Jacob J. Wilhelm and Dina Battisto.
Description: New York : Routledge, 2020. | Includes bibliographical references and index. |
Identifiers: LCCN 2019023437 (print) | LCCN 2019023438 (ebook) | ISBN 9780367075217 (hbk) | ISBN 9780367075224 (pbk) | ISBN 9780429021169 (ebk)
Subjects: LCSH: Architecture—Health aspects. | Health facilities—Design and construction. | Hospital buildings—Design and construction. | Environmental health.
Classification: LCC RA967 .A6995 2020 (print) | LCC RA967 (ebook) | DDC 725/.51—dc23
LC record available at https://lccn.loc.gov/2019023437
LC ebook record available at https://lccn.loc.gov/2019023438

ISBN: 978-0-367-07521-7 (hbk)
ISBN: 978-0-367-07522-4 (pbk)
ISBN: 978-0-429-02116-9 (ebk)

Typeset in Avenir
by Apex CoVantage, LLC

Printed in the UK by Severn, Gloucester on responsibly sourced paper

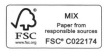

Contents

Foreword — viii

Acknowledgments — ix

Key Terms — x

1. Introduction: Discovering an Architecture for Health — 1

   Dina Battisto and Jacob J. Wilhelm

Part 1 Individual Health

2. Healthcare Facilities for Children: Designing for Distinct Age Groups — 25

   Allen Buie

3. Elderly Autonomy Through Architecture: Building a Fifth-Generation Residential Care Home — 43

   Dietger Wissounig and Birgit Prack

4. Advancing Rehabilitation: Design that Considers Physical and Cognitive Disabilities — 57

   Brenna Costello

5. Design Attributes for Improved Mental and Behavioral Health — 75

   Mardelle McCuskey Shepley and Naomi A. Sachs

6. Renewing the Human Spirit Through Design: Celebrating Maggie's Centres — 98

   Jamie Mitchell

Part 2 Community Health

7. Creating Healthy Communities Through Wellness Districts and Health Campuses — 115

   Shannon Kraus, Kate Renner, Dina Battisto, and Brett Jacobs

8. Superhospitals: The Next Generation of Public Hospitals in Scandinavia — 140

   Klavs Hyttel

9. A Rebirth of the Consolidated Health Campus: The New
   Parkland Hospital   152

   Matthew Suarez and James J. Atkinson

10. Defining a Project Method: Ensuring Project Success
    with Pre-Design Planning   169

    Harm Hollander

11. The Efficacy of Healing Gardens: Integrating Landscape
    Architecture for Health   181

    Katharina Nieberler-Walker, Cheryl Desha,
    Omniya El Baghdadi, and Angela Reeve

12. Lean Design: The Everett Clinic at Smokey Point   196

    Barbara Anderson, Melanie Yaris, and Julia Leitman

13. Employee Wellness: The Dan Abraham Healthy Living
    Center at Mayo Clinic   213

    Peter G. Smith and Stephen N. Berg

14. From Vice to Wellness: Defining a New Typology in
    Healthcare Retail Design   229

    Megan Stone

Part 3 Global Health

15. Outdoor Oncology: A Nature-Inclusive Approach to
    Healthcare Delivery   247

    Bart van der Salm

16. Living Buildings: The Bullitt Center   260

    Steve Doub, Jim Hanford, Margaret Sprug,
    Chris Hellstern, and Katherine Misel

17. Regenerative Architecture: Redefining Progress in the
    Built Environment   280

    Robin Guenther

18. A Blueprint for Using Renewable Energies in
    Remote Locations   296

    Christopher W. Kiss and Keith Holloway

19. Integrating LEED with Biophilic Design Attributes:
    Toward an Inclusive Rating System   311

    Stephen Verderber and Terri Peters

20. Connecting to Context: Place-Based Approaches to
    Biophilic Healthcare Design   328

    Mara Baum

21. The Anti-Prototype: Why Community Health Requires
    Local Solutions   343

    Michael Murphy, Amie Shao, and Jeffrey Mansfield

22. Epilogue: The Future of an Architecture for Health   359

    David Allison, Eva Henrich, and Edzard Schultz

About the Editors   380

List of Contributors   381

Index   393

Foreword

As a book lover, I always eagerly await the arrival of an anticipated release, especially when it occurs in the realm of environmental design for health. Our narrow and emerging field can always benefit from relevant new material. This book, Battisto and Wilhelm's editing of *Architecture and Health: Guiding Principles for Practice*, is just such a long-anticipated volume. Their explorations of design for human health, community health, and global health are each introduced with position statements followed by explanatory case studies from around the world, described by internationally respected authors.

The early premise for a book on healing environments was initiated by Wolfgang F. E. Preiser, a respected pioneer in architectural programming and design research with a doctorate in man-environment relations. Originally a co-editor, along with Battisto and Wilhelm, this title was to add to the extensive collection of publications realized by Preiser until his death in 2016. The adjustments that followed extended the production, but for the editors, this is in many ways an homage to Preiser's robust contributions to the field.

There is an evolving shift in the conceptual framework of architecture for health. The early thinking about research-informed design focused on hospital and clinic architecture, along with long-term care and dementia care. We have been moving away from the understanding that design for health entails only healthcare architecture, and toward the recognition that *every* design may have an impact on health at all levels. We need the work of Battisto, Wilhelm, and their invited authors to help us grasp the extraordinary range of the influence of architecture on health.

How, after all, is architecture for health any different from other types of architecture? Is it important that we identify the differences? One might propose that *all* architecture impacts health in one way or another, and that architecture created in the conscious effort to improve human health may serve a higher purpose.

Here we find Battisto and Wilhelm offering something of a sorely needed practical manifesto to raise our awareness of contemporary thinking related to architecture and health. Health has long been seen as encompassing body (physical or biological health), mind (intellectual health), and spirit (psychological or emotional health). The editors' and authors' perspectives fit nicely with the shift in thinking that recognizes designs to enable and promote health, protect health, and restore injured or failing health. This book explores their new conceptual framework in a form aligned with socio-ecological theory in that its focus progresses from the intimate micro scale of an individual's personal health to groups, systems, and communities, and ultimately to design for global and ecological health in the macro context. The important ideas that shaped the development of this book are now in place and available to all of us. I encourage you to join Battisto and Wilhelm in their challenging exploration of the new and exciting range of ways to think about architecture and health.

D. Kirk Hamilton, PhD, FAIA, FACHA, FCCM
Julie & Craig Beale Professor of Health Facility Design
Texas A&M University, College Station

Acknowledgments

While today not uncommon, working on a publication of this scope from opposite ends of the country brings its challenges. Located in South Carolina (Dina Battisto) and Colorado (Jacob J. Wilhelm), editing consisted of countless emails, phone calls, debates, and discoveries, all on the conversation of architecture and health.

This conversation would not have matured into written word without Wolfgang F. E. Preiser, whose early inspiration for a book on this topic is present at multiple levels. His mentorship and drive provided a springboard for ideas to become actions. His openness to a diverse range of practitioners and academics expanded thinking on who and what could be featured. And it was his ability to bring together diverse voices in the architectural sphere that introduced the two editors and many of their collaborators. It was this spirit that allows the conversation to now be shared with readers of all backgrounds, and contribute to a larger dialogue.

Additional appreciation is due to our plethora of contributing authors, who have shared their time, experience, and insights, allowing for this anthology to have the depth and range needed in professional discourse today. Identified for their inventive work and curiosity toward architecture and health, each author has reached across boundaries of culture, geography, and architecture to make their voice heard. Their collaborative energy and ability to adapt to the evolutions required for timely literature have been invaluable to realizing this book.

A special thanks is given to our publishers at Routledge, who have been instrumental in guiding the delivery and production of this text, including Krystal LaDuc and Julia Pollacco. In addition, thank you to Jennifer Bonnar and her team at Apex CoVantage for their copyedits of the manuscript.

Furthermore, we thank all those who contributed either directly or indirectly to the book, as reviewers, sounding boards, or motivators. This includes our colleagues, students, families, and friends, as well as Brett Jacobs and Xiaowei Li, whose input was greatly valued. The support of all of these individuals allowed the space for long nights of tracked edits, coordination of authors around the globe, image curation, and final touches. Their patience with the demands of publishing is appreciated both during and after print.

Key Terms

Health

A fluctuating state of being that is the summation of multiple determinants, including genetics, lifestyle behaviors, social and economic factors, mental well-being, the physical environment, and access to medical care. To promote health is to support an individual's ability to leverage these determinants for the purpose of improving health and well-being.

Wellness

The optimal state of well-being, encompassing an entire human experience, that stems from maximized physical, mental, and social functioning. In this state, a person feels healthy, happy, and productive; has meaningful and supportive relationships; and has access to healthful environments, programs, and natural resources.

Sickness

A state of being in an unhealthy condition of the body and/or mind that may stem from an illness, injury, or disease.

Individual Health

Individual health refers to the health and well-being of an individual by addressing a person's unique characteristics, behaviors, preferences, and abilities. The built environment can recognize and address these unique characteristics as well as unite individuals with similar sociodemographic and health needs.

Community Health

Community health refers to public health and the welfare of multiple populations organized under shared goals. The built environment, programs, partnerships, and policies aim to promote healthy behaviors and lifestyles, a high quality of life and healthful building practices. "Communities" can encompass businesses, geographic areas, and membership organizations.

Global Health

Global health refers to the general welfare of living organisms and ecosystems worldwide. The built environment that addresses global health recognizes that human civilizations, man-made environments, and policies have consequences intended and unintended that reach beyond a single site.

Salutogenesis

A model of health where programs, services, and environments focus on understanding multiple determinants of health and one's resilience for the purpose of achieving well-being.

Pathogenesis

A model of health where programs, services, and environments focus on understanding the cause of disease for the purpose of treating people who are sick.

Architecture for Health

Architecture for health is a collaborative mind-set and approach used to plan and design built environments for the purpose of promoting, maintaining, and restoring the health and well-being of individuals, communities, and natural ecosystems.

Chapter 1

Introduction
Discovering an Architecture for Health

Dina Battisto and Jacob J. Wilhelm

1.1 Introduction

Architecture and other design disciplines have long lagged behind in driving the social, political, financial, and environmental arguments for creating spaces that promote health and healing. Discoveries in modern medicine, presumably because of their emphasis on measurable outcomes, have ushered in the dominance of the hard sciences over design and the definition of health. After decades, centuries, and even millennia of partial understandings of what health is, we are finally beginning to expand its definition to include well-being, a noticeable shift from an emphasis on "sickness" to "wellness". With the myriad of testing possibilities and big data available to the twenty-first century, and evolved understandings of healthcare practice, architecture can regain agency in its interactions with health in all forms. Accompanying this opportunity is the expectation that the built environment cannot be a passive actor in contributing to the improvement of health. This reinstatement of responsibility warrants new design responses that address a broader view of health, encompassing physical, psychological, emotional, social, and environmental influences.

The purpose of this book is to provide a way forward for those who are interested in understanding how the built environment is connected to this broader view of health. To illustrate this concept, a collection of case studies has been compiled to show how to plan and design environments that contribute to the health of individuals, organizations and communities, and larger natural ecosystems. Each case study explores the intersection of design and health for a diverse range of building types, scales, and contexts.

1.2 Influence of the Built Environment on Health

Studies and public discourse centered on longevity (one of the most cited indicators of health) accurately identify it as the sum of an individual's lifestyle, social context, and more (Buettner 2012). Undoubtedly, factors relating to diet, physical activity, genetics, and access to medicine and technology affect health outcomes. But, as suggested in the seminal paper "We Can Do Better—Improving the Health of the American People", pathways to better health outcomes do not generally depend on better medical care (Schroeder 2007). In fact, the major determinants of health extend far beyond the provision of organized healthcare services, which themselves ironically have been estimated to account for only 10% of health outcomes. By comparison, the largest share contributing to health outcomes is attributed to individual behaviors (40%) and secondly, to social and environmental factors (20%) (McGinnis et al. 2002; Schroeder 2007). When we consider that individual behaviors rely partially on what the social environment affords, it becomes evident that the built environment's contribution to health, insofar as it shapes lifestyle, is highly significant. A comparison of four commonly referenced models that quantify health outcomes as a result of five different determinants shows that between 55% and 80% of overall health is driven by lifestyle behaviors and social/economic factors; between 5% and 20% is driven by environmental exposure, between 10% and 30% is driven by access to healthcare services; and between 10% and 30% is driven by genetics (Figure 1.1).

While the four different models break down health into five determinants, it is not always clear what constitutes each determinant. To help understand these further, a list of factors that commonly align with each is presented in Figure 1.2.

The influence of the built environment on health is vast, yet it is frequently subjugated to other concerns. Of course, healthcare services are essential for treating and curing the sick and will persist. However, it is imperative to broaden our perspective and recognize that biological, social, economic, and environmental factors—and their interrelationships—all contribute to health. Social services, public health programs, and environmental infrastructure, like quality housing, schools, daycare, parks, and even sidewalks and bike lanes, are necessary complements to organized healthcare facilities. A broader perspective of health means we need to think about how to design physical environments in conjunction with programs and services, recognizing that healthcare isn't provided in just one specific setting.

1.3 Healthcare Spending: An Impetus for Change

According to the Centers for Medicare and Medicaid Services, the U.S. channeled 53% of its annual healthcare budget in 2018 to hospital care, and physician and clinical services (Figure 1.3). By comparison, the government spent less than 3% of the healthcare budget on matters pertaining to public health, significantly less than the 10% spent on retail prescription drugs. When you look at spending patterns in relation to health determinants, the misallocation of resources is clear. While we put 3% of our healthcare budget toward the chunk of healthcare determinants that account for 60% of health outcomes, we put 53% of these resources toward organized healthcare services that account for only 10% of health outcomes.

Determinants of health.
Source: Dina Battisto and
Eva Henrich

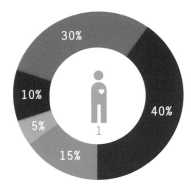

New England Journal of Medicine
Schroeder 2007

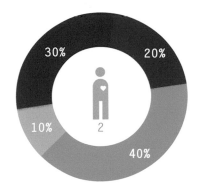

University of Wisconsin
Population Health Institute and Robert
Wood Johnson Foundation
County Health Rankings and Roadmaps, 2019

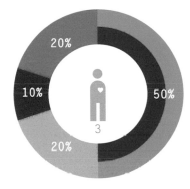

The New England Healthcare Institute
and The Boston Foundation
Hubbard, 2007

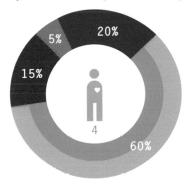

Annals of the New York
Academy of Science
Tarlov 1999
Note: Numbers are estimated

■————— Determinants of Health - 4 Models —————■

Lifestyle Behaviors   Social & Economic Factors   Genetics

 Medical Care   Environmental Exposure

The U.S. spends nearly $10,750 a year on healthcare for each American, accounting for almost 18% of the total gross domestic product (GDP) in 2017 (CMS.gov). Even though the U.S. spends twice the amount compared to other countries on healthcare, we continue to lag on health indicators, such as mortality and life expectancy (OECD). While this huge investment in organized healthcare services reduces mortality rates in the U.S., preventative diseases, such as congestive heart failure, asthma, hypertension, and type II diabetes, are on the

Lifestyle Behaviors
• Diet and nutrition
• Physical activity / exercise
• Substance abuse – i.e. drugs, alcohol consumption, etc.
• Tobacco use and vaping
• Risk-taking behaviors
• Sleep patterns – insufficient sleep
• Sexual activity
• Mental health and coping strategies

Genetics
• Relates to the genes or heredity of a living organism which is transferred from a parent to offspring
• An inherited increase in the risk of developing a disease

Social & Economic Factors
• Family and social support
• Violence and community safety
• Housing instability/homelessness
• Transportation
• Food access and insecurity (hunger and nutrition)
• Education
• Employment and income
• Utility needs
• Childcare and Eldercare

Medical Care
• Access to and quality of healthcare services
• Healthcare insurance
• Healthcare costs - affordability
• Hospital care (i.e. preventive, primary acute, emergency, etc.)
• Professional health services – Primary, specialty, and urgent care
• Other organized healthcare services – residential care, home care, long-term care
• Retail prescription drugs and medical equipment

Environmental Exposure
• Environmental hazards – toxic agents, microbial agents, structural hazards
• Environmental pollutants, air pollution, gases and airborne pollutants
• Chemical contaminants – food, water, commercial products, etc.
• Infectious disease

▲ Figure 1.2

Factors that contribute to the five determinants of health.
Source: Dina Battisto

rise. Moreover, costly chronic conditions are the largest contributors to high hospital admission rates. Many of these preventative diseases are chronic, lasting a lifetime, and are closely tied to individual behaviors and social factors. These

Dina Battisto and Jacob J. Wilhelm

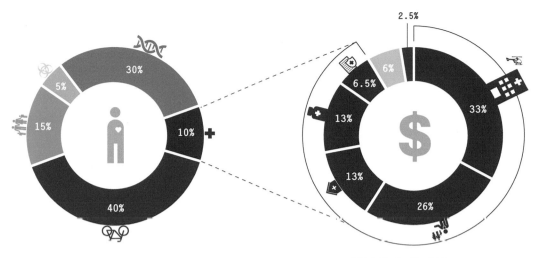

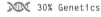

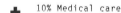

Determinants of Health

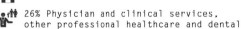

Determinants of Health	2017 U.S. Healthcare Expenditures
40% Lifestyle behaviors	33% Hospital care
30% Genetics	26% Physician and clinical services, other professional healthcare and dental
15% Social and economic factors	13% Other health, residential, home care and long term care
10% Medical care	13% Prescription drugs and medical products
5% Environmental exposure	6.5% Net cost of health insurance
	6% Other-government administration and investment
	2.5% Public health activities

Source: Schroeder, Steven A. "We Can Do Better - Improving The Health Of the American People." *New England Jornal of Medicine* 357, no 12 (2007): 1221-1228

Source: Centers for Medicare and Medicaid Services, Office of Actuary, National Health Statistic Group (2017)

▲ Figure 1.3

U.S. healthcare spending in relation to health determinants.
Source: Dina Battisto and Eva Henrich

preventative diseases, and the costs associated with treating them, could be curbed with health promotion efforts and better designed environments.

In tandem with health status, well-being is the root of a person's happiness. According to the World Happiness Report, which is a global ranking of happiness levels across 156 countries, the United States is not even in the top ten. As of 2019 the U.S. ranks nineteenth and has continued to drop in rankings over the last two years. Jeffrey Sachs, Columbia University professor and director of the Center for Sustainable Development, provides an explanation claiming "America's subjective

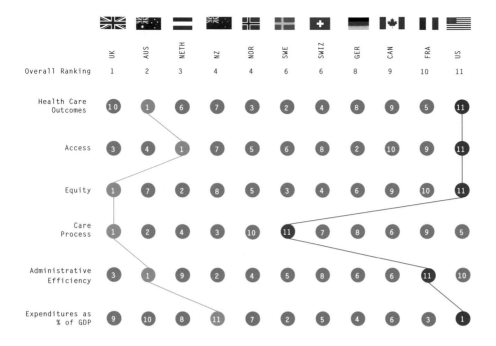

	UK	AUS	NETH	NZ	NOR	SWE	SWIZ	GER	CAN	FRA	US
Overall Ranking	1	2	3	4	4	6	6	8	9	10	11
Health Care Outcomes	10	1	6	7	3	2	4	8	9	5	11
Access	3	4	1	7	5	6	8	2	10	9	11
Equity	1	7	2	8	5	3	4	6	9	10	11
Care Process	1	2	4	3	10	11	7	8	6	9	5
Administrative Efficiency	3	1	9	2	4	5	8	6	6	11	10
Expenditures as % of GDP	9	10	8	11	7	2	5	4	6	3	1

Source: Adapted from Exhibit 2 in Schneider, Eric C., D. O. Sarnak, D. Squires, A. Shah, and M. M. Doty. "Mirror, Mirror 2017: International Comparison Reflects Flaws and Opportunities for Better US Health Care." The Commonwealth Fund, July 2017

Rankings based on 2014 data

▲ Figure 1.4

Healthcare system performance rankings.
Source: Dina Battisto and Eva Henrich

well-being is being systematically undermined by three interrelated epidemic diseases, notably obesity, substance abuse (especially opioid addiction), and depression" (Sachs 2018, p. 147). When you look at the top-ranking countries, like Finland, Denmark, Switzerland, and Canada, you see they perform noticeably well in six key variables: "income (GDP per capita), healthy life expectancy, social support, freedom, trust (absence of corruption), and generosity" (Helliwell, Layard, and Sachs 2019, p. 22). Five of these six variables address dimensions of health beyond organized medical care. Clearly, we in the U.S. are missing something.

1.4 Models of Health and Their Architectural Response: A Brief Retrospective

An examination of the past helps reveal how we've veered so far off course in pinpointing a formula for better health outcomes. Different eras have addressed

► Figure 1.5

Healthcare spending as a percentage of GDP, 1980–2014.
Source: Dina Battisto and Eva Henrich

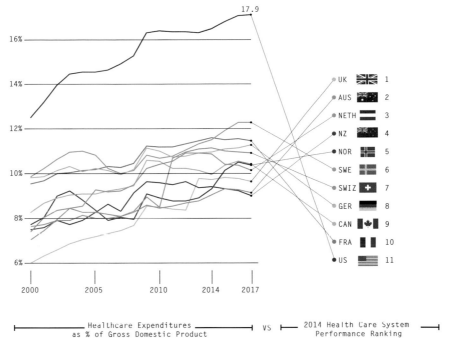

Source:: The Organisation for Economic Co-operation and Development (OECD) Data accessed 07 Feb 2019

Source: Adapted from Exhibit 1 in Schneider, Eric C., D. O. Sarnak, D. Squires, A. Shah, and M. M. Doty. "Mirror, Mirror 2017: International Comparison Reflects Flaws and Opportunities for Better US Health Care." The Commonwealth Fund, July 2017

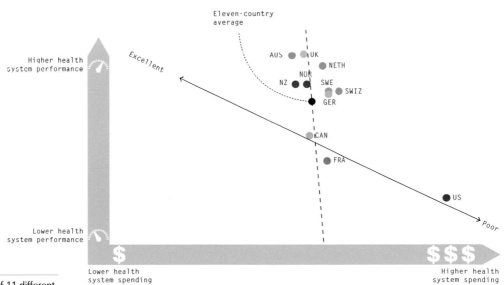

► Figure 1.6

Performance of 11 different healthcare systems in relation to spending.
Source: Dina Battisto and Eva Henrich

Source: Adapted from Exhibit 5 in Schneider, Eric C., D. O. Sarnak, D. Squires, A. Shah, and M. M. Doty. "Mirror, Mirror 2017: International Comparison Reflects Flaws and Opportunities for Better US Health Care." The Commonwealth Fund, July 2017

Rankings based on 2014 data

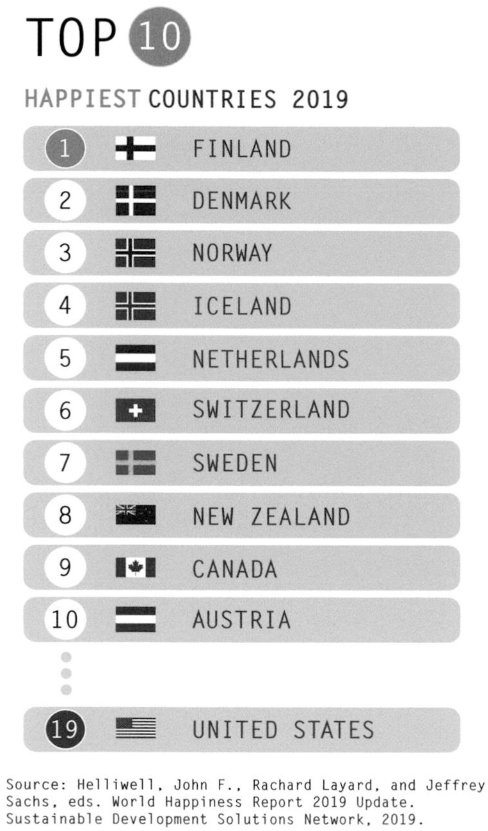

◀ Figure 1.7

World happiness rankings, 2019.
Source: Dina Battisto and Eva Henrich

TOP ⑩

HAPPIEST COUNTRIES 2019

①	✛	FINLAND
2	✚	DENMARK
3	✚	NORWAY
4	✚	ICELAND
5	▬	NETHERLANDS
6	✚	SWITZERLAND
7	≡	SWEDEN
8	※	NEW ZEALAND
9	❖	CANADA
10	▬	AUSTRIA
⑲	☰	UNITED STATES

Source: Helliwell, John F., Rachard Layard, and Jeffrey
Sachs, eds. World Happiness Report 2019 Update.
Sustainable Development Solutions Network, 2019.

health in unique ways, using architecture to varying degrees and effectiveness. Within the beliefs and motivations of a given era, a model of health describes the method in which health services are delivered. Models of health, whether salutogenic or pathogenic in nature, lead to architectural responses that serve as precedent in improving the health and welfare of populations.

1.4.1 Salutogenesis: Ancient Civilizations and Civic Wellness

All timelines tracking a focused and concerted effort to care for the needs of humans begin with ayurvedic approaches, recognized today as healthcare. Some historians have traced what is considered to be the first deliberate creation of space for the purpose of caring for individuals as existing through the ayurvedic tradition (Rannan-Eliya and De Mel 1997). Chinese medicine, evolving in Asia some centuries later, combined similar uses of herbs and rituals to balance the body, and likewise was passed along through tradition and scattered practices.

While many of these ancient systems are today largely considered pseudoscientific and at best among the protosciences, it is important to note the emphasis they all had on a holistic view of health that included physical, social, mental, and spiritual health. Greek cities, like Epidaurus, included a mix of wellness-oriented programs in therapeutic surroundings: a library

Dina Battisto and Jacob J. Wilhelm

for intellectual pursuits, a theater for entertainment and social interactions, a gymnasium for exercise and fitness, and healing temples for connecting to the gods. In all cases, a clear link is made between health and architecture: healing occurs in places of spiritual sanctity as well as in daily life, whether that be in monumental sanctuaries or socially active baths and markets (Thompson and Goldin 1975).

These approaches to health are closely tied to salutogenesis, a concept later defined by the sociologist Aaron Antonovsky in 1979 in his book *Health, Stress and Coping*. The end goal of salutogenesis is to achieve a state of wellness, or optimal health, by harnessing people's resources and their capacity to move toward health. Seen from a preventative health orientation, it utilizes the interrelated physical, mental, social, and spiritual resources needed to achieve wellness, rather than simply reacting to disease.

1.4.2 Pathogenesis: Miasma Theory, Germ Theory, and Modern Medicine

Many physicians maintained a belief in systems developed during ancient times, yet fused their beliefs with emergent "scientific" revelations. The miasma theory, or belief that disease was spread by airborne means from "bad air", exemplifies a model of health that spanned many cultural systems and geographic locations. This medical theory is perhaps the most prescient in terms of its connection between health and the environment. For centuries, the miasma theory would persist, informing design decisions of urban environments, landscapes, buildings, and approaches to healthcare. While the miasma theory, like the germ theory, viewed health from a pathogenic (reactive/treatment-based) worldview, its priorities were entirely different. In the era of miasma, environmental strategies were believed to be effective in treating sickness. However, when the germ theory became widespread, environmental factors got left behind in favor of a narrower, biomedical approach to health.

1.4.2.1 Pathogenesis: Pre-modern Medicine Era and the Miasma Theory

Halting the spread of contagion was forefront in the minds of the public as epidemics, such as the bubonic plague, devastated Europe in the fourteenth century (Loudon 1997). As a result, this conception of pathogenesis prescribed the exile of the ill, leading to the beginnings of a public health system and quarantine laws. Gradually as correlations between the environment and sickness became clear, plague hospitals, pest houses, lazarettos, and leprosaria isolated the sick with outward symptoms. The floorplans and exteriors of these buildings often manifest this isolation, while simultaneously expressing the system (often religious) that they were built within. At both the urban and building scales, architectural thinking was guided by a desire to counteract miasmas.

Urban design projects like Haussmann's renovation of Paris in the mid-nineteenth century show a visible connection to miasma theory. Boulevards and avenues were planned to create pedestrian-centric streetscapes; parks and squares were designed to bring fresh air and sunlight into the center of the city; and new public infrastructure, including sewers, fountains, and aqueducts, transformed the supply of clean water and waste management.

At the building scale, new typologies that embodied evolving perspectives on treatment, sanitation, and mental health began to reinterpret existing models in more specialized ways by health reformers, including Florence Nightingale and Thomas Kirkbride. Nightingale, credited as the founder of modern nursing, advocated for a pavilion plan concept to combat miasmas. With separate, low-height structures connected by external breezeways, pavilions allowed for isolation of patients by illness. Furthermore, separate buildings enabled windows on multiple sides of nursing wards, providing patients with access to plenty of sunlight, fresh air from cross ventilation, and visual and physical connections to the outdoors. Access to sunlight, fresh air, views, and nature was documented and celebrated for its sanitizing and therapeutic effects (Nightingale 1969). Similar strategies were applied in the Kirkbride plan, which grew in popularity as a more humanitarian alternative to the century's prevalent criminalization of mental health through asylum architecture. Drawing from the philosophies of moral treatment and environmental determinism, Thomas Kirkbride pushed to humanize mental health institutions (Kirkbride 1880). While the primary drivers and overall translations into architecture for each reformer were different, both Nightingale and Kirkbride understood the role of the environment in contributing to patient health.

1.4.2.2 Pathogenesis: Modern Medicine Era and the Germ Theory

Following the Enlightenment and its associated advancements in the hard sciences during the seventeenth and eighteenth centuries, a true shift in healthcare took place (Cunningham and French 1990). The rational, neoclassical architecture of this period was the foundation of later movements in that it redefined the architectural tradition as born from the sciences as opposed to non-measurable factors. After acceptance of the germ theory, there was a burst of scientific activity that solidified pharmacology, or the broader pathogenics, as a more effective model of health (Loudon 1997). Discoveries like vaccinations, antibiotics, antiseptics, and X-rays collectively fueled a momentum that positioned science as the panacea through which illness could be cured. Some facilities, like the Paimio Sanatorium (1929), designed by Finnish architect Alvar Aalto, were designed according to modernist tenets still anchored to the miasma theory. Aalto claimed "the main purpose of the building is to function as a medical instrument" (Woodman 2016), but physicians had already long outpaced architects in the healthcare hierarchy. As soon as the drug streptomycin was discovered and proven effective on mycobacterium tuberculosis in the late 1940s, the approach to caring for those with tuberculosis changed dramatically, another marked shift away from treating disease with edits to the environment.

Hospitals and related healthcare typologies served as laboratories for the experimentation of medical treatments, the development of new clinical technologies, and the delivery of coordinated healthcare services. It is this iteration of pathogenesis that has become the primary driver in shaping the modern hospital, medical school education, medical insurance reimbursement models,

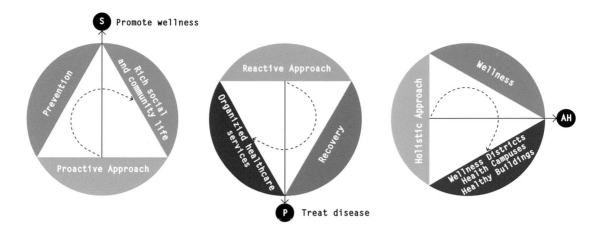

▲ Figure 1.8

Three models of health.
Source: Dina Battisto and Eva Henrich

governmental program allocations, and the priority of healthcare providers. Current connotations of "healthcare architecture" exhibit this scientific response to disease. "Healthcare architecture" and large institutions have become symbols of scientific power housing state-of-the-art technologies. Federal funding programs, like the National Institutes of Health (NIH) and National Science Foundation (NSF), reinforce this reactive approach by allocating resources to treatment-oriented studies. Under this reactionary mind-set, "built healthcare environments" serve merely as the backdrop for modern medicine.

1.5 A Path Forward: An Architecture for Health

At this point in history, it would appear the pendulum has swung too far toward the science of medicine, away from past precedents of holistic health. The physical, social, and emotional needs of humans have always been intertwined and nonlinear in their influence over architecture. In the past these needs were largely provided by systems of religion and spirituality, which continued to affect the motivations behind architecture in the twentieth century (Hejduk and Williamson 2011). Further proof lies in the West's resurgence of interest in Eastern medicine and homeopathic remedies as a continually developing field, showing social, emotional, and spiritual needs running in parallel with physical needs. These necessities have been met with varying levels of success through different architectural movements, but this reality has been made clear: Architecture has been embedded in both salutogenic and pathogenic models of health throughout history.

A new era is upon us that warrants a renewed purpose. The integration of pathogenic and salutogenic models of health is becoming more important as

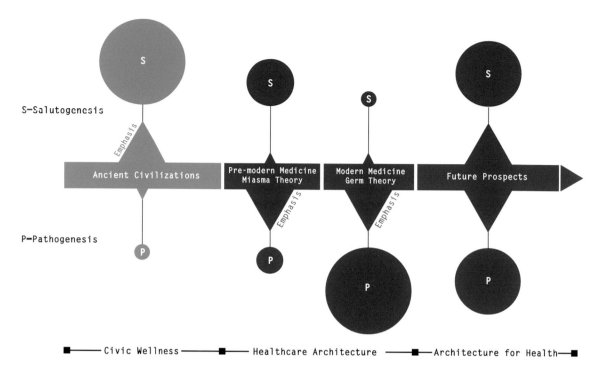

S—Salutogenesis

P—Pathogenesis

Ancient Civilizations

Pre-modern Medicine
Miasma Theory

Modern Medicine
Germ Theory

Future Prospects

Emphasis

■———Civic Wellness————■——— Healthcare Architecture ———■—Architecture for Health—■

▲ Figure 1.9

Timeline of architecture and health eras.
Source: Dina Battisto and Eva Henrich

the present state of healthcare becomes less and less sustainable. Perhaps moving resources upstream by designing environments and programs that promote healthy lifestyles can mitigate the need for greater resources downstream. With more attention to promote wellness on the front end, we can reduce the need to treat sickness on the back end.

Rather than creating "healthcare architecture", we must create "architecture for health". This is no mere semantic discrepancy. Instead, it represents two entirely different schools of thought. "Healthcare architecture" is a specialty area in architecture for the care of the sick, whereas "architecture for health" is an attitude, a mind-set. While "healthcare architecture" attempts to heal sick people with an emphasis on pathogenesis, "architecture for health" attempts to promote wellness through salutogenesis as well as cure diseases through pathogenesis (Figure 1.9). Interestingly, this shift represents a paradigmatic difference in what the intent of architecture should and arguably must be. Architecture for health should not be a niche subject. It should be part of every conversation on architecture.

1.6 Three Domains of an Architecture for Health

As our understanding of the diverse determinants of health expands, our architectural responses must also evolve. Using case study projects from around the world, this book attempts to kick-start the process of rethinking the relationship

Dina Battisto and Jacob J. Wilhelm

Three domains of an
architecture for health.
Source: Dina Battisto and Eva
Henrich

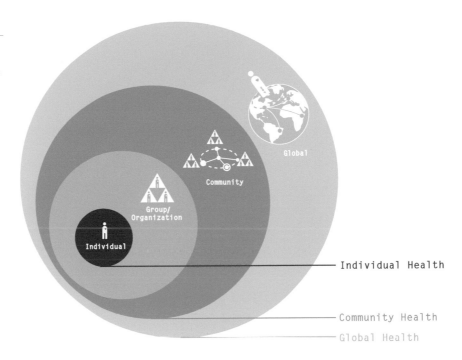

between architecture and health in such a way that it more accurately reflects the
contemporary understanding that health is not merely the absence of disease
but is instead the promotion of wellness. Along these lines, various domains of
consideration are defined. This book is divided into architectural responses to
three domains: health for definable population groups at the level of the individual; health for organizations and communities made of multiple and diverse
groups; and finally, global health viewed from the macro lens of societal and
ecological wellness.

The definitions for these domains are defined here:

1. Individual Health
   Groups (G) equal the sum of individuals (I) with common health characteristics
   $G = \sum I$
2. Community Health
   Communities (C) equal the sum of groups (G)
   $C = \sum G$
3. Global Health
   Ecosystems (E) equal the sum of communities (C)
   $E = \sum C$

Each domain provides a filter to understand how to design an architecture for
health through spaces, buildings, campuses, communities, and larger ecosystems. While each domain provides a unifying theme following a broad approach
to health, each chapter has different goals and solutions. With clearly stated
goals, we have a means of evaluating architecture.

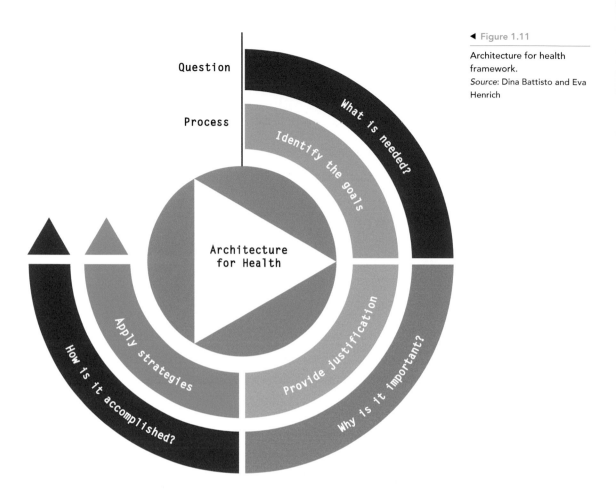

◀ Figure 1.11

Architecture for health
framework.
Source: Dina Battisto and Eva
Henrich

Question

Process

What is needed?

Identify the goals

Architecture
for Health

Apply strategies

How is it accomplished?

Provide justification

Why is it important?

1.6.1 Individual Health

The first domain is based on the belief that the design of built environments
should elevate the health of individuals. As such, this domain focuses on planning and designing buildings, spaces, and landscapes for individuals who are
defined by a social group with similar characteristics and health needs. To
improve the health of individuals, it is important to observe and understand
the patterns of behaviors, needs, preferences, and distinguishing characteristics of individuals defined by a group. This can be achieved through a variety
of ways, from observations and interviews to a review of existing literature
and data sources. Despite differences, there are some commonalities across
groups like children, the elderly, and people with mental illness, physical disabilities, and cancer. Case studies have been selected to show how architecture takes a personalized approach to address the needs and characteristics
of these groups. The goals in each project case study are interpreted into
actionable design strategies and specific design solutions based on project
requirements, constraints, and context. Table 1.1 displays a breakdown of the
populations covered in the first domain and an overview of each corresponding chapter.

Table 1.1 Overview of individual health domain

Chapter	Population	Characteristics	Design intent
2	Children	Dependent on family Need stimulation (education, play, socialization) Developing Confused, fearful, possibly traumatized Angry, possibly impulsive Self-conscious	Design of a hospital that considers children of all ages, along with their specific needs for play, education, and family support
3	Elderly	Deteriorating physical and cognitive health Fragile Socially isolated May be financially vulnerable Loss of autonomy	Design of a residential care model for seniors with deteriorating cognitive health due to dementia that supports autonomous living
4	People with physical or cognitive disabilities	Physical limitations May be psychologically distressed Self-conscious Socially isolated May be dependent on others	Design of rehabilitation centers to help people manage the physical, cognitive, and social challenges of living with debilitating illness post-injury or trauma
5	People with mental or behavioral health challenges	Diverse, non-homogenous group Human needs are exaggerated Vulnerable, stigmatized or perceived as outcasts or "other" Loss of autonomy Anxious and or depressed Frequently self medicating Reactive aggression possible	Design of inpatient and outpatient settings tailored around the needs of people who suffer from mental illness or behavioral health issues
6	People living with cancer	Sudden devastation; crisis Life-altering Lost, vulnerable, and at risk Scared, alone, and isolated Fear the unknown	Design of multiple cancer support centers providing a comprehensive program of nonclinical support activities for people and families affected by cancer within a domestic environment

Source: Dina Battisto and Jacob J. Wilhelm

1.6.2 Community Health

The second domain focuses on designing built environments for multiple groups of people with a goal of improving occupant well-being, promoting public health, and preventing chronic diseases for a defined community. Grouping individuals based on shared beliefs, principles, or goals establishes them as part of a larger organization or community. The stakeholder group, whether a business, health-care provider, religious group, or nonprofit agency, needs to strive for optimal health to continue functioning at full capacity and efficiency. Members of these groups largely join by choice, as they are gaining something of value by being a part of a larger group. To provide this value, organizations need to continually ask themselves how their practices, programs, and environments influence the health of the groups they serve. Buildings designed for organizational and community health can encourage participation of its members, whether they are employees, donors, or patients, to live healthier lives. Ideally, architecture that understands organizational and community health can lead to longevity for the specific organization or group, improving it over time.

Recognizing this, health provider organizations are starting to think beyond the walls of their hospitals and satellite healthcare facilities to consider "health campuses" and "wellness districts". They are offering services beyond medical care, like fitness programs, health fairs, farmers markets and grocery deliveries in food desert areas, educational programs on nutrition, and access to transportation for doctor visits (Pollack et al. 2019). Hospitals are also screening for social determinants, like housing quality, family and social support, violence in the home, education, and income to gain a more complete understanding of the factors influencing health outcomes (Lee and Korba 2017).

Case studies have been selected to show how architecture has the power to elevate organizations and communities. Table 1.2 displays a breakdown of the chapters covered in the second domain, the stakeholders involved, and an overview of each chapter.

1.6.3 Global/Ecological Health

The third domain focuses on how to design built environments across multiple communities with the understanding that our actions affect more than just ourselves. The role of the built environment in protecting, preserving, and improving the natural environment is an overpublished yet seldom actionable objective of many projects today. The world in which we live is a constellation of integrated systems, a network, supporting a circle of life that consists of several codependent living organisms and ecosystems. Built environments consume an enormous amount of nonrenewable resources from our finite supply, contribute to deforestation and climate change, and force ecological disruptions and possible extinctions. Buildings are large consumers of fossil fuel energies that contribute to the greenhouse gases that have been known to affect ecosystems, biodiversity, and human welfare (USGBC 2008). These realities solicit all new and existing buildings to consider global health by clearly identifying what issues a project can confront and then apply relevant design strategies in response.

New programs and advocacy groups are tackling the macro problems caused by man-made developments. Programs like LEED, BREAM, WELL Building, and Living Building Challenge all have established criteria for measuring sustainability and health. Now that we have entered the twenty-first century, architects are moving beyond their past notions of what is "green". Concepts for living buildings, regenerative architecture, biomimetic design, and biophilic design are imposing new demands on projects. Impacts from buildings and

Dina Battisto and Jacob J. Wilhelm

Table 1.2 Overview of community health domain

Chapter	Stakeholder	Characteristics	Design intent
7	Multiple stakeholders (USA)	Nonprofit public health systems, community groups, nonprofit organizations and investors	Creating health campuses or wellness districts through master planning to improve public health
8	Danish Health Authority (Aarhus, Denmark)	Public university hospital supported by the Ministry of Health	Creating a model for a public university hospital that centralizes healthcare services on a campus to express the community's values of democracy, access, and transparency
9	Parkland Hospital (Dallas, Texas, USA)	Public health system	Creating a large-scale health campus that serves as a community anchor by providing state-of-the-art healthcare services, encouraging healthy lifestyles, and improving access to care
10	Queensland Children's Hospital (Queensland, Australia)	A public hospital supported by the Australian government	Creating a project vision for a large-scale, public hospital for children that is integrated into the urban fabric
11	Queensland Children's Hospital (Queensland, Australia)	A public hospital supported by the Australian government	Creating a series of distinct healing gardens as therapeutic interventions in hospitals for patients and their families
12	The Everett Clinic (Smokey Point, Washington, USA)	Physician-owned private group offering primary and specialty healthcare services	Creating a new prototype for a multi-specialty clinic that uses Lean methodologies to streamline care and enhance the patient experience
13	Mayo Clinic (Rochester, Minnesota, USA)	Nonprofit academic medical center focused on integrated clinical practice, education, and research	Creating a healthy living center to improve the health and wellness of employees working in the healthcare system, their families, and the surrounding community
14	Private business owners (multiple locations, USA)	Individual retailers	Creating medical and recreational cannabis retail locations that consider patient health, education, safety, and the cultural impacts of design

Source: Dina Battisto and Jacob J. Wilhelm

landscapes are felt much longer than their intended function, potentially compromising the health and well-being of future generations.

For this domain, case studies have been selected to show how architecture is approached beyond the scope of the project itself, conscious of the global context that is home to us all. Table 1.3 displays a breakdown of the chapters covered in the third domain, the stakeholders involved, and an overview of each chapter.

Table 1.3 Overview of global health domain

Chapter	Stakeholder	Characteristics	Design intent
15	Tergooi Hospital (Hilversum, Netherlands)	Dutch healthcare system	Creating an opportunity to receive chemotherapy treatment outdoors with respect to native ecosystems
16	Bullitt Foundation (Seattle, Washington, USA)	Environmental nonprofit organization	Creating a new approach to human ecology through the concept of a living building; Bullitt Center has been claimed to be the greenest commercial building in the world
17	Various case studies (multiple locations, USA)	Varies	Creating buildings, whether for private, for-profit businesses or for healthcare organizations, that incorporate regenerative design principles for a more restorative built environment
18	United States Military Health System	U.S. government–operated military hospitals and installations for training soldiers	Creating self-sufficient hospitals in remote or rural regions that incorporate principles of energy conservation, environmental sustainability, and economic viability
19	Residential care providers (multiple locations, North America)	Varies	Creating a composite environmental sustainability-biophilia scoring system for residential facilities for the elderly
20	Eskenazi Health Main Campus, (Indianapolis, Indiana, USA); Ng Teng Fong General Hospital & Jurong Community Hospital (Singapore)	Public health systems	Creating hospitals that are responsive to climate, context, and cultural expectations of patients
21	Redemption Hospital (Caldwell, Liberia); African Center for Excellence in Infectious Diseases (Ide, Nigeria)	Humanitarian-focused organizations and infrastructure	Creating context-specific solutions beyond the universal prototype to improve public health in developing areas where access to organized healthcare is scarce

Source: Dina Battisto and Jacob J. Wilhelm

1.7 Conclusions

An architect has cultural, social, and political agency through the medium of architecture. Each chapter of this text demonstrates a use of this medium that exercises this agency in one of the three presented domains of individual health, community health, and global/ecological health. It is important to note that while the strategies presented cannot always feasibly be executed simultaneously, they do not necessarily compete in terms of priority or inclusion. Rather, a combination of strategies or recommendations from multiple authors may be amalgamated into a new design framework for any future project. It's in this vein that each chapter becomes like a tool on the designer's toolbelt: a loose prescription of strategies that may apply to the project at hand. Ideally, however, any built work can benefit from perspectives at each level or domain presented, creating a holistic way to provide better health outcomes.

As Norman Foster said, "Architecture is an expression of values—the way we build is a reflection of the way we live" (Rosenfield 2014). Many people are drawn to architecture as a pathway to make the world a better place. If architects were only craftsmen, concerned only with formal, material, and spatial explorations, we would lose perhaps the most valuable of our responsibilities—the responsibility to help people. Designers give shape to reality, and while we can choose to acknowledge this in its full complexity, it remains true that our collective decisions influence the health of not only individuals but also communities and ecosystems. This responsibility is too great to not take seriously.

Bibliography

Antonovsky, Aaron. *Health, Stress, and Coping*. San Francisco, CA: Jossey-Bass, 1979.

Buettner, Dan. *The Blue Zones: 9 Lessons for Living Longer from the People Who've Lived the Longest*. Washington, DC: National Geographic Society, 2012.

Centers for Medicare and Medicaid Services, and Centers for Medicare and Medicaid Services. "NHE Fact Sheet." Washington, DC: CMS, 2017. www.cms.gov/research-statistics-data-and-systems/statistics-trends-and-reports/nationalhealthexpenddata/nhe-fact-sheet.html.

Cunningham, Andrew, and Roger French, eds. *The Medical Enlightenment of the Eighteenth Century*. Cambridge: Cambridge University Press, 1990.

Dilani, Alan. "A New Paradigm of Design and Health in Hospital Planning." *World Hospitals and Health Services: The Official Journal of the International Hospital Federation* 41, no. 4 (2005): 17–21.

Givens, Marjory, Keith Gennuso, Amanda Jovaag, Julie W Van Dijk, and Sheri Johnson. *County Health Rankings: Key Findings 2019*. University of Wisconsin Population Health Institute, 2019. www.countyhealthrankings.org/reports/2019-county-health-rankings-key-findings-report.

Hejduk, Renata J., and James Williamson, eds. *The Religious Imagination in Modern and Contemporary Architecture: A Reader*. New York: Routledge, 2011.

Helliwell, John F., Peter R. Layard, and Jefferey D. Sachs. *World Happiness Report 2019*. New York: Sustainable Development Solutions Network, 2019. Last modified March 20, 2019. https://worldhappiness.report/ed/2019/.

Hubbard, Thomas. *The Boston Paradox: Lots of Health Care, Not Enough Health*. Boston Foundation and the New England Healthcare Institute, June 2007. www.tbf.org/tbf/56/hphe/~/media/BBCC5400440E4D14A8ADCE51D3F45CDC.pdf.

Kirkbride, Thomas Story. *On the Construction, Organization, and General Arrangements of Hospitals for the Insane: With Some Remarks on Insanity and Its Treatment*. Philadelphia: J. B. Lippincott, 1880.

Lee, Josh, and Korba Casey. *Social Determinants of Health: How are Hospitals and Health Systems Investing in and Addressing Social Needs?* New York: Deloitte Center for Health Solutions, 2017. www2. deloitte. com/content/dam/Deloitte/us/Documents/noindex/us-lshc-addressing-social-determinants-of-health.pdf.

Loudon, Irvine, ed. *Western Medicine: An Illustrated History*. New York: Oxford University Press, 1997.

Martin, Anne B., Micah Hartman, Benjamin Washington, Aaron Catlin, and National Health Expenditure Accounts Team. "National Health Care Spending in 2017: Growth Slows to Post—Great Recession Rates: Share of GDP Stabilizes." *Health Affairs* 38, no.1 (2018): 10–1377. www.healthaffairs.org/doi/10.1377/hlthaff.2018.05085.

McGinnis, J. Michael, and William H. Foege. "Actual Causes of Death in The United States." *JAMA* 270, no. 18 (1993): 2207–2212. www.healthaffairs.org/doi/full/10.1377/hlthaff.21.2.78.

McGinnis, J. Michael, Pamela Williams-Russo, and James R. Knickman. "The Case for More Active Policy Attention to Health Promotion." *Health Affairs* 21, no. 2(2002): 78–93.

Nightingale, Florence, 1820–1910. *Notes on Nursing: What It Is, and What It Is Not*. New York: Dover Publications,1969.

OECD. 2017. "Health at a Glance 2017." https://doi.org///doi.org/10.1787/health_glance-2017-en.

Organisation for Economic Co-operation and Development (OECD). www.oecd.org/.

Pollack, Rick, Brian Gragnolati, Nancy Howell Agee, and Eugene A. Woods. "2019 Environmental Scan. Report." *American Hospital Association, 2019*. www.aha.org/center/emerging-issues/market-insights/year-in-review/2019-environmental-scan-innovation-and-coordination.

"Press: Benefits of Green Building." *USGBC*. https://new.usgbc.org/press/benefits-of-green-building.

Rannan-Eliya, Ravi P., and Nishan De Mel. "Resource Mobilization in Sri Lanka's Health Sector." *Harvard School of Public Health & Health Policy Programme, Institute of Policy Studies* (1997): 19.

Rosenfield, Karissa. "Norman Foster's Interview with the European: Architecture is the Expression of Values." *ArchDaily*. October 31, 2014. https://www.archdaily.com/563537/interview-norman-foster-on-the-role-of-architecture-in-modern-society.

Sachs, Jeffrey D. "Chapter 7: Americas Health Crisis and the Easterlin Paradox." In *World Happiness Report 2018*, edited by John F. Helliwell, Peter R. Layard, and Jefferey D. Sachs, 146–159. New York: Sustainable Development Solutions Network, 2018.

Schneider, Eric C., D. O. Sarnak, D. Squires, A. Shah, and M. M. Doty. *Mirror, Mirror 2017: International Comparison Reflects Flaws and Opportunities for Better US Health Care*. The Commonwealth Fund, July 2017 (2017): 1532121939–394285837. https://interactives.commonwealthfund.org/2017/july/mirror-mirror/.

Schroeder, Steven A. "We Can Do Better—Improving the Health of the American People." *New England Journal of Medicine* 357, no. 12 (2007): 1221–1228.

Tarlov, Alvin R. "Public Policy Frameworks for Improving Population Health." *Annals of the New York Academy of Sciences* 896, no. 1(1999): 281–293.

Thompson, John D., and Grace Goldin. *The Hospital: A Social and Architectural History*. New Haven: Yale University Press, 1975.

U.S. Green Building Council Inc. (USGBC). *Buildings and Climate Change*, 2008. www. eesi.org/files/climate.pdf.

U.S. Green Building Council Inc. (USGBC). *Green Buildings for Cool Cities: A Guide for Advancing Local Green Building Policies*, 2011. www.usgbc.org/sites/default/files/ GreenBuildingsGreenCities.pdf.

Woodman, Ellis. "Revisit: 'Aalto's Paimio Sanatorium Continues to Radiate a Profound Sense of Human Empathy'." *The Architectural Review*, November 17, 2016. www. architectural-review.com/buildings/revisit-aaltos-paimio-sanatorium-continues-to-radiate-a-profound-sense-of-human-empathy/10014811.article.

Part 1 | **Individual Health**

This domain is based on the belief that the design of architectural settings should elevate the health of individuals defined by a social group with similar characteristics and health needs. As such, designed environments address the health needs of identifiable groups, such as children, the elderly, and people living with mental illness, physical disabilities, or cancer. Case studies selected show how architecture must take a tailored approach to address the needs of a specific population.

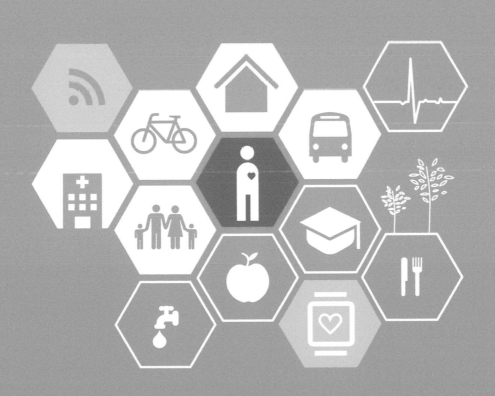

Chapter 2

Healthcare Facilities for Children
Designing for Distinct Age Groups

Allen Buie

2.1 Introduction

Pediatric healthcare facilities must respond to the unique medical, social, and emotional needs of children of all ages and their families. All too often, healthcare services for children are fragmented in different locations and are provided by different caregivers, resulting in challenging experiences for children and their families. While basic organizational concepts for "adult" hospitals apply to children's hospitals, there are distinct needs that have to be recognized when the primary user group is children: children need to play, socialize, and continue to learn, and deserve a healthcare environment that can support these functions.

2.2 A Varied Patient Population With Complex Needs

Time in the hospital can significantly disrupt children's development by interfering with their ability to play, learn, and grow through the same means as their peers not undergoing treatment. Typically, specialized outpatient clinics and inpatient units are dedicated to different patient types and respond to their specific needs for diagnosis, treatment, and therapy. Complex medical issues that are commonly treated in children's hospitals include:

- Congenital issues, such as heart defects
- Respiratory issues, such as asthma and bronchiolitis
- Neurological issues, including cerebral palsy and seizures
- Blood disorders, such as sickle cell anemia
- Childhood cancers

While a children's hospital may treat a range of conditions, it is important to recognize that children are not a homogenous group and have distinct needs according to age. The pediatric population ranges from newborns to teenagers and can extend to patients in their early twenties depending on diagnosis and treatment. Children at each stage of development perceive their environment differently, communicate differently, and are still growing physically, cognitively, and emotionally. For example, babies may not have conscious awareness of their surroundings or need spaces for socialization, but are sensitive to light, temperature, and noise. Young children can be fearful and confused by what's happening to them, while teenagers can have anger, self-consciousness, or even a sense of invincibility. Young children need spaces dedicated to playing and learning in addition to private space. Teenagers need privacy, but also enjoy spaces that allow them to socialize with peers. Important for both populations is maintaining a sense of connection with their world outside of the hospital in addition to the sense of community they build within the hospital. A brief summary of these particular considerations can be found in Figure 2.1.

In addition to age-specific needs, pediatric inpatient stays are often longer in duration and can be repetitive, meaning that many patients return to the same team over an extended period of time, whether at the same location or across specialized facilities. Hospitals can provide a less fragmented experience with appropriate staff, technology, and settings that allow children to stay connected and continue schooling remotely.

AGE RANGE	CHARACTERISTICS
INFANTS 0 - 18 MONTHS	Newborns not conscious of surroundings Sensitive to light and temperature
TODDLERS 1 - 3 YEARS	Fear separation from parents Fear of being hurt Desire to explore environment
PRESCHOOL 3 - 6 YEARS	Regression Fear pain, blood, etc. Aggresive responses
SCHOOL AGE 6 - 12 YEARS	Fear loss of control, pain, and death Bodily harm concerns Understand effects of treatments
ADOLESCENT 12 - 18 YEARS	Fear loss of control and death Concern for body function and appearance Feel separation from peers

◀ Figure 2.1

Patient age groups and characteristics.
Source: Author

2.2.1 Design With Family in Mind

Although family members may or may not be involved in the care of adult patients, pediatric patients are always accompanied by guardians. Caregivers work closely with a child's guardian and effective communication is vital to the care process. Parents or legal guardians are the primary advocates for children, yet their needs are generally not deemed necessary in general hospitals. Spaces for these auxiliary users vary depending on the length of the visit, and may include sleep rooms, laundry facilities, family kitchens, and flexible lounges that can be reserved for occasions like meals or birthday parties.

Surgical and diagnostic procedures can take many hours, so spaces should provide options for families to work, eat, and get outdoors, while remaining informed about the progress of their child's procedure. Waiting areas should be much more than rows of chairs. Comfortable seating, tables, and ample and easily accessible power outlets are vital to keeping parents productive during a long wait. Mobile technology increasingly allows people to continue working remotely, so having access to reliable wireless networks and business centers allows parents to remain productive at the hospital. These technologies also allow parents to stay informed during the procedure, even if they move around

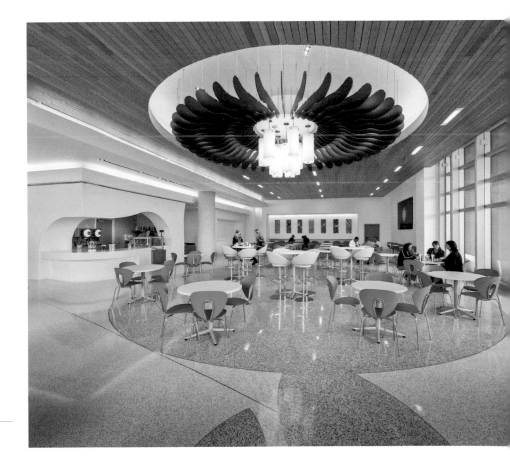

▶ Figure 2.2

Café.
Source: Jonathan Hillyer

the building as necessary. Access to food and drink is also important during these times, so a café nearby is ideal.

In addition to parents, siblings often accompany patients to the hospital and must be considered since they have emotional and social needs possibly similar to the patient. Because the sick child receives so much attention, siblings can feel marginalized. Caregivers and child-life specialists understand this and respond to it. For example, one children's hospital system gives a toy to a sibling when the patient receives one for completing a treatment. Waiting spaces typically integrate play areas among the seating that can be used by both patients and siblings.

2.3 Multidisciplinary Caregiver Teams

Pediatric caregivers are specially trained to understand the physical and emotional needs of children and are able to communicate with them in ways they understand. Caregivers read cues from patients and family members that inform how they will communicate. In response, exam rooms must be designed to allow for providers to sit face-to-face with patients and guardians in ways that promote clear communication and build trust.

Inpatient units should provide a variety of work and respite spaces for staff. Because of the fragility of many child patients, close and prolonged observation of the patients is essential. Moving supplies and charting closer to the point of care is ideal for maximizing time spent observing and caring for patients. Collaborative workspaces also must be located near patient rooms. In addition, lounge and respite spaces near the units are just as important as having appropriate workspaces, and allow staff to recharge from stressful work responsibilities.

In addition to physicians, nurses, and various medical staff, child-life specialists are integral to the provider team. These specialists help patients and families cope with medical treatment, diagnosis, and hospitalization through play, preparation, education, and self-expression. A variety of therapies are used to help children cope and heal, including art, music, and other creative therapies. Caregivers need access to spaces they can use with a single child or with a group, storage space for supplies and toys, and the ability to clean toys. Dishwashers are often provided in or near child-life spaces for sanitizing items.

2.4 Nemours Children's Hospital

Established in 1936, the Nemours Foundation is dedicated to fostering the health of children and operates a system of hospitals and clinics in Delaware and Florida. In 2005, the Nemours Foundation began planning a new acute care hospital to improve access to pediatric healthcare services in Central Florida. The site for the new hospital is located two miles south of the Orlando International Airport and was one of the first major sites developed in the Lake Nona Medical City development. Lake Nona is a mixed-use development that collocates major hospital buildings, research and education facilities, retail, hotel

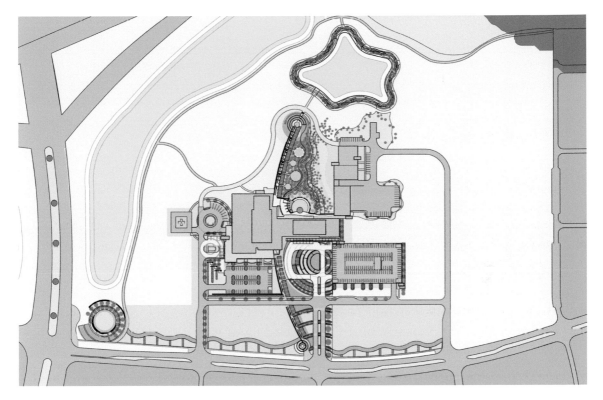

▲ Figure 2.3

Campus site plan.
Source: Stanley Beaman & Sears; Perkins and Will (SBS/PW)

accommodation, and housing to create a "medical city". Nemours purchased a 60-acre greenfield site for the new hospital in Phase 1, while allowing for future expansion of inpatient and outpatient services and the growth of ancillary support buildings.

The hospital is 630,000 square feet and includes 95 inpatient beds, 76 ambulatory clinic exam rooms, six operating rooms, full diagnostic imaging services, an emergency department, and an on-site lab, pharmacy, and sterile processing. It also includes a shelled inpatient floor for future expansion. Additional buildings include a central energy plant, data center, and parking garage. The landscape is a mix of tailored gardens and low-maintenance native grasses, and overall the project achieved LEED Gold certification. It is organized vertically with Logistics, Emergency Services, and Imaging at the lowest level, and public and clinical space on upper levels, as seen in Figure 2.4.

A key objective of the campus was to create a simple and integrated clinical experience for patients and families who typically receive care at multiple locations. The building combines inpatient, outpatient, and diagnostic and treatment services organized along key service lines. Additionally, creating an efficient and supportive environment for caregivers was paramount, so that they can maximize their time with patients.

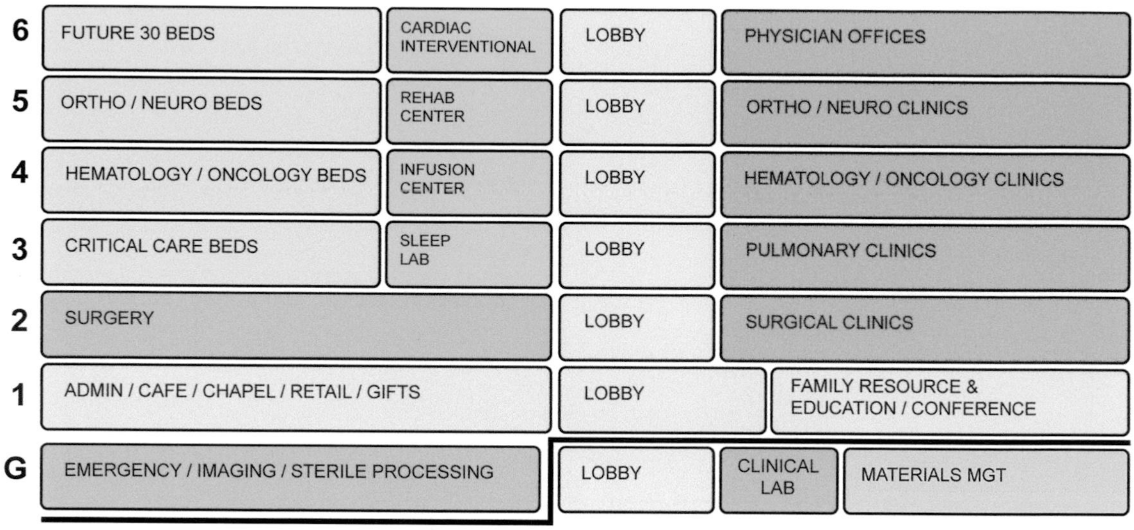

6	FUTURE 30 BEDS	CARDIAC INTERVENTIONAL	LOBBY	PHYSICIAN OFFICES
5	ORTHO / NEURO BEDS	REHAB CENTER	LOBBY	ORTHO / NEURO CLINICS
4	HEMATOLOGY / ONCOLOGY BEDS	INFUSION CENTER	LOBBY	HEMATOLOGY / ONCOLOGY CLINICS
3	CRITICAL CARE BEDS	SLEEP LAB	LOBBY	PULMONARY CLINICS
2	SURGERY		LOBBY	SURGICAL CLINICS
1	ADMIN / CAFE / CHAPEL / RETAIL / GIFTS		LOBBY	FAMILY RESOURCE & EDUCATION / CONFERENCE
G	EMERGENCY / IMAGING / STERILE PROCESSING		LOBBY	CLINICAL LAB / MATERIALS MGT

▲ Figure 2.4

Nemours functional stacking.
Source: Author

2.5 A Patient-Focused Design Process

As this was a new hospital, there were no existing clients to reach out to for user feedback. To compensate for this, Nemours assembled user groups of caregivers at their Delaware hospital, national experts, and a family advisory council to provide guidance to the design team. To ensure an inclusive and informed design process with the patient at the center, different processes were defined at the onset.

2.5.1 Design an Experience

In order to integrate operations and technology into the physical environment, Nemours engaged multiple consultants to identify a patient-centered model of care as well as define how the patient could be supported by a seamless brand experience. During concept and schematic design, Nemours retained global design and innovation company IDEO to develop an innovative and patient-centered experience for the new hospital. The patient journey was used as a framework to understand key experience touchpoints and patient/family needs. Some of the concepts developed included clinical concierge greeters at every floor, multiuse family lounges, and integrated "smart bracelets" and "smart rooms", which welcome patients to their rooms and identify caregivers to patients via media panels. IDEO helped to interpret these touchpoints into architectural concepts, which the design team took forward as it developed reception points, room entries, and lounges.

2.5.2 Engage Children and Families

Meetings between the design team and a family advisory council were fundamental to keeping the design focused on children's needs. The council, including

Allen Buie

a group of parents and children who were patients in the Nemours system, met monthly alongside clinical user group meetings. The design team gained insight into how to best design public areas, waiting spaces, gardens, and patient rooms for the children. Overall, patients and families expressed preferences for simple but engaging spaces that weren't tied to a juvenile theme.

The group discussed the patient room extensively because of its importance as a healing space where patients and families spend large amounts of time. Consistent with studies that show pediatric patients' need for a sense of control (Lambert et al. 2014), the children in the advisory council expressed interest in having a level of control over their environment, which became a strategy used later in the project. Additionally, patient and family feedback directly influenced the design of storage for clothing, luggage, and toys, as well as the technology that allows for connectivity to the Internet and access to power outlets.

2.5.3 Mock Up and Simulate Clinical Experience

Mock-ups of key rooms were vital for developing and refining the design of repetitive spaces, including emergency department exam rooms, clinic exam rooms, and inpatient rooms. User group meetings were held in the mock-up rooms and provided clinicians with a deeper understanding of space, flow, and usability. Using hospital equipment, users simulated situations like a code to understand if and how the space provided would work. Using props like outlet covers, photographs, and cardboard, users directly configured elements like headwalls and handwashing zones in the rooms to ensure that room elements were functional and ergonomic. The results of these simulations were translated into the drawings for the project.

Once key room designs were refined using these simulated environments, Nemours constructed a preview center, which contained fully finished inpatient room, clinic exam room, and emergency exam room mock-ups. This center not only raised awareness of Nemours in the community but also was a valuable resource for recruiting and training caregiver staff, who would ultimately deliver care in the new hospital.

2.6 Project Goals, Concepts, and Design Strategies

The patient-focused design process, combined with the opportunity of a greenfield site, enabled Nemours and the design team to develop a campus unencumbered by existing buildings or care models. Four key goals drove the design and provided a framework for concepts and strategies that focus on the human experience:

1. Provide a positive experience for patients and families
2. Ensure a safe and secure environment for children's needs
3. Create an efficient and effective workplace for multidisciplinary care teams to provide coordinated care
4. Design a flexible and adaptable environment that allows for program evolution and future expansion

2.6.1 Goal 1: Provide a Positive Experience for Patients and Families

Typical healthcare environments can be confusing and overwhelming for patients, resulting in a stressful and negative experience. Nemours provides a positive experience by creating an environment that is easy to navigate and keeps families comfortable and connected to the outdoors.

2.6.1.1 Create Simple, Direct, and Dedicated Circulation Pathways

Many large hospital campuses are characterized by complicated corridor systems that confuse and stress patients. Although Nemours is over 600,000 square feet, the hospital is designed to create clear and straightforward pathways for families. The building and campus are organized to consolidate vertical transportation and minimize the horizontal distance families must travel to reach their destinations. Upon entering the campus, the entry door is clearly visible, and patient/family parking is directly adjacent. Families can park and walk under a canopy directly to the front door, highlighted by a reception/security desk that acts conceptually as the porch light for the hospital that glows day and night.

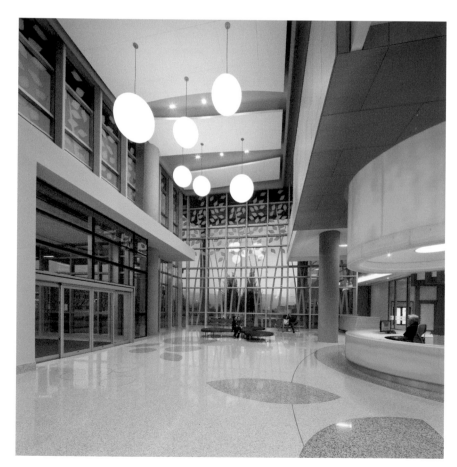

◀ Figure 2.5

Main entrance lobby.
Source: Jonathan Hillyer

Allen Buie

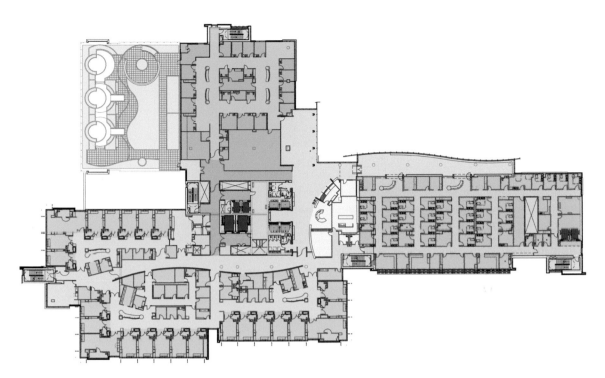

▲ Figure 2.6

Nemours typical tower-level
plan.
Source: Stanley Beaman &
Sears; Perkins and Will (SBS/
PW)

This concept of the glowing lantern repeats on every level of the hospital, so
that a round, backlit desk is identified as an information and arrival point immediately outside of public elevators. Therefore, despite the size of the facility,
patients and families are always greeted by a person with dedicated pathways
to inpatient, outpatient, or shared services.

Contributing to the simplified clinical experience is the organizational and
operational idea of the "medical home". This concept organizes inpatient, outpatient, and shared services horizontally along specialty service lines across one
level, simplifying patient wayfinding and improving staff efficiency. Returning
patients then always come back to the same floor and have easy access to other
providers in the same building and site as needed. As an example, the hematol-
ogy/oncology floor includes the inpatient bed unit, ambulatory clinics, and an
infusion center that can be accessed from an outpatient entry, while inpatients
have direct access via a back corridor.

Conceptually, the major public circulation is designed as an internal extension of the gardens outside. Hence, the hospital in a garden becomes a garden in
the hospital. Instead of conventional corridors, circulation pathways are defined
with curvilinear walls, furniture that recalls hedges and flowers, and built-ins that
allude to garden walls. Major destinations, such as public elevators, reception
points, and departmental entries, are highlighted as destinations along these
pathways with color, portal frames, and lighting.

Color is a strong element that distinguishes each floor by function, and
the spectrum of colors is inspired by flowers in the garden. Elevators open to a
lobby defined by the floor color, which is repeated at each major control point in
the inpatient unit and ambulatory clinic. Elevator buttons correspond in color to
each floor number, continuing the wayfinding system on a smaller scale.

2.6.1.2 Provide Comfort and Control for Families

To accommodate families with multiple children, family members, strollers, and bags, circulation and waiting spaces are larger at Nemours than in typical hospitals. During design, the team asked where strollers would be parked when stopping at exam rooms or information areas. The design team began to treat this open space as program space, so that it would be included in the final solution. Ample space to move around creates a smoother flow of patients and families.

Whereas many healthcare waiting spaces consist of row after row of chairs, Nemours waiting areas include access to power outlets and Wi-Fi, so that parents can work remotely while waiting during a procedure or appointment. Workstations allow for access to patient educational resource materials, and hidden cabinets store toys that can be distributed to patients. The inpatient floors provide work and respite space for families in the rooms and on the units. Each patient floor has a family lounge.

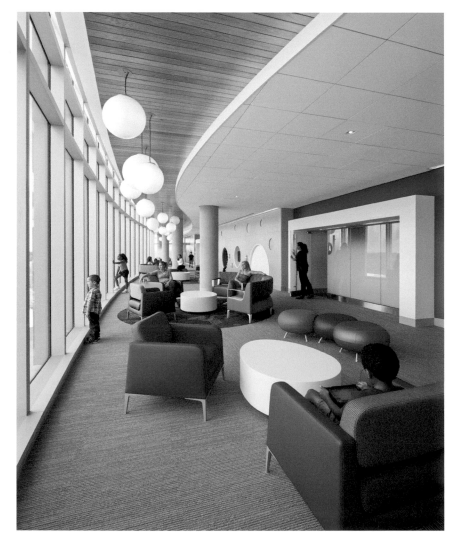

◀ Figure 2.7

Clinic waiting area.
Source: Jonathan Hillyer

2.6.1.3 Provide Access to Daylight, Views, and Exterior Respite Space

Evidence supports the therapeutic benefit of natural light and views for patients. Nemours prioritizes access to natural light and exterior views, beginning at the entrance. The main lobby has glass on the north and south sides, allowing views into the gardens upon entering. All upper-floor lobbies look down to the gardens on the north, reorienting visitors with design features seen upon entry.

As a hospital in a garden, the campus is designed to provide opportunities for patients and families to have easy access to the outdoors and nature. Surgery and clinic waiting areas have full-height glass walls to bring light in, while surgery waiting areas have direct access to a rooftop garden and play area that act as a grand porch for the facility. Portions of this roof garden are recessed under the bed tower above, providing opportunity to be outdoors even during rainstorms. The infusion center has direct access to a second rooftop garden that is designed as a respite space as well as a therapeutic environment for rehabilitation patients.

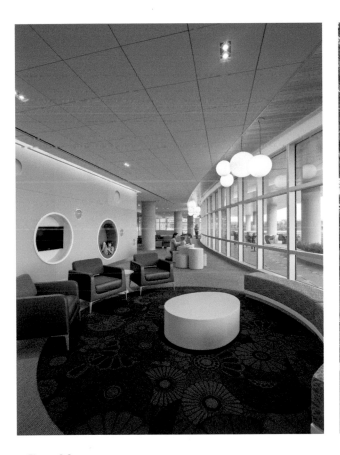

▲ Figure 2.8

Surgery waiting area.
Source: Jonathan Hillyer

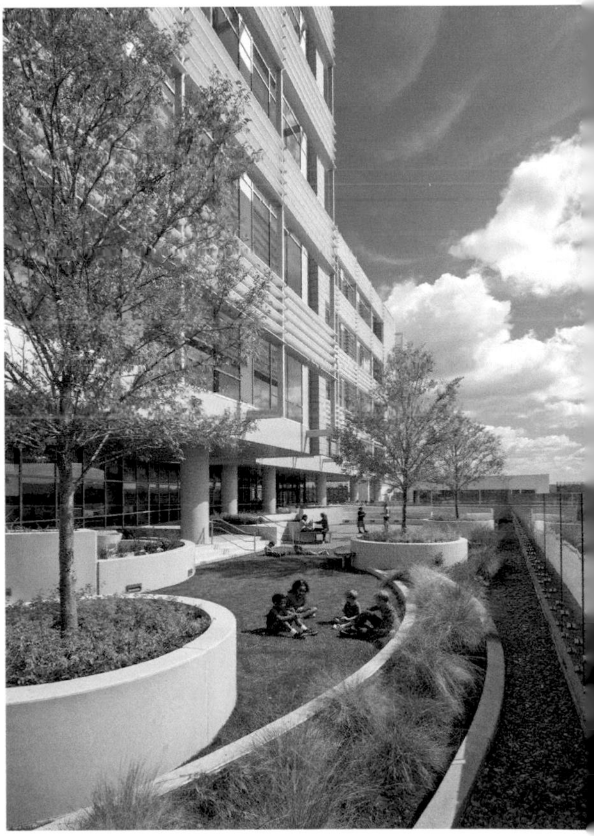

▲ Figure 2.9

Surgery-level roof garden.
Source: Jonathan Hillyer

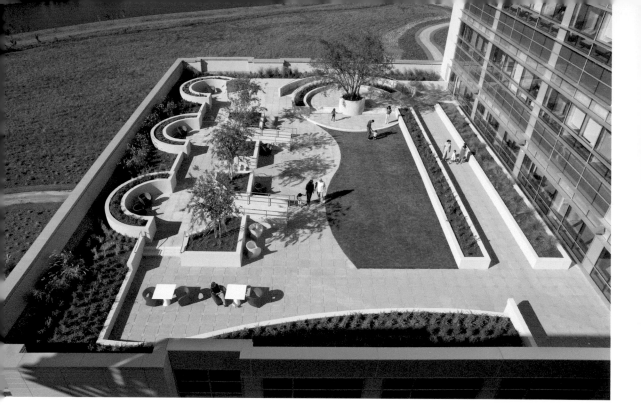

▲ Figure 2.10

Level 4 roof garden.
Source: Jonathan Hillyer

Every patient room has floor-to-ceiling glass and high ceilings that bring natural light deep into the room. Potential glare from the Florida sun is mitigated by both exterior metal sunshades and interior roller shades.

Additional sensory gardens are located on the north side of the building along the garden wall and are designed to engage patients with textures, scents, sounds, and visual distractions.

2.6.2 Goal 2: Ensure a Safe and Secure Environment That Meets Children's Needs

Because children are still developing physically and cognitively, the healthcare environment must respond with space that creates a sense of safety and provides opportunities for learning and play. Nemours utilizes concepts and strategies that focus on scale and engagement to provide a child-centered environment.

2.6.2.1 Provide Age-Specific Spaces for Child-Life and Educational Activities

To support the psychosocial, educational, and recreational needs of children, Nemours incorporates a variety of child-life and family spaces into the inpatient units. A dedicated child-life room for younger children is provided adjacent to the inpatient units and can be used for a variety of social and educational activities led by child-life staff. Teenagers have a dedicated "Teen Center" on Level 3 that caters to their needs for socialization without mixing with younger patients. Family lounges at the end of each inpatient unit have both comfortable seating for respite

Allen Buie

Chapel.
Source: Jonathan Hillyer

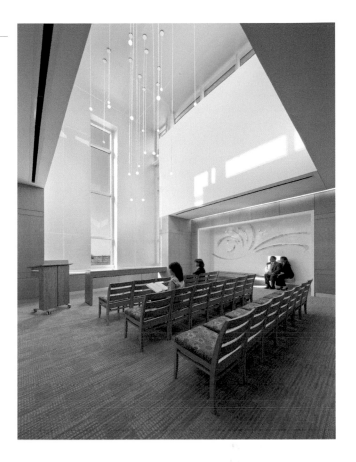

and dining furniture so that families can dine together or host a birthday party. A chapel and spaces with minimal levels of sound allow for more quiet respite.

Other spaces are provided throughout the hospital to support activities for larger groups. The auditorium on the main level can be used for performances or movies for patients when not being used by staff for conferences, grand rounds, or meetings. An outdoor amphitheater space is also available in the north garden for large-scale activities.

2.6.2.2 Utilize Playful Elements That Respond to Children's Sensibilities

The concept of the hospital in a garden provides a framework for a design language that responds to children without becoming cartoonish, utilizing variations in scale, color, and form to create positive distractions for patients.

Waiting spaces incorporate seating elements that recall elements of the gardens outdoors. Seating areas include custom serpentine benches inspired by hedges in a garden and serve to organize more conventional loose seating. Bright, floral, circular patches of carpet organize colorful seating into "picnic blankets" spread across a field of light green carpet that alludes to grass in a park. In addition, long walls of translucent material have recessed circular seats with cushions, sized for smaller patients. The idea of these "habitable walls" was to provide a space scaled to children that provides a sense of comfort and safety.

Almost every waiting space has exterior exposure with access to daylight and views. The only waiting space that does not have exterior access is the imaging department due to its location on the lower level of the building. In this case, a 1,500-gallon saltwater aquarium provides positive distraction for waiting patients and families. All occupants of the hospital also have access to this waiting space to enjoy the aquarium.

Throughout waiting and public spaces are interactive, with multimedia elements that serve to both educate and entertain patients and families. The main lobby showcases a grand luminous portal, with a field of color-changing LED light panels that can be programmed to create abstracted static or kinetic forms.

Patient care areas are designed with the child in mind. The patient room is a place for rest and recovery, but it is important to note that in pediatric facilities it is also considered a safe space for the patient. Procedure rooms are provided on the inpatient units to be a space for more clinical interactions. To further provide a sense of comfort and control for the patients and give them a sense of ownership over their space, the team developed patient rooms that can be painted with light to the patient's preference. Color-changing LED lighting in the ceiling is controlled by the patient's pillow speaker and gives the opportunity to wash the room in colored light. Due to the floor-to-ceiling windows in every room, the façade of the hospital becomes a colored mosaic at night, each color representing the choice of a patient inside.

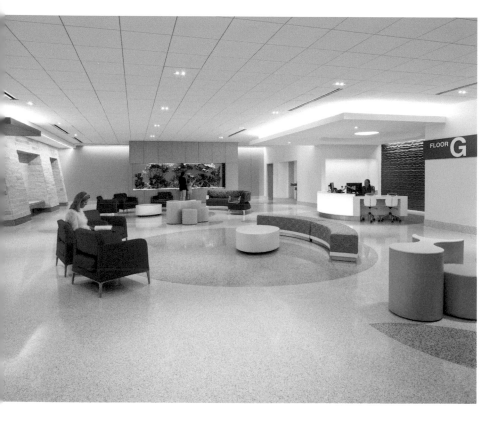

◀ Figure 2.12

Imaging waiting with aquarium.
Source: Jonathan Hillyer

Nemours inpatient room.
Source: Jonathan Hillyer

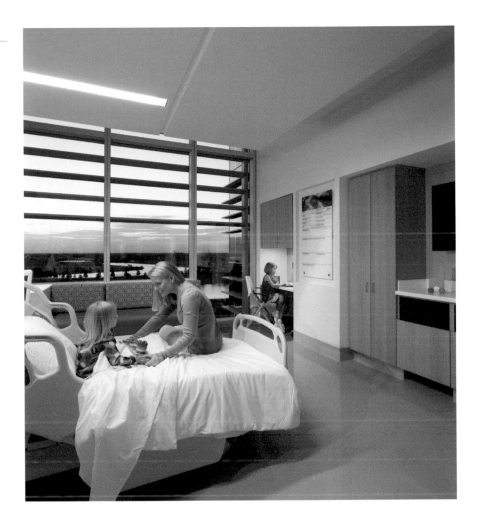

Nemours exterior at night.
Source: Jonathan Hillyer

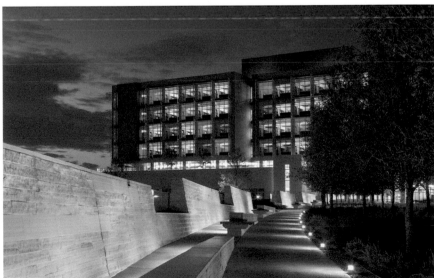

2.6.2.3 Organize Inpatient Beds Into Neighborhoods

The concept of creating neighborhoods of beds benefits patients as well as staff. Clustering beds reduces the scale of the hospital for children, so that the environment is not overwhelming and provides a greater sense of security and privacy. The 27 beds per floor are organized as three 9-bed neighborhoods, each with a team work center, pneumatic tube, medication room, nourishment room, clean and soiled utility, equipment storage, and a huddle space. An L-shaped arrangement of the patient rooms allows staff to minimize walking distance and maximize time spent at the bedside.

2.6.3 Goal 3: Create an Efficient and Effective Workplace for Caregivers

Just as the environment responds to the needs of children and parents, it must also respond to the needs of staff. The arrangement of space, from whole departments to supply locations, directly influences how effectively caregivers can meet their patients' needs. Nemours achieves operational efficiency with strategies by creating linkages between services, putting supplies near the patient, and separating public and staff flows.

2.6.3.1 Directly Link Staff Spaces Between Inpatient and Outpatient

Just as the horizontal alignment of departments by specialty creates a simple flow for patients and families, it also creates an efficient workflow for staff. Because inpatient bed units are directly connected to outpatient clinics, doctors and other caregivers can easily navigate between the two, monitoring inpatients and seeing outpatients. Additionally, the direct connection of the inpatient unit to a specialty space (infusion center, rehab center) further improves caregiver communication across the service line. Staff shares a single lounge area, strategically located at the knuckle between inpatient and outpatient areas to further enhance their versatility.

2.6.3.2 Provide Supplies at the Point of Care

A key operational element to achieve this goal is the idea of moving common supplies directly to the point of patient care. Supply carts in every patient room hold commonly used items, while less common items are in the clean supply room that supports only nine beds. A computer is placed at each bedside as well, for charting and medication administration. Personal protective equipment (PPE), including gowns, masks, and gloves, is provided in a cabinet at every patient room entry, along with a linen hamper for disposing of the PPE items. Rooms also integrate conventional signage and digital signage that can indicate patient precautions for the room.

2.6.3.3 Separate Onstage and Offstage Flow

The campus separates public, patient, staff, and materials flow through the campus and building itself. This strategy allows patients and families to have direct pathways to clinical areas, which improves the experience. Staff and materials can then move separately in an efficient offstage corridor system.

The building and site are organized by a garden wall that originates at the campus entry point, extends through the main lobby of the building, continues out toward the rear, and leads to a series of sensory discovery gardens. This wall is an aesthetic, functional, and wayfinding element that also acts as a retaining wall to elevate the main public entry above a walk-out basement level, which cannot be underground due to groundwater constraints. This lower level includes loading docks, materials management, a laboratory, central sterile processing, and staff support areas in spaces not accessible to patients and visitors. These offstage flows happen in wide corridors that connect to dedicated material movement elevators. Patients and families access the emergency department only at this lower level, while primary public arrival and circulation occur on Level 1 in a totally separate flow.

Like the corridor system, the vertical circulation is split into separate flows. Public elevators are completely separated from service elevators, which are further divided into two trauma-sized elevators for patient movement and two hospital-sized elevators for staff and materials movement. Regarding horizontal circulation, the upper levels provide for distinct flows of outpatients, inpatients, and staff in separate areas.

2.6.4 Goal 4: Design a Flexible and Adaptable Environment for Program Evolution and Future Expansion

Healthcare delivery changes over time as delivery models, technology, treatments, and patient populations evolve. Facilities must be designed to anticipate change and flex to accommodate it. Nemours is planned to change over time while maintaining clear organization, flow, and wayfinding.

2.6.4.1 Plan the Campus for Clear Growth Avenues

The campus is designed to provide for future expansion of both inpatient and outpatient wings while maintaining the major circulation and building access points. A future inpatient wing could be added north of the diagnostic and treatment block, which would build on an extension of the main lobby and follow the path set by the garden wall. A future outpatient wing would grow at the northeast corner of the existing clinic building, continuing the pattern of waiting spaces that overlook rear gardens. The emergency and imaging departments are strategically located on the ground level with an expansion zone to the south. Building on the initial wayfinding framework, the campus will be able to significantly expand while remaining easily understood by patients and families, and efficient for logistics and staff flow.

2.6.4.2 Organize Clinics as a Flexible, Modular Chassis

Ambulatory clinics are organized into clusters of rooms that allow for flexible use over both the short and long term. As needs change in either a day or a year, a modular layout allows staffing and operations to adapt without need for renovations. On floors that require specialty spaces, like radiology, these spaces are placed at the edge of the clinic versus in the middle, so that the continuity of the clinical modules is maintained.

2.6.4.3 Utilize Universal Layouts to Allow Uses to Change With Patient Population

Because patient populations can shift over time, the inpatient units and rooms at Nemours were designed to be universal and adaptable for different patient types and acuities. The inpatient room was designed to accommodate intensive care clearances, while the inpatient neighborhoods are similar across all floors. This will allow the facility to redefine unit types based on changes in the patient population without doing wholesale renovations.

2.7 Conclusions

Healthcare facilities for children must respond to a complex patient population that spans a large range of ages and levels of mental, physical, and social development. Additionally, parents, siblings, and other auxiliary individuals that accompany the child to the hospital must be considered as users, participating in care and interacting with caregivers. Multidisciplinary teams of caregivers are trained to respond to all of these complexities and treat the medical issues while making sure each child's development and growth can continue. All these forces demand a complex physical environment that is playful, sophisticated, adaptable, flexible, efficient, and therapeutic. Nemours has taken these complex forces and given its patients and families a setting that is simple to navigate, connects to nature, and ensures that it can change over time with medical and technological advancement.

Acknowledgments

Special thanks to EYP (Stanley Beaman Sears), Design Architect and Architect of Record, as well as project team members Perkins and Will, TLC Architecture, AECOM (Glatting Jackson), Skanska, IDEO, and Bowen & Briggs.

Bibliography

Lambert, V., J. Coad, P. Hicks, and M. Glacken. "Social Spaces for Young Children in Hospital." *Child: Care, Health and Development* 40, no. 2 (2014): 195–204.

Chapter 3

Elderly Autonomy Through Architecture
Building a Fifth-Generation Residential Care Home

Dietger Wissounig and Birgit Prack

3.1 Introduction

In German-speaking countries, the residential care of elderly people has changed tremendously in recent decades—and thus also the planning and design of residential care facilities. Modern care concepts and architectural spatial planning are no longer based on the hospital model, but rather on the individual requirements of the elderly as well as the increasing number of people suffering from dementia.

The Erika Horn Residential Care Home in Graz, Austria, designed by Dietger Wissounig Architekten, is presented as an exemplar of this new trend in residential care. Named after an Austrian gerontologist, this multiple award–winning project is classified according to the definition of the Kuratorium Deutscher Altershilfe (Committee on German Care for the Elderly, or KDA) as a care facility of the fourth generation, which, as such, meets state-of-the-art geriatric care standards. This advancement in the understanding of the needs of those affected by dementia, along with what constitutes a future fifth-generation care facility, is outlined in this chapter to help guide projects intended for specialized populations, specifically the elderly.

3.2 Designing for Dementia: Establishing the Relationship Between Resident and Care Home

According to the World Health Organization (WHO), dementia is a condition that is chronic or progressive in nature, resulting in an irreversible decline and deterioration in cognitive functioning and mental ability that alters one's behavior, personality, and memory. People who suffer from dementia typically are challenged with everyday tasks, and have confusion in familiar environments, difficulties with words and numbers, memory loss, and changes in mood and

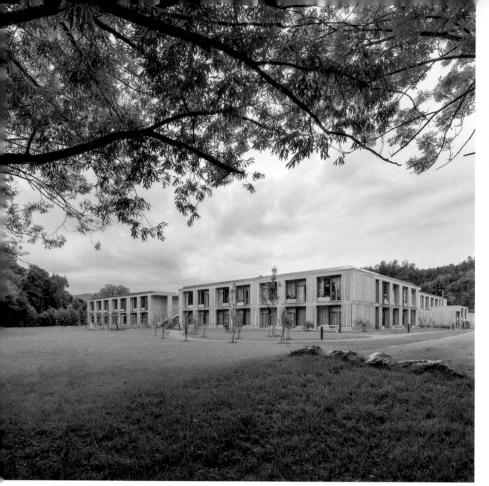

◀ Figure 3.1

The residential care home
Erika Horn. Exterior view,
Graz (2015).
Source: Helmut Pierer, pierer.
net

behavior (World Health Organization 2017). Dementia affects each person differently depending on a variety of factors and is best understood by three stages. The early-stage symptoms of dementia are often overlooked because the onset is gradual, whereas the middle-stage signs and symptoms become clearer and limit one's ability to perform activities of daily living. During this middle stage, if proper care and support are not available at home, a person suffering from the symptoms of dementia often needs to seek more supportive housing options. In the late stages of dementia, memory loss and physical signs are more obvious and often lead to total dependence and inactivity. According to current estimates, there are between 115,000 and 130,000 people living with dementia disease in Austria. Of these, Alzheimer's is the most frequently occurring dementia disorder. Due to the continuously increasing life expectancy, this number is expected to double by the year 2050 (Höfler et al. 2015). Understanding the signs and symptoms that correspond to the three stages is important for designing environments around the specific needs of dementia.

3.2.1 Environmental Press and the Elderly

How the elderly relate to their environment, especially those with dementia, can be understood through Powell Lawton and Lucille Nahemow's environmental

1940 -1960	1940 -1960	Since 1980	Since 1995
Model: Detention Center	**Model: Hospital**	**Model: Dorm**	**Model: Family**
Inmate is kept	Patient is being treated	Resident is activated	Residents experience security and normality

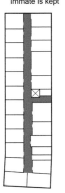 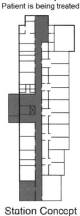 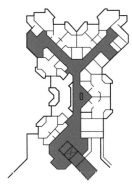 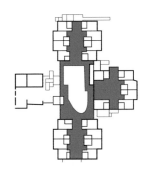

| Agency Concept | Station Concept | Living Area Concept | House Community Concept |

▲ Figure 3.2

Models of care are reflected in the plans associated with each generation of care home.

Source: Xiaowei Li

press model (1973). This understanding of the interaction between person and environment posits that a person's "competence", or ability to perform physical or mental tasks, can be either challenged or supplemented by the built environment, the combination of which results in their behavior. Disability, sensory loss, poor health, or a condition such as dementia changes an individual's competence, which forces him or her to adapt to the existing environment. If the environment is not designed in a way that can support changes in health over time, a person is forced to adapt his or her behavior in positive, negative, or neutral ways. This is the "environmental press" that can either improve an individual's competence or suppress it in a way that does not allow the person to exercise his or her competence to its full potential. For example, a patient with dementia may be experiencing memory loss, trouble with orientation and wayfinding, and accompanying physical weakness. If a person's care home has confusing circulation paths and no landmarks for reference, then the person is less able to orient him- or herself and can become lost. Conversely, if the care home has unstimulating circulation paths and no separation of space in a floorplan that is overtly clinical or open, the resident could find little interest in moving around. Both scenarios can lead to the maladaptive behavior of the person staying locked away in his or her room, not participating in the community the care home should provide, which furthers the deterioration of the individual's physical and mental capacities. Ideally, a care home's level of environmental press matches residents' changing needs and competence, encouraging them to care for themselves while providing support when needed.

Several scientific studies draw similar conclusions and show how the physical environment within care facilities can have a positive effect on the well-being and behavior of residents, especially those suffering from dementia disorders (e.g., Zeisel et al. 2003; Marquardt, Bueter, and Motzek 2014). Typically occurring behavioral dysfunctions, like anxiety, agitation, aggression, and apathy, as well as social withdrawal and psychotic symptoms, can be reduced by specific design elements. Through analyzation and combination of design guidelines from existing studies, John Zeisel (2013) developed a set of eight design performance criteria:

1. Exit controls (on doors, windows, and garden fences to allow residents their independence and reduce elopement attempts)
2. Walking paths (with place-defined landmarks and meaningful destinations that enhance the person's sense of place and thus his or her sense of self)
3. Common spaces (to support appropriate social behavior)
4. Privacy and personalization (reducing aggression and agitation and improving sleep)
5. Secure garden access (to feel comfortable and in control in that space and to have a sense of time and season)
6. Residential-ness (to provide a strong and recognizable feeling of being at home)
7. Sensory comprehension (colors, sound, smells, and textures must be coherent to all the senses at once and be within the comprehension range of each person)
8. Support for capacity (to remain independent for as long as possible)

Both the environmental press model and Zeisel's identified strategies for improved environments for those with dementia establish a clear link between residents and their environments, one that is intensified with age.

3.3 Improving the Nursing Home Typology: Past to Future

Since 1962, the KDA has been one of the leading institutions in Germany that work for a better quality of life for elderly people. The care concept of the City of Graz Geriatric Health Care Centres—the operator of the presented building—is largely oriented toward applying the knowledge of the KDA. The KDA has developed the following chronology of nursing home types:

- The first generation of care facilities (developed about 1940–1960) was simply a "storage institution" without any care or living concept, which offered just a sleeping and dining area for elderly people. The occupation density was very high and there was only one common sanitation facility.
- The second generation of care facilities (developed about 1960–1980) was designed and based on the model of the hospital. It included geriatric knowledge and offered reactive care. The nursing rooms were furnished with a washbasin.
- The third generation of care facilities has been present since the 1980s and is based on models of residential homes. Care and living requirements both are considered, with a focus on individuality and activating care. Every room has its own separate bathroom.
- The fourth generation of care facilities developed since about 1995 is based on the model of family. Family-like houses offer a spacious kitchen and living area, a high range of primarily single rooms, and handicapped-accessible

baths designed as a feel-good oasis. The goal is to preserve and support the skills and autonomy of the residents. This model also orientates toward an improvement of life quality and security of residents, with an emphasis on normality.

- An emerging fifth generation is underway, building on the strengths of the fourth generation, through the building organization of so-called district houses. The Erika Horn Residential Care Home, operated by KDA, serves as a first prototype of this evolving concept. The KDA "district houses" are care homes that have a sophisticated range of systems and are located near an area referred to as the "quarter"—a relatively restricted social area for residents. Each "quarter" has its own identity and environmental demarcations, such as a central square or community plaza. All permanent necessary supplies exist inside each "district house" and are accessible for the elderly. A further significant feature is the integration of multiple generations and the promotion of laymen assistance to help those suffering from dementia. The KDA "district houses" will give further access to people who choose to live life within the greater community, thereby protecting their rights to privacy and self-determination (Mitchell-Auli and Sowinski 2012). The guiding principle of normality, which is described as living in contact with community, is the basis for the evolutionary thinking on residential care facilities for people with dementia.

▼ Figure 3.3

Axonometric view (2017). Source. Dietger Wissounig Architects

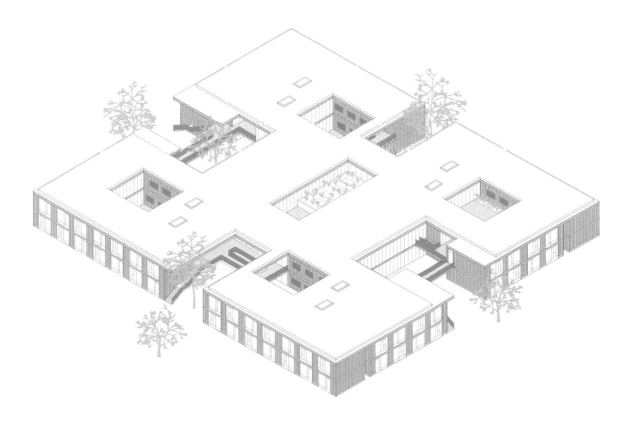

3.4 The Erika Horn Residential Care Home

The Erika Horn Residential Care Home accommodates 105 elderly residents suffering from typical age-related diseases, such as dementia, Parkinson's disease, and cardiovascular diseases. Residents on average live at the care home for one and a half years. For most residents, the care home is the final place of stay in their lives (Pojer and Hartinger 2017).

3.4.1 Defining Project Goals

To find the optimal design for the Erika Horn Residential Care Home, an architectural competition on the part of the client (Gem. Wohn- u. Siedlungsgenossenschaft Ennstal reg. Gen.m.b.H. Liezen) was announced in 2012. From the onset, the competition defined exact specifications and goals in terms of quantitative values (e.g., program, areas, and room adjacencies) and described qualitative expectations (e.g., the level of familiarity residents might feel in connection with their residence). Out of ten architectural offices, Dietger Wissounig Architekten won the competition for this new home for senior citizens. The barrier-free, passive design residence was erected in 2015 on a parklike site amid natural surroundings in the urban periphery. The home is designed using a mix of timber and reinforced concrete construction. While the floors and partitions in the rooms are made of reinforced concrete, all other structural elements are of timber.

3.4.2 Programming

Knowledge was gained through the realization of eight previously built care homes. The Peter Rosegger nursing home, which was completed in Graz in 2014, has been the most significant model, and informed the proposal for the new care home. With both projects, the clients were similar, and the floor plans were organized in a four-leafed clover layout because of comparable programmatic requirements. Like the Peter Rosegger nursing home, the two-story building consists of four wings, with a total of seven residential groups of 15 residents (13 single rooms and 1 double room) and one caregiver each. Each wing also has a shared living room with a dining area, and an integrated kitchen to support the residents of that wing. The single rooms are equipped with floor-to-ceiling glazing and an alcove to sit in, a window and door combination, and a French balcony. Similarly, the combination kitchen and living rooms are naturally lit by spacious glazing on two sides. From there, access to the outdoors is provided via balconies, terraces, or gardens. The atriums, which are furnished with raised garden beds, not only act as light wells but also offer protected leisure areas for residents.

The four wings are grouped around a semipublic central "village square", which is used for various events, and where residents from the four different housing wings can come together. The glazed entrance space opens to a foyer and adjoining reception area. Various amenity rooms for the residents include a hairdresser, a small chapel, a doctor's room, a physiotherapist, and a chiropodist. In addition, a main office and a room to store supplies and technical equipment are centrally located to the "village square". Due to difficult soil conditions

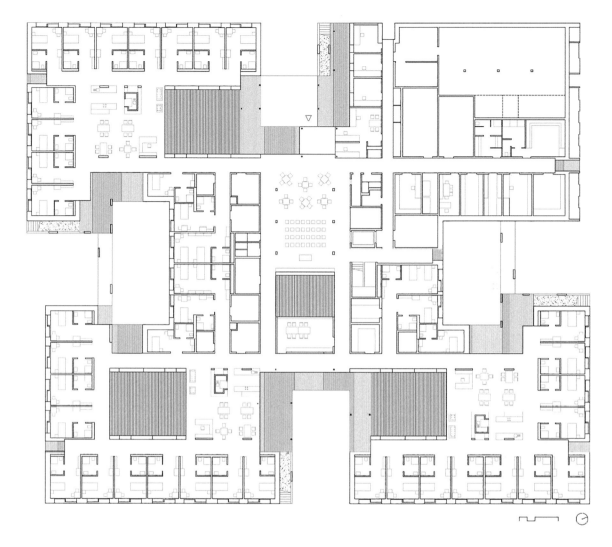

▲ Figure 3.4

Ground floor (2017).
Source: Dietger Wissounig
Architects

and the proximity to the adjacent brook, the Andritzbach, the building was not equipped with a cellar.

What was regarded as vital for a quality environment was to create an atmosphere of friendliness and brightness throughout the entire complex, which is reinforced by the views throughout the building. A special focus was put on the design of green and leisure areas afforded by the courtyard typology of the complex. In addition to a garden in the north, residents can enjoy a protected garden in the south. There is a vineyard in the east that provides a transition to the park. Finally, there is a wooden platform built above the water that creates an additional place to linger.

3.4.3 Design Principles of the Residential Care Home

In order to execute the fifth-generation care concept, it was imperative that there was regular communication between the architects, the client, and the

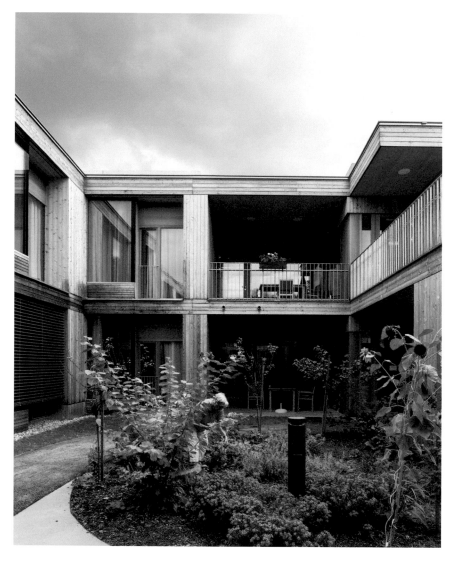

◀ Figure 3.5

Atrium view (2016).
Source: Simon Oberhofer

operators from the beginning of the project until its completion in 2015. Many in-depth discussions and constructive conversations occurred in regular meetings between all members of the project team, which included the operating staff of the facilities (project managers, carers, organizational staff, building services, logistic teams, and even laundry and housekeeping employees). This led to the final design of a building that was thought out in every detail. Responsibilities were clearly defined from the outset. The architects were responsible for the design and architecture, while the operators provided insight into activities involving caregiving. Over the course of time, this led to an enhancement of understanding and knowledge on both sides. For example, minimum clearances defined in city design standards were not always preferred or supported by care staff, and room sizes could be adjusted to better fit the reality of providing assisted living.

Dietger Wissounig and Birgit Prack

The purpose of the care home was to emphasize meaningful activities and quality of life; therefore, caregiving aspects were to remain in the background. The planning and design of the built environment was designed to counteract general symptoms of disease (e.g., disorientation, passivity, fear, restlessness, and perception disorders) suffered by residents, many of which could be overcome with the replicable design strategies outlined ahead:

- Connect the residential care home to nature: The building should be situated in green surroundings even when located in an urban setting. The natural areas surrounding the building and the urban context should serve as a recreation area for visitors, staff, and exterior services. These gardens or park spaces encourage social contact with others, physical activity through walks, and everyday exchanges for the residents. The site should also allow for access to public transportation services (Welter, Hürlimann, and Hürlimann-Siebke 2006).
- Allow for personal autonomy and comfort preferences: The design should promote a sense of normality by providing a residential community model as well as a person-centered care approach. When people with dementia feel at home, they are less likely to exhibit anxiety, agitation, aggression, and apathy (Zeisel 2013). Thus, a homelike environment should be created through a familial, small group of 15 residents to promote intimacy and avoid institutional character. The kitchen and living room are combined to create an open place to eat and participate in day-to-day activities and hobbies as well as a place to meet with people. As frequently as possible the residents are encouraged to be involved in daily living activities, like cooking or setting the table, according to their individual preferences, abilities, and needs. Even passive participation in everyday events has positive effects. People with dementia orient themselves to sounds, such as the clatter of dishes, or smells, such as the aroma of coffee, proving activity plays an important role in wayfinding and normalization. In addition, a pleasant atmosphere consistent with the rest of the living space is needed in specially equipped bathrooms. Bathrooms are an extension of the private quarters of a resident and therefore should be designed to foster well-being, not just to meet hygienic and accessibility requirements.
- Program a floorplan that balances both resident needs and staff needs: The home should be organized to support the residents as well as the care staff, who should work autonomously to a certain extent. Care support areas and all other adjoining rooms required for caregiving should be adjacent to each other and easily accessed to ensure a smooth and efficient operation. Alongside the regular staff, "everyday carers" act as contact persons for the seniors. In consultation with residents, they organize the daily program, provide support to regular staff, and take care of household duties—not unlike a homemaker in a large family.
- Create communal hubs to foster socialization: In the semipublic area, the "village square", participation and social integration are welcomed and encouraged. The rooms offer enough space for privacy and retreat and can also be furnished individually, thus fostering a feeling of participation and adaptability. Areas can be programmed with varying degrees of specificity, to act as simple lounges or event spaces, to establish a link to the resident's previous life.

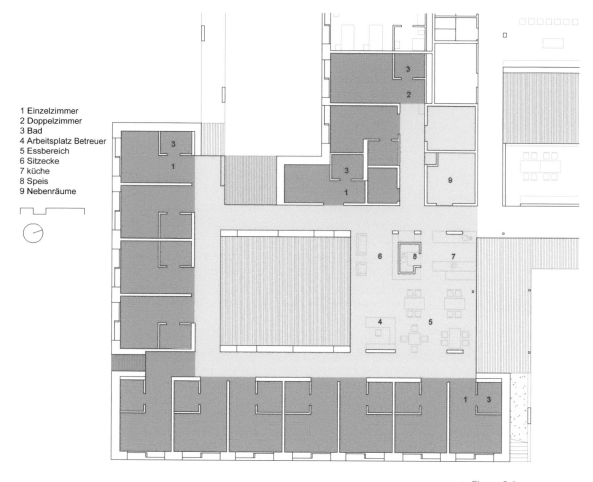

1 Einzelzimmer
2 Doppelzimmer
3 Bad
4 Arbeitsplatz Betreuer
5 Essbereich
6 Sitzecke
7 küche
8 Speis
9 Nebenräume

▲ Figure 3.6

Program distribution.
Source: Dietger Wissounig
Architects

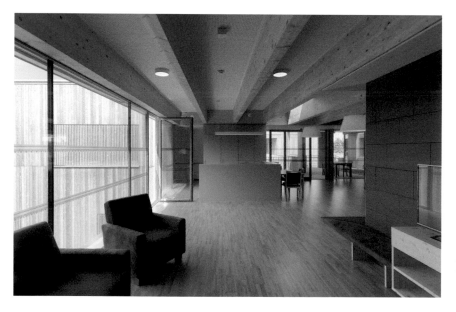

◀ Figure 3.7

Community area (2015).
Source: Paul Ott photografiert

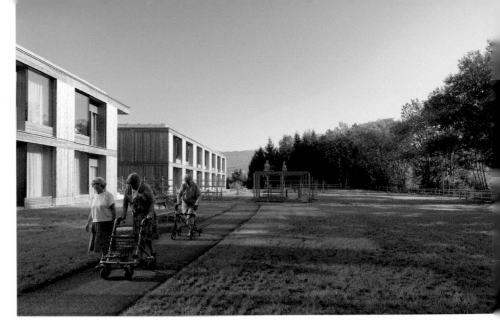

Courtyard (2015).
Source: Paul Ott photografiert

- Design to encourage independence for residents: Acknowledging the past lives of residents, senior citizens living here are treated as individuals with their own specific social and cultural backgrounds. In addition, the self-help capacity of older people is supported. Living in a community conveys the sense of security and protection that a person suffering from dementia needs. The aim of the care and support concept is to strengthen the existing abilities of elderly people and create a maximum degree of living quality and personal freedom, while at the same time providing adequate assistance. The work of the team is aimed at helping residents (especially those suffering from dementia) to continue to participate in activities and feel capable of acting independently (Pojer and Hartinger 2017).
- Create legible wayfinding: Spatial orientation, which can be mentally and physically difficult for those with dementia or those with impaired vision, is facilitated by a clearly organized sequence of rooms and walkways. Walkabouts (especially in bad weather) in corridors, loggias, atriums, and protected gardens provide space for exercise and a wealth of sensory experiences (smells, colors, sounds, and a variety of shapes). Additionally, various seating options invite residents to actively take in what is happening around them or just have a rest. Different colors utilized as effective design elements create different moods or act as unconscious orientation aids. While, for instance, general areas are furnished with parquet flooring, a reddish-brown linoleum floor was laid in the rooms to mark the transition. From public to private areas in the same way, the white doors stand out from the timber walls to aid orientation and to find entrances more easily.
- Provide access to natural light: Plenty of natural light and views of the countryside are supplied by generous glazed surfaces in different designs. In this way, residents can experience the course of the day and seasons from their beds. Natural light conveys stimulation and supports spatial and temporal orientation. A resident's circadian rhythm, which can be negatively impacted as a result of dementia, is also allowed to function naturally. Recurring rhythms give structure and bring back memories (Welter, Hürlimann, and Hürlimann-Siebke 2006).

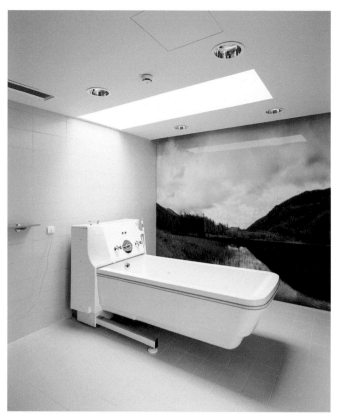

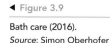

◄ Figure 3.9

Bath care (2016).
Source: Simon Oberhofer

- Select materials to create a warm, inviting area: Wood is a natural material used in walls, floors, furniture, ceilings, shutters, sunshade lamellas, and paneling to generate a warm and cozy atmosphere in living areas. However, quite apart from that, wood also has positive hygienic properties since its surface is antibacterial. In places where strong cleaning substances must be used, wood should not be used since it is a porous material.

- Promote safety and security: The scale and layout of the building are designed to help elderly residents feel safe. There is barrier-free accessibility and wheelchair-friendly design throughout the entire building, including outdoor areas. Entrances and doors don't have thresholds, which can prove hazardous, and there are walkways throughout the green area. In addition, there are senior-friendly bathrooms and kitchens to increase safety and reduce the risk of falling as well as making caregiving easier. Grab rails, handles, and handrails as well as other safety measures, such as the application of stickers to slippery surfaces, are provided to increase safety and orientation (Welter, Hürlimann, and Hürlimann-Siebke 2006).

- Promote sustainability: The building combines ecologically sustainable, energy-efficient technology. The passive house design is equipped with a solar and photovoltaic system as well as a ventilation system with heat recovery and air temperature control through earth-tube collectors. Sustainable energy management and the environmental policy of operators were studied, such as the EU Green Building Programme Award and klima:aktiv certification.

Including sustainability goals as part of care home planning allows for such facilities to be less reliant on expensive mechanical equipment, allows them to not place a burden on their surrounding community and world, and is a powerful expression of their mission to help residents be at peace with their surroundings.

3.5 Conclusions

When planning a residential care facility today, architects are faced with the complex task of creating a place tailored to the needs of residents in their last years of life. The design of residential care facilities should foster an individual's quality of life, autonomy, and personal competencies. In addition, a residential care home needs to be designed to balance practical and architectural requirements to provide staff and family members with an appropriate environment for caring for those with dementia. Once the building is optimized according to those requirements and its interior architecture exhibits clearly recognizable frameworks that convey a feeling of security, then it will contribute decisively to the well-being of residents and, ultimately, to that of caregivers and visitors, too. In the end, environmental strategies may have beneficial effects on the cost of medical care through the mitigation of the symptoms of dementia that can be life-altering and debilitating.

Above all, social and demographic changes and medical progress will proceed quickly, necessitating a new model of living and caring for older adults in planned communities. The reasons for this are diverse: the increasing life expectancy, multi-morbidity and accompanying dementia symptoms, dissolution of traditional family structures, declining social security systems, higher demands of the patients and their relatives, and the major shortage of trainees and qualified staff (Heil 2011). Therefore, it will be increasingly important to design surrogate homes for people with dementia, so they are able to live with dignity and respect for the remaining years of their lives.

Bibliography

Blasi, Ivan, and Giralt, Anna Sala. "Residential Care Home Erika Horn." *EU Prize for Contemporary Architecture—Mies van der Rohe Award 2017*. Barcelona: Fundació Mies van der Rohe, 2017.

Blezinger, Sylvia. "Das Alters- und Pflegeheim der Zukunft." *Heime und Spitäler*, no. 2 (2016).

Christophe, Hespel. "Dietger Wissounig: Maison de Retraite." *AMC. Hors-Série: Bois*. Paris: Le Moniteur, 2017.

"Dementia." World Health Organization. Last modified December 12, 2017. www.who.int/news-room/fact-sheets/detail/dementia.

Dietger Wissounig Architekten. "Nursing Home, Graz." *Arquitectura Viva: Senior Housing* 196, no. 7–8 (2017), Palermo.

Dore, Marta. "Senior Housing." *Platform: Architecture and Design*, no. 12 (2017).

Fabach, Robert, and Hebenstreit, Martin. "Pflegeheime und Architektur. Ein Leitfaden für eine bewohner- und pflegegerechte Planung." In *Gesellschaft für Pflege und Gesundheit*, Bregenz: Connexia, 2008.

Gregoric, Tina, and Markus Bogensberger. *Pragmatisch Und Poetisch: Pragmatic and Poetic.* Basel: Birkhäuser Verlag GmbH, 2017. Doi:10.1515/9783035610574-002.

Heil, Günther. "Altenpflege Morgen: Das Pflegeheim der Zukunft." *Die Schwester Der Pfleger. Die führende Fachzeitschrift für Pflegeberufe* 50 (2011): 1–151.

Höfler, Sabine, Theresa Bengough, Petra Winkler, and Robert Griebler. "Österreichischer Demenzbericht 2014." *Bundesministerium für Gesundheit und Sozialministerium* 7 (2015), Vienna.

Lawton, M. P., and L. Nahemow. "Ecology and Aging Process". In *The Psychology of Adult Development and Aging*, edited by C. Eisdorfer and M.P. Lawton, 619–674. Washington, DC: American Psychological Association, 1973.

Marquardt, Gesine, Kathrin Bueter, and Tom Motzek. "Impact of the Design of the Built Environment on People with Dementia: An Evidence-Based Review." *HERD: Health Environments Research & Design Journal* 8, no. 1 (2014): 127–157.

Mitchell-Auli, Peter, and Christine Sowinski. *Die 5. Generation: KDA-Quartiershäuser.* Berlin: Kuratorium Deutsche Altershilfe, 2012.

Pflegewohnheim Erika Horn, Andritz. *Best Architects Award, Zinnobergruen Gmbh, Best Architects*, 2017.

Pojer M., and C. Hartinger. "Köln: Kuratorium Deutsche Altershilfe." *Participation in Everyday Life: The Care Concept* (2017): 52.

Residential Care Home Andritz. *Architektur & Detail: Concept*, no. 3 (2016).

Sütterlin, Sabine, Iris Hoßmann, and Reiner Klingholz. *Demenz-Report: Wie sich die Regionen in Deutschland, Österreich und der Schweiz auf die Alterung der Gesellschaft vorbereiten können.* Berlin: DEU, 2011.

Tragatschnig, Ulrich. "Dietger Wissounig: Pflegewohnheim in Graz Andritz. Bauen für die Generation Z." *Architektur Aktuell: The Art of Building*, April, 2016.

Welter, Rudolf, Matthias Hürlimann, and Katharina Hürlimann-Siebke. *Gestaltung von Betreuungseinrichtungen für Menschen mit Demenzerkrankungen: Arbeitsbuch für Trägerschaften, Leitungen von Heimen und Pflegewohngruppen, Behörden, Architekten, Innenarchitekten sowie Bauausführende.* Zurich: Demenzplus Hürlimann, Welter, K, Hürlimann-Siebke, 2006.

Zeisel, John. "Improving Person-Centered Care Through Effective Design." *Generations* 37, no. 3 (2013): 45–52.

Zeisel, John, Nina M. Silverstein, Joan Hyde, Sue Levkoff, M. Powell Lawton, and William Holmes. "Environmental Correlates to Behavioral Health Outcomes in Alzheimer's Special Care Units." *The Gerontologist* 43, no. 5 (2003): 697–711.

Chapter 4

Advancing Rehabilitation
Design that Considers Physical and Cognitive Disabilities

Brenna Costello

4.1 Introduction

The design of rehabilitation facilities can help people manage the myriad physical, psychological, cognitive, and social challenges of living with debilitating illnesses or injuries. There are many types of rehabilitation facilities, including inpatient and outpatient rehab facilities, as well as long-term acute care rehab. Each facility has different licensing requirements based on the population and length of stay. An inpatient rehabilitation facility (IRF) typically has a length of stay from 3 to 28 days, whereas a long-term acute care hospital (LTACH) specializing in rehabilitative medicine can range from two to six months for an average length of stay.

This chapter introduces the health needs of individuals who have physical disabilities and cognitive disorders, describes the history of rehabilitative medicine and design, outlines key design concepts for rehab facilities, and presents case studies that utilize these concepts.

4.2 Recognizing Health Needs

4.2.1 Conditions

There are several types of injuries or disorders that lead people to require rehabilitative care. Physical and cognitive disabilities can be caused by brain damage, orthopedic injury, stroke, amputation, or a serious wound. There are also many chronic diseases that interfere with physical mobility and cognition, such as multiple sclerosis, epilepsy, cerebral palsy, Parkinson's disease, and Alzheimer's disease. Some of these conditions, such as craniosynostosis and spina bifida, cause physical disabilities that are present from birth, while others represent a significant life change after injury or diagnosis. In all cases, patients often require lifelong therapies to regain some of their independence. Unfortunately, the number of patients facing these conditions is increasing. The U.S. outpatient rehabilitation market is estimated to grow 5% or more, with the inpatient rehabilitation population growth projected at 3% annually. As more and more services are offered in outpatient settings, outpatient volumes will continue to increase faster than inpatient volumes.

4.2.2 Comorbidities

Individuals with an incapacitating illness or injury frequently experience multiple medical conditions, known as comorbidities. For example, physical disabilities that severely limit movement and physical activity often prevent people from performing cardiovascular exercise. A lack of exercise can lead to heart or lung disease, weight gain, obesity, and diabetes. Limited mobility can make skin vulnerable to breakdown and pressure ulcers. Someone who has experienced a stroke, amputation, or injury that affects one side of the body may develop an irregular gait to compensate for the side that does not function properly; this, in turn, can cause hip or knee problems or other adverse reactions. Psychological disorders, like depression and anxiety, are commonly experienced by rehab patients as well. Rehabilitation medicine covers a broad spectrum of these linked health needs.

4.3 History

Warm Springs, Georgia, where Franklin Delano Roosevelt sought regular treatment for polio beginning in the 1920s, is largely recognized as one of the first facilities in the U.S. to offer comprehensive rehabilitation care. During this time, therapies included sunlight therapy, exercise, massage, and orthotics, as well as occupational and recreational therapies. Less than a decade later, Temple University Medical School in Philadelphia created the first university department dedicated to this type of medicine in 1929. The department was founded by Dr. Frank Krusen, who noticed the physical effects of inactivity in himself and other bedridden patients treated at a tuberculosis sanatorium. In 1935, Dr. Krusen moved to Mayo Clinic in Rochester, Minnesota, to study treatments for physically disabled military personnel and other rehab patients. Throughout the latter half of the twentieth century, the science of rehabilitation medicine continued to expand beyond physical therapies and pain management. Other therapies began to emerge, such as psychological counseling, vocational therapy, and therapy using early stages of robotics (Atanelov, Stiens, and Young 2015).

4.4 Evolution of Care

Advancements in medicine, science, and technology continue to change the nature of rehabilitation medicine. More people are surviving accidents, injuries, and medical emergencies that would have proved fatal in the past. Patients with complex health needs, such as a person with a spinal cord injury coupled with internal bleeding, often require access to medical expertise from multiple disciplines, different care protocols, and a range of state-of-the-art medical equipment and technologies. Given the rapid advances in rehabilitation medicine, rehab facilities need to be designed to support not only the medical science of today but also what is on the horizon. Examples include high-tech biomechanical limbs with Bluetooth technology to track and enhance mobility, which are supplanting earlier prosthetics shaped and colored to look much like the body part they were built to replace. Advanced imaging technologies are also being used to aid in diagnosing complex injuries. Motion capture cameras and virtual reality simulators are being used to help rehab patients recondition their bodies and minds. All of these advanced technologies create the need for architecture to be flexible and adaptable to future needs. Raised floors, larger data centers, and simulator labs that can be easily converted from single spaces to large-team virtual reality (VR) settings are just a few examples of how a building can grow over time as new therapeutic products are released. The continuum of care has also evolved to include a broad network of services that goes beyond taking someone from the onset of trauma to independent living. While no single facility uses a scripted program for delivering care, many facilities have a few common therapy spaces, such as physical therapy, occupational therapy, speech therapy, and nursing care spaces. Table 4.1 provides basic rules of thumb for common injuries and disorders requiring rehabilitation services. It is important to note, however, that rehabilitation care is delivered by teams of different care providers, such as physical therapists, occupational therapists, pharmacists, nutritionists, and speech therapists (Gans, Pomeranz, and Riggs 2016).

4.5 Design Objectives

Rehab facilities help people with physical disabilities develop personal autonomy and find a pathway toward independent living. The design of these facilities must strike a balance between the spatial and infrastructure needs of advanced technologies and the humanistic needs of patients. Patients are typically in a facility for an extended period; therefore, the facility becomes a patient and his or her family's home for several months.

4.6 Key Concepts

To create rehab facilities that serve as effective therapeutic vehicles for recovery, designers need to keep the six key concepts outlined ahead in mind.

4.6.1 Design Should Support Multidisciplinary Care

Workspaces should be collaborative, shared, and open (with minimal private offices), to support team-based care models. Patients can see upwards of 12–15 specialists during their recovery journey, so it is imperative that these providers work together for the benefit of the patient.

Table 4.1 Overview of needs for rehabilitation care

Injury/disorder	Average length of stay	Specific program needs	Staffing model (nurses only)
Brain injured	1–4 months, but varies depending on severity of injury; years of outpatient follow-up	Low-stimulus environments, intensive speech, psychology, and occupational therapy (OT), physical therapy (PT)	1:3–5 ratio; team based—occasional one-on-one supervision needed
Spinal cord injured	1–6 months, but varies depending on the severity of injury; years of outpatient follow-up	Mobility training devices, assistive technologies, casting/splinting areas	1:4–5 ratio; team based
Orthopedic	3–28 days; months to years of outpatient follow-up	Mobility training devices, casting/splinting areas	1:5–6 ratio; team based
Stroke	3–28 days; months to years of outpatient follow-up	Cognitive therapy of all forms, general OT and PT	1:5 ratio
Birth disorders	Varies; typically a few months at a time over various times of their lives; continuous outpatient follow-up	Varies	1:4–6 ratio; team based—occasional one-on-one supervision needed
Sensory (blind, deaf rehab)	Varies; but usually this is combined with another impairment	Blind rehab training areas and vision testing areas	1:4–5 ratio; team based
Aging population	Varies	Similar needs and environment as all mentioned earlier, but less robust equipment due to age of patient	1:4–6 ratio

Note: Not all patient populations are included in this chart.

Source: SmithGroup and RTA Associates

4.6.2 Design Should Help Patients Regain Independence

To facilitate greater independence, patients often use equipment like voice activation software or other assistive technology that enables them to control devices through the motor functions available to them. Private patient rooms with adaptive controls for elements like lighting, room temperature, and window shades give patients in rehab facilities more control over their personal environment. A variety of spaces outside the patient room are also needed to encourage autonomy. Rehab patients often feel more comfortable in different types of settings during their recovery process. Creating a range of environments, from

Brenna Costello

sheltered areas to livelier spaces, promotes independent choice and individual well-being. As an example, many patients with post-traumatic stress disorder (PTSD) who have recently been injured by someone or something approaching them from out of their line of sight need to see all entry points of a space from where they are sitting to feel safe. Alternately, people injured by a sporting accident or perhaps born with an impairment are more at ease in larger public spaces. Keep in mind that every patient is different and may often be suffering from more than just the physical impairment seen by the eye.

4.6.3 Design Should Empower Patients

Rehab facilities utilize a wide range of diagnostic and treatment spaces, equipment, and technology to help patients regain mental and physical capabilities. These facilities must accommodate several therapies intended to strengthen patients' minds and bodies through spaces like meditation rooms, therapy pools, rehab gyms, and places to practice daily living skills. These may also include highly technical environments, like computerized gait labs or virtual reality simulators (Figure 4.1).

4.6.4 Design Should Optimize Safety

Rehab facilities should be accessible and easy to navigate. Illness or injury can adversely affect rehab patients' physical mobility, vision, balance, concentration, and wayfinding abilities. Designs that respond with sensitivity to patients' needs

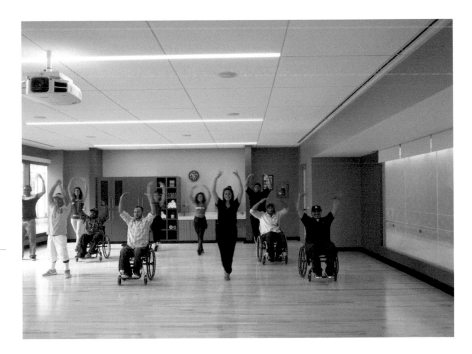

▶ Figure 4.1

Dance therapy at Rancho Los Amigos National Rehabilitation Hospital to promote a healthy cardio lifestyle.
Source: John Edward Linden Photography

help them navigate a facility safely and with greater independence. Clear sight lines and other safety features, like patient lifts, also help caregivers prevent injuries. Staff should be consulted to understand care processes, technology requirements, and spatial adjacencies. Staff are the front line in caring for rehab patients, so they need to understand patients' needs and act on their behalf when necessary.

4.6.5 Design Should Inspire Occupants

Rehab facilities should instill confidence, hope, serenity, and stability in patients, staff, and visitors. The facilities should be beautiful and uplifting to encourage healing. Designers should utilize materials, forms, and features like natural light and landscaping to help reduce stress.

4.6.6 Design Should Enhance Personal Connections

Designs that help strengthen family bonds, promote group interaction, and engage the larger community aid patients in healing and encourage their integration into society. Spaces that support family and group togetherness and communication, or that invite community members into the facility, reinforce social ties. Café spaces, family lounges, and gaming areas provide interaction among patients and families, building camaraderie.

It is important to note that rehabilitation services have expanded outside the patient room to every area of a rehab facility. Corridors, gyms, dining rooms, gardens, social spaces, and high-tech simulated settings are all for rehabilitation care. The following case studies demonstrate how rehab facility design concepts can be put into practice.

4.7 Case Studies

4.7.1 Craig Hospital, Englewood, Colorado

Craig Hospital, located in the Denver suburb of Englewood, is consistently ranked among the top ten rehabilitation hospitals in the United States. The hospital specializes in advanced care for people with traumatic brain injuries and spinal cord injuries. In designing an expansion and renovation of the facility, project team members immersed themselves in hospital operations through a week-long shadowing exercise that included night-shift observations. These nightly observations provided insight into how rehabilitation care and culture were either enhanced or hindered by spatial conditions. This exercise helped to identify ways in which the design could help patients with cognitive and physical impairments regain independence after a catastrophic event (Frasca et al. 2013).

The Craig Hospital leadership team's primary goal for the expansion was to create a cohesive campus from the existing but separate buildings (Figure 4.2).

Craig Hospital expansion with new drop-off and plaza connecting two buildings to create a campus.
Source: Cooperthwaite Productions

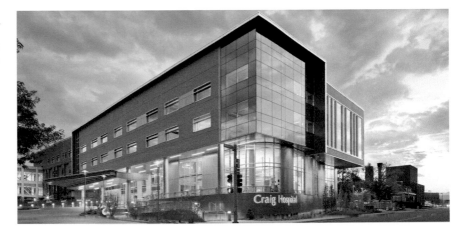

Craig Hospital patient room with full-coverage lift system.
Source: Cooperthwaite Productions

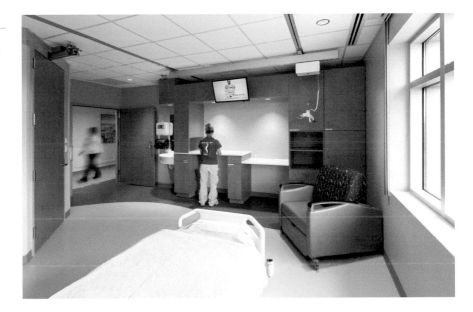

Their defined program required private occupancy patient rooms, therapy spaces that allowed for the most state-of-the-art technologies, and flexibility for potential growth in outpatient services. Through a series of vision sessions, an immersion process, and collaboration with patient advocacy groups, the project started to unfold in clear directions. The expanded hospital is designed with two new inpatient units housing 52 private, generously sized patient rooms to allow for private family interactions and consultations with the care team. All patient rooms have a full-coverage lift system that continues from bed to bath, providing safety to both the patient and staff members. The lift system also provides standing support for daily habits training at the patient sink, encouraging patients to be independent (Figure 4.3). To facilitate care for complex patients, outlets for medical gases are located on both sides of the patient bed. To give patients more control over their personal environment, light switches, television remotes, and electronic window shades can be operated by a tablet device.

Places of respite outside the patient room are provided to prevent patients from feeling isolated. Group settings vary in size to allow patients to choose environments that make them feel most comfortable, from minimal noise and distraction to progressively higher levels of social interaction. Each unit features a light-filled gathering space and main bistro. In addition, there are small alcoves off the corridor for one-on-one communication, spaces for groups of four to six patients to mingle, and large group rooms.

The new inpatient units at the hospital adjoin an intensive therapy zone with space for physical therapy, occupational therapy, assistive technologies, and a daily living suite, where patients can learn to accomplish routine tasks. Clinic support spaces are included here as well. The therapy zone also houses an aquatic therapy pool and the hospital's PEAK (Performance, Exercise, Attitude, and Knowledge) Center, a health and wellness program where members of the community can access rehabilitation therapy and use adaptive equipment for fitness and strength training (Figure 4.4).

A post-occupancy evaluation at Craig Hospital revealed a 10% reduction in patients' length of stay compared to the existing facility's average rating over the previous four years; for quadriplegics, this percentage represents a two-week reduction. The evaluation also showed a 100% increase in patient satisfaction with respect to privacy compared to the previous four years, much of which is attributed to the new private patient rooms, the reduction of noise throughout the facility, and the inclusion of spaces that allow family and patients to build camaraderie.

▼ Figure 4.4

Craig Hospital's PEAK (Performance, Exercise, Attitude, and Knowledge) Center.
Source: Cooperthwaite Productions

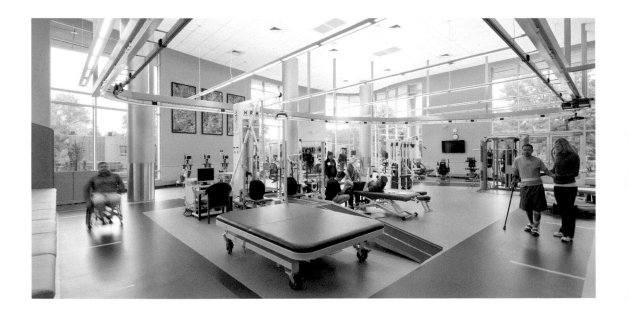

Brenna Costello

4.7.2 Center for the Intrepid, San Antonio, Texas

The Center for the Intrepid (CFI) is a 65,000-square foot, four-story building designed for the care of military patients and veterans with severe extremity injuries, amputations, and burns. The most critically injured patients, many of whom were wounded in Iraq or Afghanistan, have experienced double or triple amputations, severe burns, head and body trauma, blindness, deafness, and partial or full paralysis. Many patients had sustained multiple concurrent traumas, or polytraumas (Department of Veterans Affairs, Polytrauma System of Care 2019).

The center is located on six acres of the Brooke Army Medical Center complex of Fort Sam Houston. In addition to the rehab center, the site contains two Fisher Houses, which are 21-unit, short-term-stay residences for families of soldiers receiving rehabilitative care. The site's landscape design creates an atmosphere of healing and welcome. A pergola planted with wisteria frames a series of indoor and outdoor rooms that include a healing garden, outdoor activity area, outdoor terrain park, and a ribbon of cypress trees. The gardens feature palms, flowering trees and shrubs, perennials, semitropical plants, and ground cover. Live oaks and cedar elms of various sizes shade the grounds.

The facility is the prototype for similar centers across the nation and worldwide. State-of-the-art technologies, like advanced prosthetics, computerized monitoring for biomechanical studies, virtual reality, robotics, and simulators, can potentially dehumanize a space. Therefore, this needed to be accounted for in the design. To give patients the best opportunity to regain their pre-injury abilities, the building provides a therapeutic environment with abundant natural light and warm materials. Besides consultation and examination rooms, the clinic includes specialized spaces for prosthetics fitting and adjustments and areas for psychological counseling, clinical nutrition, social work, physical and occupational therapy, gait studies, telemedicine, and research. The therapy zone features a full-coverage lift system to ease patients on and off the mat tables for treatment, a rock-climbing wall for upper-body strength training and mobility, and other advanced therapy equipment (Figure 4.5).

The Center for the Intrepid has some of the most advanced rehabilitative technologies currently available. There is a Gait Lab fitted with 24 motion capture cameras mounted on a custom-fitted truss. There is also a Computer Assisted Rehabilitation Environment (CAREN), an advanced technology focusing on vestibular and balance coordination while being fully immersed in a virtual environment. It features a 21-foot-diameter dome with a 300-degree screen capable of displaying multiple virtual realities to help patients relearn real-world skills in safety, like walking on different terrains (Figure 4.6). The hospital also has a state-of-the-art Firearms Training Simulator (FATS) that allows patients who wish to return to active duty to practice and qualify with military-standard weapons systems. In addition, an activities of daily living (ADL) apartment and vehicle training simulator provide patients with realistic environments in which to practice everyday skills.

The building's training and exercise center features a cantilevered running track, a 21-foot climbing tower, and custom-designed elevating parallel bars. Gait lanes, uneven terrain and obstacle simulations, and specialized equipment for strength, balance, agility, and motor skill therapy are included as well. The two-story, light-filled space for rehabilitation training and exercise spans the

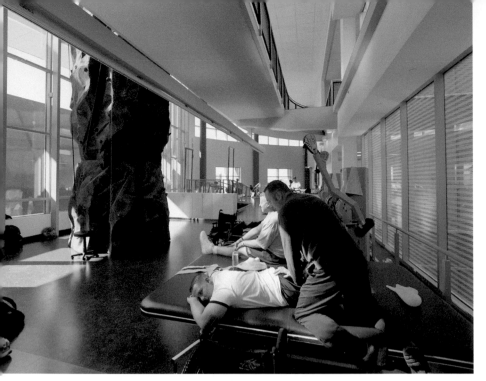

◀ Figure 4.5

The Center for the Intrepid
therapy zone.
Source: Timothy Hursley

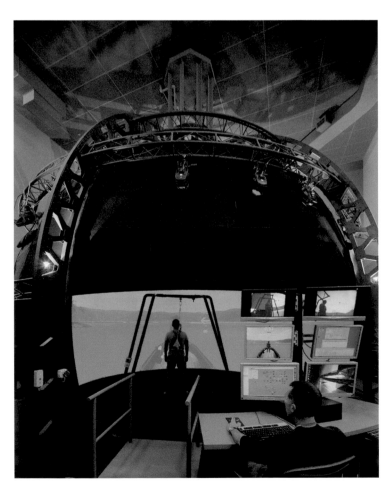

◀ Figure 4.6

The CAREN at the Center
for the Intrepid.
Source: Timothy Hursley

Brenna Costello

entire front of the building. The elongated, expansive design allows multiple rehabilitation activities to be conducted simultaneously within and adjacent to this area, facilitating visibility and interaction between patients, families, and caregivers. The openness and transparency enable people to encourage and sustain one another when the going gets tough. A swimming pool, wave pool, coffee/Internet lounge, and several outdoor recreation areas, including a basketball court with a custom-designed cushioned surface, are provided as recreational therapy and social spaces for patients and their families (Beringer 2004).

4.7.3 National Intrepid Center of Excellence, Bethesda, Maryland

The National Intrepid Center of Excellence (NICoE), located at the Walter Reed National Military Medical Center, is a 72,000-square-foot outpatient rehabilitation facility for military personnel with mild to moderate traumatic brain injury (TBI), PTSD, and other psychological health issues (Figure 4.7). The center provides imaging, assessment, diagnostic, and treatment services in an environment designed to meet the physical, emotional, and spiritual needs of patients, families, and caregivers.

The NICoE encompasses each of the key concepts previously discussed, with the addition of a few other design principles focused around patient- and family-centered care. These include sensitivity to how light fills the building and the use of materials that are contextual to the military base. Given the mission

▼ Figure 4.7

National Intrepid Center of Excellence façade detail and exterior uplighting.
Source: Maxwell MacKenzie

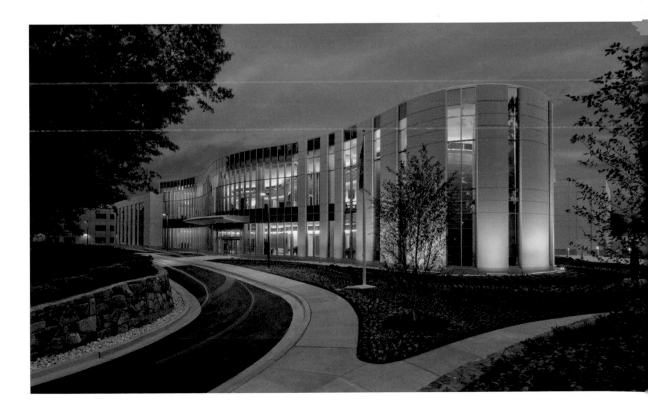

of the NICoE of focusing on invisible wounds—wounds not seen by others but those that impact the brain and psyche of a human—the building needed to reflect understanding and compassion in the design (Collicutt McGrath 2009). For this reason, the building was intended to be an inward-facing building, one that is less pronounced on the exterior, focusing most of its importance and emotion inward.

Multidisciplinary, collaborative workspaces, known as "beehives", are strategically located within each department to enhance staff collaboration and cross-pollination of medical knowledge. A dedicated patient intake room, located near the front of the clinic, provides a space for patients to meet with their entire care team of professionals and discuss their specific ailments at the start of their stay. The team is able to ask questions pertaining to their respective specialty and learn about all of the patient's issues as they are covered by each discipline in the room; the team can then better collaborate on the best diagnostic and treatment care plan for each patient (Figure 4.8).

The building was designed analogously to the way a brain functions (Figure 4.9). The right brain, the more whimsical, free-flowing side, is represented in the virtual reality areas, education spaces, and physical therapy gym. Representing the left brain, the more structured and orthogonal side of the brain, are the imaging suite, exam rooms, and diagnostic areas. To diagnose complex brain injuries, the NICoE facility houses advanced imaging technologies that include a 3-Tesla magnetic resonance imaging (MRI) machine, a 64-slice positron emission tomography–computed tomography (PET-CT) scanner, an Elekta Neuromag magnetoencephalography (MEG) scanner, and a functional transcranial Doppler spectroscopy (fTCDS), each with its own spatial requirements.

A CAREN virtual reality environment, FATS firearm training simulator, and a motor vehicle simulator, like those available at the National Center for the

▼ Figure 4.8

The National Intrepid Center of Excellence operational model for collaborative diagnostic and treatment planning.
Source: SmithGroup

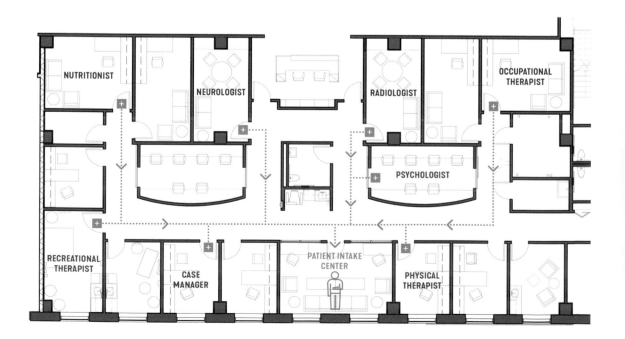

Brenna Costello

Concept diagram of the NICoE building describing the functional layout of the building.
Source: SmithGroup

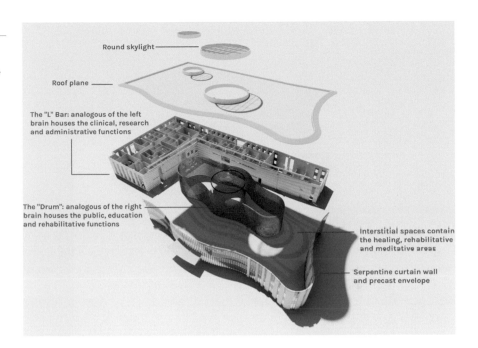

Round skylight

Roof plane

The "L" Bar: analogous of the left brain houses the clinical, research and administrative functions

The "Drum": analogous of the right brain houses the public, education and rehabilitative functions

Interstitial spaces contain the healing, rehabilitative and meditative areas

Serpentine curtain wall and precast envelope

Intrepid in San Antonio, Texas, also are provided at the NICoE. In addition, there is a 900-square-foot virtual reality environment laboratory that is dedicated to researching virtual reality as a tool to help patients overcome post-traumatic stress and improve cognitive abilities.

The importance of indirect and uniform levels of lighting in a facility of this kind cannot be understated. Patients recovering from brain injuries have a difficult time adjusting to contrast, especially when it comes to bright light vs. dark spaces. A beautiful ray of light shining through a building and casting a shadow on the wall or floor becomes a hurdle for these patients to navigate. At the NICoE, lighting levels are even throughout the building, with smooth transitions from light to dark as opposed to sharp contrasts. The building is sited to take advantage of northern light—the softest, least intense natural light—as much as possible. Very few spaces are lit only with artificial light; floor-to-ceiling glass and clerestory windows bring natural light into the building. This is supplemented with indirect uplighting.

In addition to the lighting, the design focuses on a series of goals encompassing the essence of how one would feel in this space: a welcoming sense of transparency, sense of stability, performance, calmness, and a feeling of hope. This is achieved through a serpentine glass curtain wall that encloses educational and therapy spaces as well as all public areas. This wall is mirrored by a wood-clad wall that runs along the main lobby. The curved curtain wall is intended to welcome patients and visitors and aid with wayfinding. The lobby and waiting areas have a variety of types of spaces, allowing patients to find their preferred place to rest and wait (Figure 4.10). Simple and warm finishes convey a sense of stability and permanence, while natural materials and warm-colored finishes provide a calming environment. A water feature near the reception/registration desk and a white noise system along the entire inner lobby mask noise from the two-story open space. Acoustical ceiling tile, carpet, textiles, and furnishings

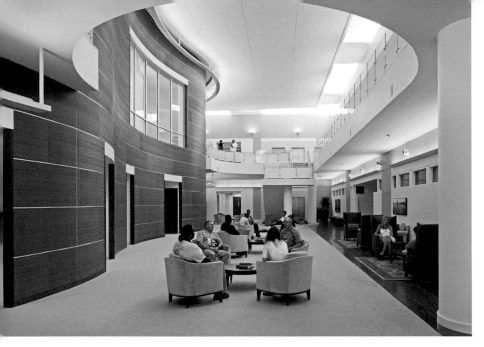

◀ Figure 4.10

National Intrepid Center
of Excellence lobby and
waiting area.
Source: Maxwell MacKenzie

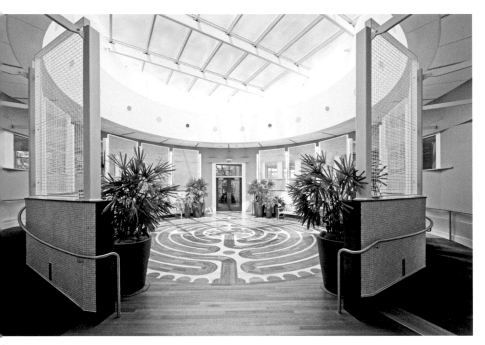

◀ Figure 4.11

Central Park at the
National Intrepid Center of
Excellence.
Source: Maxwell MacKenzie

in the inner lobby help absorb noise, while the curved surfaces deflect noise in multiple directions, allowing it to dissipate.

The free-form spaces created within the undulating walls are meant to evoke feelings of confidence in a purposefully non-institutional environment. A variety of ceiling heights and widths, as well as numerous cutouts and overlooks, gives users a rich spatial experience and access to light and views from any vantage point.

An open, sky-lit space known as Central Park provides room for music and art therapy, meditative activities, and theater performances (Figure 4.11). Central Park is a light-filled multi-purpose space providing patients with terrain challenges

Brenna Costello

around the perimeter and calming labyrinth training in the middle. The staff also use this space for weekly yoga classes, music therapy, and family respite space. In addition, there is a state-of-the-art multimedia conference room that allows staff members to brief visitors, communicate with other facilities, and provide patients with a direct link to remote family members. Other spaces at the facility designed for family interaction include a family lounge and an outdoor seating area with patio tables and chairs; a children's play structure, swing set, and sandbox; and a putting green, a basketball court, and badminton court.

A post-occupancy study was completed a year after opening. This study combined data from patient satisfaction surveys issued by the facility, along with operational shadowing and workshops to analyze the functional use, efficiency, and satisfaction with the performance of the building. The facility received an overall satisfaction rate of 99% from people surveyed about the design, with 92% responding that they feel more hopeful after coming to the building.

4.7.4 Ranchos Los Amigos National Rehabilitation Center, Downey, California

Ranchos Los Amigos National Rehabilitation Center provides inpatient, outpatient, and wellness services for individuals with brain injuries, orthopedic disabilities, stroke damage, neurological disorders, physical and developmental disorders, and adult or pediatric spinal cord injuries. The facility, which was established in 1888, is the longest continuously operating rehab facility in the U.S. and is now owned and operated by the County of Los Angeles.

In a project totaling 209,250 square feet, the existing inpatient hospital was renovated and expanded while a new outpatient building and aquatics center were constructed. The design of the renovation and expansion project focuses on four key factors. First, create an intuitive environment through wayfinding and navigation. Second, promote opportunities for social interaction and rest for recovering patients and family support teams. Third, create an environment that is bright, joyful, and comfortable. And lastly, support an inclusive community that allows for continued involvement. The newly constructed outpatient center entry connects to the newly constructed wellness center with a seamless architectural fabric. With these two additional buildings, Rancho now provides the full continuum of rehabilitative care to its patients and community (Figure 4.12).

To orient patients and family members in the building, a central, double-height concourse in the outpatient building leads to the clinics, wellness center, therapy gyms, and inpatient facility. Along the 150-foot-long, light-filled space, there are small alcoves and niches for interaction and rest for recovering patients. The interior is defined by warm wood tones, neutral stone, and bright graphics. Layered materials, including glass screens, acoustical panels, and mosaic tile, combine to create an uplifting, healing environment. Sliding window walls in the double-height therapy gym blur the border between indoor and outdoor spaces.

With community engagement being the spirit of Rancho, the leadership team wanted the design to express the ebb and flow of people on-site. To encourage this flow, several site improvements were completed on the exterior, including a parking structure, healing gardens, therapy gardens, and a

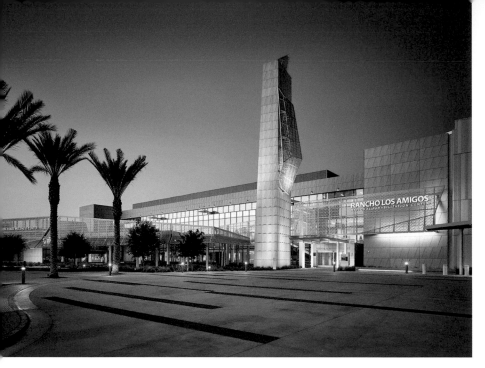

◀ Figure 4.12

Rancho Los Amigos
National Rehabilitation
Hospital.
Source: John Edward Linden
Photography

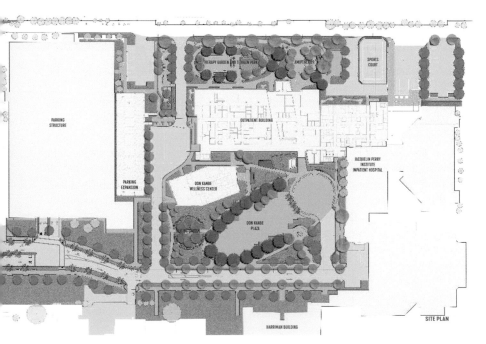

◀ Figure 4.13

Site plan of Rancho
Los Amigos National
Rehabilitation Hospital
Campus.
Source: SmithGroup and
Taylor Associates

terrain park. In addition to these spaces, the grand plaza, which connects all the buildings, is designed to host a weekly farmers' market, special events, and the annual wheelchair games. An iconic tower references the historical design vernacular and provides a dominant wayfinding cue. A series of interconnected gardens surround the facility, providing a parklike atmosphere. These outdoor gardens serve a dual purpose as clinical and meditative spaces, and are programmed specifically, as is the case with the terrain park (Markus and Sachs 2014) (Figure 4.13).

Brenna Costello

4.8 Conclusions

As rehabilitation technologies and assistive devices continue to progress, rehabilitation environments will need to evolve to support the model of care being delivered. To accommodate the rapid changes in care delivery, raised floors, flexible simulation labs, and open therapy areas with multiple storage closets may be considerations in future designs. Certain technological innovations, such as the development of robotic exoskeletons that assist seriously injured people in standing and walking, may diminish comorbidities associated with limited bodily movement, but will be able to be utilized only if the space is supportive of this new technology. In this case, a long, clear floor space, or gait lane, is needed, where a patient can wear the device and practice walking on an unobstructed path.

In closing, rehabilitation facilities need to deliver high-level care for patients working to rebuild their lives. It is important to address not only the physical needs but also the psychosocial needs by increasing family and care partner involvement. Open workstations or collaborative workspace and digital wall displays that enable care teams to talk through challenges together, combined with more private consultation rooms and phone rooms, will help teams deliver more effective, multidisciplinary care. Holistic spaces that give caregivers a place of respite, as well as work areas that allow them to collaborate on complex cases, will continue to be critical in the design of these facilities.

Bibliography

Adevi, Anna A., and Fredrika Mårtensson. "Stress Rehabilitation Through Garden Therapy: The Garden as A Place in the Recovery from Stress." *Urban Forestry & Urban Greening* 12, no. 2 (2013): 230–237.

Atanelov, Levan, Steven A. Stiens, and Mark A. Young. "History of Physical Medicine and Rehabilitation and Its Ethical Dimensions." *AMA Journal of Ethics* 17, no. 6 (2015): 568–574.

Beringer, Almut. "Spinal Cord Injury and Outdoor Experiences." *International Journal of Rehabilitation Research* 27, no. 1 (2004): 7–15.

Campagnol, Gabriela, and Mardelle McCuskey Shepley. "Positive Distraction and The Rehabilitation Hospitals of João Filgueiras Lima." *HERD: Health Environments Research & Design Journal* 8, no. 1 (2014): 199–227.

Collicutt McGrath, Joanna. "Post-Acute In-Patient Rehabilitation." *Psychological Approaches to Rehabilitation After Traumatic Brain Injury* (2009): 39–64.

Davis, Brad E. "Rooftop Hospital Gardens for Physical Therapy: A Post-Occupancy Evaluation." *HERD: Health Environments Research & Design Journal* 4, no. 3 (2011): 14–43.

Department of Veterans Affairs. *Polytrauma Rehabilitation Center Design Guide.* 2014, December. www.cfm.va.gov/til/dGuide/dgPRC.pdf.

Department of Veterans Affairs. *Polytrauma System of Care: VHA Directive 1172.01.* 2019, January. www.va.gov/OPTOMETRY/docs/VHA_Directive_1172-01_Polytrauma_System_of_Care_1172_01_D_2019-01-24.pdf.

Frasca, Diana, Jennifer Tomaszczyk, Bradford J. McFadyen, and Robin EA Green. "Traumatic Brain Injury and Post-Acute Decline: What Role Does Environmental Enrichment Play? A Scoping Review." *Frontiers in Human Neuroscience* 7 (2013): 31.

Gans, Bruce M., Bruce A. Pomeranz, and Richard V. Riggs. "Avoiding Harm and Achieving Good in Rehabilitation Hospitals and Units." *American Journal of Physical Medicine & Rehabilitation* 95, no. 11 (2016): 787–788.

Goto, Seiko, Thomas J. Gianfagia, John P. Munafo, Eijiro Fujii, Xuting Shen, Minkai Sun, Bertram Emil Shi, Congcong Liu, Hiroshi Hamano, and Karl Herrup. "The Power of Traditional Design Techniques: The Effects of Viewing a Japanese Garden on Individuals with Cognitive Impairment." *HERD: Health Environments Research & Design Journal* 10, no. 4 (2017): 74–86.

Han, Ah-Reum, Sin-Ae Park, and Byung-Eun Ahn. "Reduced Stress and Improved Physical Functional Ability in Elderly with Mental Health Problems Following a Horticultural Therapy Program." *Complementary Therapies in Medicine* 38 (2018): 19–23.

Horowitz, Sala. "Therapeutic Gardens and Horticultural Therapy: Growing Roles in Health Care." *Alternative and Complementary Therapies* 18, no. 2 (2012): 78–83.

Logan, P. A., M. F. Walker, and J. R. F. Gladman. "Description of an Occupational Therapy Intervention Aimed at Improving Outdoor Mobility." *British Journal of Occupational Therapy* 69, no. 1 (2006): 2–6.

Markus, Clare Cooper, and Naomi A. Sachs. *Therapeutic Landscapes: An Evidence-Based Approach to Designing Healing Gardens and Restorative Outdoor Spaces.* Hoboken, NJ: Wiley, 2014.

Souter-Brown, Gayle. *Landscape and Urban Design for Health and Well-Being: Using Healing, Sensory and Therapeutic Gardens.* New York, NY: Routledge, 2014.

Spring, Josephine Anne. "Design of Evidence-Based Gardens and Garden Therapy for Neurodisability in Scandinavia: Data from 14 Sites." *Neurodegenerative Disease Management* 6, no. 2 (2016): 87–98.

Ulrich, Roger S., Robert F. Simons, Barbara D. Losito, Evelyn Fiorito, Mark A. Miles, and Michael Zelson. "Stress Recovery During Exposure to Natural and Urban Environments." *Journal of Environmental Psychology* 11, no. 3 (1991): 201–230.

Wagenfeld, Amy, Connie Roy-Fisher, and Carolyn Mitchell. "Collaborative Design: Outdoor Environments for Veterans with PTSD." *Facilities* 31, no. 9–10 (2013): 391–406.

Williams, Brian J., Pratik Gandhi, and Arthur Jimenez. "Poster 169 Assessment and Discussion of Acute Care Hospital Readmission Etiologies from Acute Inpatient Rehabilitation Units: A Quality of Care Analysis." *PM&R* 9, no. 6 (2014): S244.

Brenna Costello

Chapter 5

Design Attributes for Improved Mental and Behavioral Health

Mardelle McCuskey Shepley and Naomi A. Sachs

5.1 Introduction

Mental illnesses are common worldwide and exceedingly complex, resulting from factors linked to biology, psychological conditions, personal choices and habits, and environmental influences. According to the U.S. Department of Health and Human Services, "mental health" is the "successful performance of mental function, resulting in productive activities, fulfilling relationships with other people, and an ability to adapt to change and to cope with adversity" (2019). While achieving mental health is an ideal state, the reality is that many people suffer from diagnosable mental disorders that can be disruptive, life-altering, and debilitating if untreated. Almost one in five adults is affected by mental illness in the United States, higher for women (22.3%) than men (15.1%), and highest among the population between the ages of 18 and 25 years old (25.8%) (SAMHSA 2017). Mental health and substance abuse disorders as a category are the leading cause of working years lost due to disability in the United States, just ahead of musculoskeletal disorders (Kamal 2016).

There are two major shortcomings with respect to the treatment of mental illness and behavioral health issues: lack of access to health services and inadequately planned and designed facilities. First, the lack of access to mental health services is due, in part, to the underfunding and shortage of qualified professionals. Second, mental and behavioral health facilities are not aligned with the needs and conditions of the diverse population they serve. Designers and providers find it difficult to simultaneously support the needs of such a wide variety of individuals, many with multiple diagnoses, sensory processing deficits, and cognitive disorders (Shepley and Pasha 2017). Furthermore, the carryovers from historical approaches to mental health design reinforce an institutional model that often contradicts basic human needs for privacy, autonomy, territoriality, socialization, and self-worth.

This chapter tackles mental and behavioral health (MBH) design and is organized into five main sections: (1) defining mental and behavioral health,

(2) an overview of MBH settings and patients, (3) an evidence-based design (EBD) MBH framework, (4) design goals and strategies for MBH facilities, and (5) three exemplary projects that showcase these design goals and strategies.

5.2 Defining Mental and Behavioral Health

Mental illnesses encompass a wide variety of mental disorders, including mood disorders, like depression and bipolar disorder; generalized anxiety disorders (e.g., obsessive-compulsive disorder, panic disorder, and social phobia); trauma-related disorders (e.g., post-traumatic stress disorder); and schizophrenia and other psychotic disorders (National Institute of Mental Health (n.d.). These disorders can be classified as any mental illness (e.g., schizophrenia, bipolar disorder or manic depression) that results in serious functional impairment and interferes with or limits the ability to perform major life activities. These health conditions involve changes in emotions, thinking, or behavior (or a combination of these) and can lead to problems with functioning in social situations, the workplace, and family relations.

Similar to other medical conditions, like heart disease or diabetes, mental disorders today are treatable by a variety of healthcare professionals at home or in outpatient and inpatient settings. Unfortunately, only about 35% of people who have been diagnosed with a mental disorder are seeking treatment, likely due to the stigma associated with the condition, and costs and other barriers that inhibit access to services (Kaiser Foundation 2017). Another reason may be that facilities are not designed around the needs of specific populations.

A related term that is often used interchangeably with mental health is behavioral health. Behavioral health is viewed separately and even as a subset of mental health. Not all mental health disorders are a result of behavioral issues, but rather are caused by brain chemistry and genetic inheritance. Behavioral health relates to choices and habits resulting in maladaptive behaviors that negatively impact one's physical and mental health (Torres and Estrine 2013). For example, schizophrenia might be defined as a mental disorder, while drug addiction might be perceived as a behavioral health issue. The line between "mental health" and "behavioral health" is blurred, and many people suffer from multiple mental and behavioral health comorbidities. For this reason, we have coupled the terms in this chapter as "mental and behavioral health (MBH)" to encompass the range of conditions.

5.3 Mental and Behavioral Health (MBH) Settings and Patients

The history of MBH facilities has shown multifarious attitudes toward mental illness, ranging from punishing the ill to treating them with compassion. As far back as the Middle Ages, caring for those with mental illness was focused on the secure incarceration of patients in hospices, workhouses, jails, and asylums. Forward in time, reports of German asylums around the 1800s described "mad cages", where patients were locked up "like animals" (Shorter 1997, p. 34–66). From the mid-eighteenth century to the nineteenth century, facilities were used

Mardelle McCuskey Shepley and Naomi A. Sachs

for custodial purposes and run by lay administrators who would seek consults from physicians. Physical restraints and extreme temperatures were used, since the common belief at the time was that the mentally ill were insensitive to pain and that extreme temperature conditions could shock them back to sanity (Talbott 1978). At this time, doctors believed that "insanity" cases were curable.

The Enlightenment brought new changes to the field and advancements in the understanding of mental health as an illness organic in nature. By the end of the nineteenth century, an enhanced understanding of mental illness led to more individualized care and better-trained attendants, which reduced reliance on medical restraints (Capland 1969). Pioneers like Philippe Pinel, William Tuke, and Thomas Kirkbride advocated for "moral treatment" of the mentally ill, which led to the banning of cruel and inhumane punishments and confinements. With this newfound mind-set, mental health disorders were treated through environmental therapies, like access to daylight, sun, nature, and the design of humanistic spaces. Tuke, for example, claimed that security could be achieved through direct observations of patients rather than the use of physical restraints. To reduce anxiety and restlessness, he recommended employing spaces such as galleries for indoor exercise, courts for outdoor exercise, and dayrooms for activity and social interaction (Tuke 1815).

Another pioneer, Dr. Thomas Kirkbride, wrote a book titled *On the Construction, Organization, and General Arrangement of Hospitals for the Insane* (1854). This book became the primary building template for asylums following a compassionate approach to care. His model included a series of designated patient wards (for different groups of patients) that were staggered to form canted wings attached to a central section of the building housing shared functions (Shepley and Pasha 2017). However, Kirkbride's belief that "moral treatment" could cure mental illness was shortsighted, resulting in an undertow of violence and chaos (Tomes 2000). The mental health profession realized over time that all mental illnesses are not the same, and that some people with severe mental disorders required more than "moral treatment" and, likely, medical interventions.

A collection of eye-opening essays published by Irving Goffman in the 1960s from his participant observation fieldwork in an asylum argued that a "total institution" (arrangement where people who are grouped based on conditions and cut off from the greater society for a considerable time) had detrimental effects on both patients and staff. Prolonged exposure to often hostile environments, ill-treatment of patients, and seclusion led to depression, anxiety, aggression, and violence. Therapies often mirrored the inhumane environments that warehoused people with mental illness. Lobotomy, electric shock therapy, and other medically based interventions were still common up until about the 1960s. Goffman's publication along with other notable studies and policies fueled a deinstitutionalization movement and community-based approaches to care. Once again, constraints, observation, seclusion, or physical restraints were reduced. Furthermore, the discovery of effective psychopharmacological agents in the 1950s enabled patients to function at a level that would allow them to be discharged, offering a promising solution to overcrowding (Talbott 1978).

In the late twentieth century, specific planning and design guidelines for mental health facilities were introduced (e.g., American Institute of Architect's first *Design Considerations for Mental Health Facilities* in 1993. Subsequent to that the first edition of the *Department of Veteran Affairs Mental Health Facilities Design Guide* and

Hunt and Sine's first edition of *Mental Health Facilities: Design Guide* published in 2010. These guidelines cover a variety of types of mental health facilities. According to Carr (2011), facilities serving MBH populations include: freestanding psychiatric hospitals, neurological/psychiatric nursing units within hospitals, facilities supporting individuals with both standard medical and mental health issues, gerontology psychiatric units, substance abuse treatment facilities (inpatient and outpatient), mental health clinics, correctional/forensic mental health facilities, ambulatory day hospitals, day treatment centers, and others (Shepley and Pasha 2017).

5.4 An Evidence-Based Design Mental and Behavioral Health (EBD MBH) Framework

Shepley and colleagues (2013) conducted a literature review and identified 17 topics related to the planning and design of MBH facilities. These 17 topics were then used in a research study that interviewed 19 psychiatric staff, facility administrators, and/or architects (Shepley et al. 2016). The researchers built upon their first study by conducting surveys with 134 psychiatric nursing organizational members to identify the features in the physical environment that are believed to positively impact staff and patients in psychiatric environments (Shepley et al. 2017). The most significant findings were used to generate an EBD MBH framework (Table 5.1). The framework is organized around

Table 5.1 **An EBD MBH framework**

All mental/behavioral health facilities	*Inpatient mental/behavioral health facilities*	
Behavioral outcomes		
Patient socialization	Patient socialization	
Patient satisfaction	Patient satisfaction	
Suicide reduction	Suicide reduction	
Pathological behavior reduction	Pathological behavior reduction	
Aggression reduction	Aggression reduction	
Staff stress reduction	Staff stress reduction	
	Patient stress reduction	
Physical environmental attributes – **Environmental qualities**		
Attractiveness and aesthetics	Ambience of patient safety	Attractiveness and aesthetics
Deinstitutionalized and homelike	Positive distraction	Deinstitutionalized and homelike
Nature connection	Ambience of staff support	Nature connection
Well-maintained environment	Social interaction	Well-maintained environment
	Autonomy and spontaneity	
Environmental features		
Proper light (daylight/electrical)	Indoor/outdoor therapy	Proper light (daylight/electrical)
Furnishings	One-on-one consult spaces	Furnishings
Noise control	Open nurse stations	Noise control
Staff support (respite and safety)	Private patient rooms	Staff support (respite and safety)

Source: Authors

Mardelle McCuskey Shepley and Naomi A. Sachs

three components: behavioral outcomes, environmental qualities, and environmental features. Behavioral outcomes relate to individuals' display of behavior, what is expected to be accomplished, and/or responses to environmental stimuli. Environmental qualities relate to high-level goals concerning ambience (e.g., attractiveness, aesthetics, deinstitutionalization, relationship to nature, and well-maintained environment). Environmental features relate to physical interventions, such as adequate light, furnishings, staff respite features, and acoustics. Inpatient MBH facilities were examined separately from outpatient because inpatients generally have a higher acuity level, spend longer amounts of time in the facilities, and have heightened issues of stress, loss of choice and control, and greater need for safety. Therefore, the framework is also separated into two categories: all MBH facilities and inpatient MBH facilities. Environmental qualities and features combined are referred to as attributes. The framework ahead is not meant to suggest a desired direction; rather it is a list of the most salient factors supported by research that should be considered in the design process and/or research studies. Presented here is a summary of the most significant findings from two studies (Shepley et al. 2016, 2017) that should be considered when designing for all MBH facilities (Table 5.2) and inpatient facilities (Table 5.3).

Table 5.2 Research on environmental qualities and features for all MBH settings

Physical environmental attributes	General findings	Related references
Environmental qualities		
Attractiveness and aesthetics	Beautiful spaces receive more positive ratings. An aesthetic environment includes appropriate lighting, comfortable furniture, positive distraction, and pleasant restrooms.	Maslow and Mintz (1956); Shepley et al. (2017)
Deinstitutionalized and homelike	Deinstitutionalized or homelike environments are generally supported by research; lack of a residential character in an environment is associated with poor evaluations.	Grosenick and Hatmaker (2000)
Nature connection	Access to nature provides psychological, physical, and cognitive benefits. Nature exposure, both real and simulated, has positive effects on pain and pulse rate.	Bailey (2002); Diette et al. (2003); Ulrich et al. (2003, 2018)
Well-maintained, orderly, and organized	Providing a well-maintained environment may decrease patient violence, improve staff mood, reduce staff absences, and support treatment.	Christenfeld et al. (1989); Grosenick and Hatmaker (2000)

(Continued)

Table 5.2 (Continued)

Physical environmental attributes	General findings	Related references
Environmental features		
Proper lighting (daylight/electrical)	Daylighting correlates with improved mood and improved sleep. Proper illumination in interior space contributes to reduced aggression.	Boubekri et al. (2014); Partonen and Lönnqvist (2000); Ulrich, Bogren, and Lundin (2012)
Furnishings (attractive, comfortable, damage-resistant)	Furniture should be attractive and damage-resistant as well as comfortable to provide psychological support and to support treatment.	Carr (2011); Davis, Guck, and Rosow (1979); Grosenick and Hatmaker (2000); Ingham and Spencer (1997); Shepley et al. (1999); Ulrich et al. (2018)
Noise control	Populations may be more susceptible to the negative effects of noise, such as headaches, anxiety, fatigue, and depression.	Brown et al. (2016); Stansfeld et al. (2000); Ulrich et al. (2018)
Staff support (respite and safety)	Staff respite areas enhance staff satisfaction and safety.	Forster, Cavness, and Phelps (1999); Martin (1995); Nejati, Rodiek, and Shepley (2016); Nejati et al. (2016)

Source: Authors

Table 5.3 Research on environmental qualities and features for inpatient MBH settings

Physical environmental attributes	General findings	Related references
Environmental qualities		
Ambience of patient safety	Patient safety, specifically suicide resistance, is a widely researched and crucial quality. It can be achieved through anti-ligature doorknobs and handles and tamperproof electrical systems.	Carr (2011); Watts et al. (2012)
Positive distraction	Positive distraction includes interventions such as views of nature, art, music, social interaction, and interactive technology. Aggression, agitation, and anxiety may be positively affected by distractions.	Cooper Marcus and Sachs (2014); Nanda et al. (2011); Shepley (2006); Ulrich, Bogren, and Lundin (2012); Ulrich et al. (2018)
Ambience of staff support	Staff respite is an environmental quality of interest, as staff can experience significant stress, especially if performing restraints or attempting to prevent self-destructive patient behavior.	Salerno et al. (2012)

Mardelle McCuskey Shepley and Naomi A. Sachs

Physical environmental attributes	General findings	Related references
Social interaction	Social interaction and community can be promoted through common areas and dayrooms allowing for interaction between patients and between patients and staff.	Davis, Guck, and Rosow (1979); Devlin (1992); Gutkowski, Ginath, and Guttmann (1992); Sidman and Moos (1973); Turlington (2004)
Autonomy and spontaneity	Spontaneity is a behavior associated with well-being.	Davis, Leach, and Clegg (2011); Sorlie et al. (2010)
Environmental features		
Indoor/outdoor therapy areas	Research supports indoor and outdoor therapy spaces. Indoor spaces are common and include group meeting spaces or spaces for art and OT; outdoor spaces, such as gardens, are less common.	Bryan, Rudd, and Wertenberger (2013); Cooper Marcus and Sachs (2014); Gjerden (1991); Sorlie et al. (2010); Ulrich, Bogren, and Lundin (2012)
One-on-one consultation	Spaces facilitating one-on-one consultation are specific recommendations aimed at encouraging interaction and community.	Gutkowski, Ginath, and Guttmann (1992); Perkins et al. (2012); Tyson et al. (2002)
Open nurse stations	Open nurse stations support patient-centered care and improve supervision. They may increase interaction with patients and improve patient self-image and satisfaction, and decreased violence.	Carr (2011); Christenfeld et al. (1989); Turlington (2004); Whitehead et al. (1984)
Private patient rooms	Private patient rooms facilitate emotional attachment and expression of ownership and provide a sense of therapeutic security and comfort.	Bailey (2002); Forster, Cavness, and Phelps (1999); Lynch, Plant, and Ryan (2005); Martin (1995); Salerno et al. (2012); Ulrich et al. (2018)

Source: Authors

5.5 Environmental Qualities and Features Most Supported by the Research

Based on the synthesis of the research for all MBH facilities (Shepley et al. 2016, 2017), three physical environmental attributes were associated with the most positive behavioral outcomes: one environmental quality (nature connection) and two environmental features (proper light and noise control):

- Nature connection: The benefits of access to nature are indisputable. Apart from our affinity for interaction with nature based on the evolutionary principles associated with biophilia, the enrichment associated with diversity in daily experience as flora and fauna continually grow and move helps to

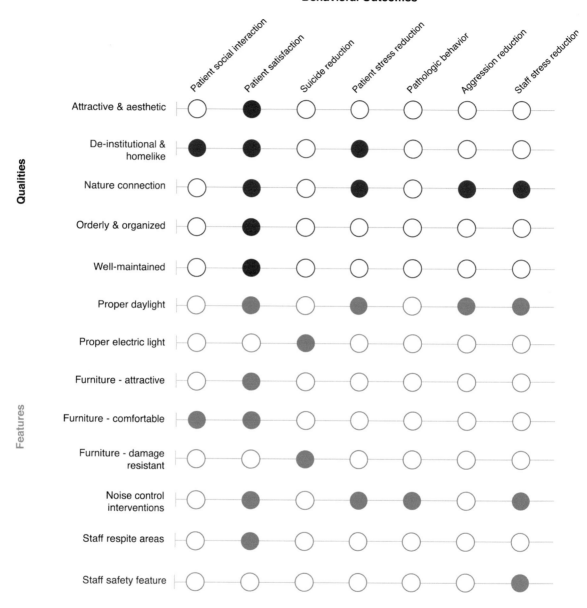

Behavioral Outcomes

Figure showing strength of relationship between environmental qualities and features (rows) and behavioral outcomes (columns).

Columns (Behavioral Outcomes): Patient social interaction, Patient satisfaction, Suicide reduction, Patient stress reduction, Pathologic behavior, Aggression reduction, Staff stress reduction

Qualities / Features (rows):
Attractive & aesthetic, De-institutional & homelike, Nature connection, Orderly & organized, Well-maintained, Proper daylight, Proper electric light, Furniture - attractive, Furniture - comfortable, Furniture - damage resistant, Noise control interventions, Staff respite areas, Staff safety feature

improve mood and reduce boredom, stress, and aggression (Cooper Marcus and Sachs 2014). Additionally, olfactory experience may stimulate cognitive processes (Warm, Dember, and Parasuraman 1991).

- Proper light (daylight and electrical): Access to daylight is a natural fit for any therapeutic environment and has been studied in other environments, including prisons and facilities for people with dementia (Balan et al. 2001;

▲ Figure 5.1

Strength of relationship between environmental qualities and features and behavioral outcomes in all MBH settings.
Source: Authors

Mardelle McCuskey Shepley and Naomi A. Sachs

Benedetti et al. 2001; McMinn and Hinton 2000). In addition to support of biological factors, such as circadian rhythms, diurnal variation, and vitamin D absorption, daylight enhances the natural rendering of color and perception of distance through shadows. Although daylight has not been studied sufficiently in MBH settings, we can assume that it would be as, if not more, important for the health of people who suffer from problems with sleep, mood, and perception. Adequate electrical light for recreational and therapeutic tasks is also necessary.

- Noise control: Proper acoustical control is clearly desirable as unwanted noise has been identified as detrimental to human health. Noise interferes with the ability to concentrate and relax due to the inherent associated lack of control. Exposure to uncontrollable or unpredicted noise can trigger stress, which can lead to undesirable behavioral outcomes like dissatisfaction and aggression, and even compromise communication between staff and patients (Brown et al. 2016; Ulrich et al. 2018).

▼ Figure 5.2

Strength of relationship between environmental qualities and features and behavioral outcomes in inpatient MBH settings.
Source: Authors

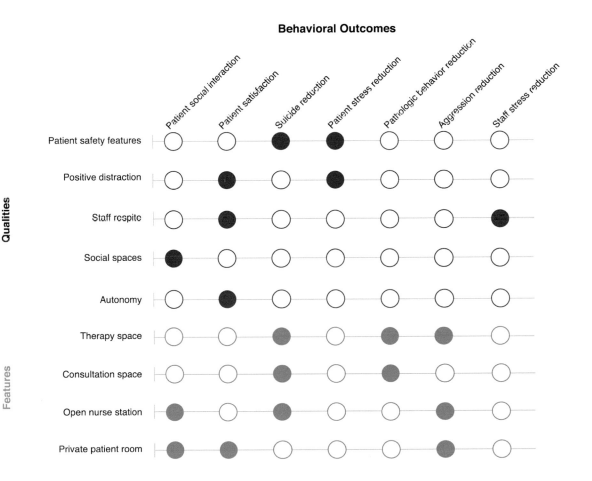

For inpatient MBH settings specifically, three physical environmental attributes, all of which were environmental features, were associated with the most frequently positive behavioral outcomes:

- Flexible therapy spaces: The inclusion of a variety of treatment venues is essential to support the various needs of individuals in both small and large group sizes. Both indoor and outdoor therapy spaces are desirable as well as one-on-one consult spaces.
- Nurse station observation: Patient observation can be achieved through the purposeful design of nurse stations for observability, safety, and control. There are trade-offs to open versus closed nurse stations. The benefits of open stations are increased visibility to patients, providing the insight required to properly care for patients in a timely manner. Open nurse stations may also feel less institutional and encourage relationships between the patients and staff. The benefit of closed stations may be more protection for staff and a more private environment for conducting focused tasks.
- Private patient rooms: The environmental feature that can help satisfy this need is the provision of patient rooms for privacy, increased control, and personal space. Regarding single-occupancy vs. shared rooms, people generally prefer private rooms because they afford more privacy, are quieter, allow for increased control, and support personalization. Private rooms also potentially reduce conflicts between individuals. People opposed to private rooms argue that the presence of a roommate serves as a deterrent to suicide and self-injury attempts and promotes socialization.

In the next section, the six physical environmental attributes defined earlier from the EBD MBH framework (environmental qualities and environmental features) will be explored through three case studies to demonstrate how these attributes are realized in practice.

5.6 Case Studies: Application of Evidence-Based Design Components

The first case study primarily serves forensic patients with mental health issues; the second facility serves general psychiatric inpatient care; and the third facility serves women recovering from domestic violence and substance abuse.

5.6.1 Vermont Psychiatric Care Hospital in Berlin, Vermont, USA

Client: VT Department of Health
Architect: architecture+
Associated architect: Black River Design
Landscape architect: Wagner Hodgson
Square footage: 50,150

Vermont Psychiatric Care Hospital is a 25-bed hospital that primarily serves individuals who have committed a crime and have been ordered by a judge to be hospitalized for mental health issues. The hospital also serves individuals whose hospitalization has been ordered by a physician due to concern of self-harm or harm to others. The hospital was built in 2014 to replace Vermont State Hospital in Waterbury, Vermont, which was badly damaged in 2011 by Hurricane Irene.

The overall design intent was to create a therapeutic environment that is safe, promotes healing, and reduces aggression. To make the hospital feel smaller, its two flexible units were arranged around two courtyards, providing a human scale and improved legibility. In turn, each unit has two separate bedroom wings with four to eight patient beds and a shared kitchenette, dining area, living rooms, quiet rooms, and comfort rooms. A library, fitness room, greenhouse, art room, and visiting rooms accommodate daytime activities. The chapel space is flexible enough to serve also as a family visiting room and a courtroom. There is a labyrinth incorporated as a mechanism for supporting psychological focus.

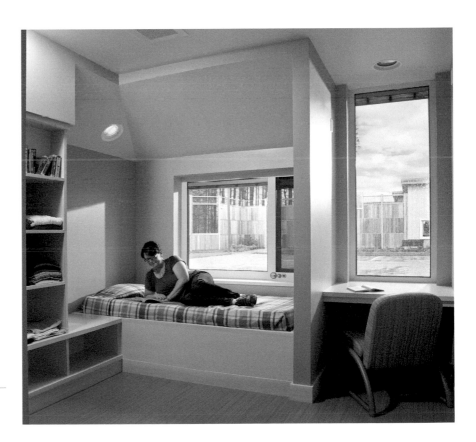

▶ Figure 5.3

Patient bedroom.
Source: architecture+; Photo by Jim Westphalen

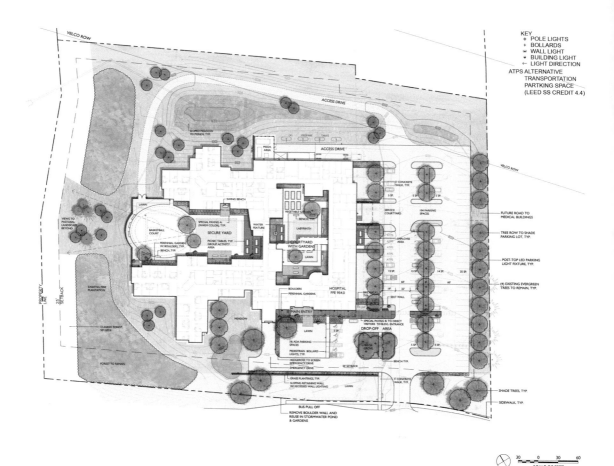

KEY
- ● POLE LIGHTS
- + BOLLARDS
- ⊟ WALL LIGHT
- ◉ BUILDING LIGHT
- ← LIGHT DIRECTION

ATPS ALTERNATIVE TRANSPORTATION PARKING SPACE (LEED SS CREDIT 4.4)

SCALE OF FEET

5.6.1.1 Specific Attributes Applied in the Vermont Psychiatric Care Hospital

- Nature connection and daylight: All the bedrooms, recovery spaces, and offices have windows that bring in light and offer views of the courtyards and/ or surrounding landscape. The windows are operable, much larger than the 4" normal for ventilating psychiatric windows, to allow for fresh air and nature sounds. Biophilic elements within the building include finishes of wood and stone, and colors inspired by the Vermont landscape.

- Nature connection and access to outdoor spaces: Areas that are physically accessible to patients include courtyards with benches and picnic benches—some of which are covered by solid shade structures—lawn areas, a small labyrinth, and decorative plantings. There are also places for solitary and group exercise—a jogging track, a half basketball court, and a volleyball court.

- Noise control: All walls between the buildings extend continuously from the floor deck to the underside of structural decks above the finished ceilings. Walls between occupied rooms are packed with sound-absorptive baffles and isolating separations between deck and framing. Ceilings and floors in major activity spaces are made of sound-absorptive materials. Absorptive felt

▲ Figure 5.4

Rendered plan of Vermont Psychiatric Care Hospital.
Source: architecture+

panels are used in upper areas of most public spaces. Ceilings in corridors, public spaces, and bedrooms frequently utilize changes in heights, and soffits coupled with alcoves to deflect sound and improve acoustic performance.

- Flexible therapy spaces: The hospital has several dedicated therapy spaces, including a special "sensory room" for individual patient-focused therapy.
- Nurse station observation: For each unit, there is an open area with a patient care desk that includes a large piece of custom-designed furniture for storing nursing resource materials. Sightlines from the desk are clear so that staff at the desk can easily observe patient activity. A secure charting station, not accessible to patients, separates the two units.
- Private patient rooms: All 25 bedrooms are private rooms with their own bathrooms. Each bedroom comes with a built-in bed, desk area, and cubbies for shelves.

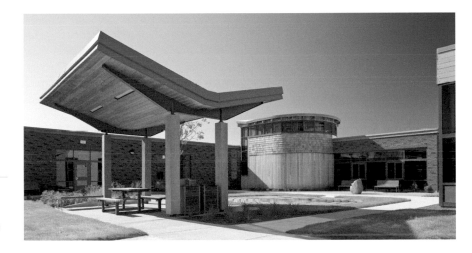

▶ Figure 5.5

Courtyard area with lawn, labyrinth, and shaded seating.
Source: architecture+; Photo by Jim Westphalen

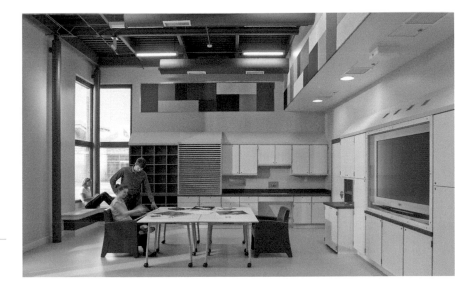

▶ Figure 5.6

Common room.
Source: architecture+; Photo by Jim Westphalen

5.6.2 Sahlgrenska University Hospital, Östra—Acute Psychiatric Ward, Gothenberg, Sweden

Client: Västfastigheter
Architect: White Architects/White Arkitekter
Landscape architect: Landskapsgruppen AB
Square footage: 193,750 (18.800 m² gross area)

Östra Acute Psychiatry Hospital, completed in 2006, provides general psychiatric inpatient care for patients with schizophrenia and affective disorders (86 beds) and addiction (32 beds). The floor plan features four repeating L-shaped departments (wards) that connect visually and physically with three outdoor courtyards. Each self-sufficient 14-bed ward has its own patient bedrooms (ten single and two double patient bedrooms), living rooms, treatment rooms, and administrative offices.

The overarching vision for the project was to create an open atmosphere and avoid any associations with power hierarchies. An open plan concept, coupled with a room-within-a-room concept, helps patients feel in control of their own personal space and connected to the outdoors or other areas in the facility. Östra is designed to minimize crowding, which has been found to increase stress and aggression. To make the facility feel welcoming and encourage independence, areas are organized into clusters or pods without corridors so patients can move around freely. The core of the ward includes a gradation of social spaces to convey a domestic character. Other communal areas are grouped around a glazed conservatory to enhance understanding of the spatial organization and provide access to natural light.

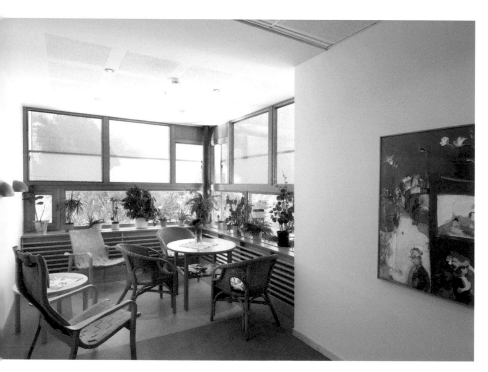

◀ Figure 5.7

The common room evokes a Swedish-style veranda. *Source*: Stefan Lundin, partner at White Arkitekter; Photo by Hans Wretling

Mardelle McCuskey Shepley and Naomi A. Sachs

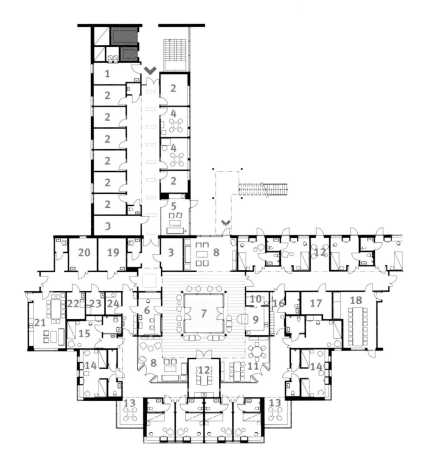

1	Recycling room
2	Office etc.
3	Services
4	Consulting rooms
5	Consultation/Team room
6	Ward station
7	Light court, glass-roofed
8	Day room/TV room
9	Kitchen
10	Larder, lockable
11	Dining alcove
12	Activity room
13	Sitting room
14	Patients' room (2 beds)
15	Patient's room, with isolation portal
16	Cloakroom
17	Store
18	Team room/conference room
19	Treatment room
20	Restraint room
21	Staff room
22	Laundry
23	Utility room
24	Drug storage

▲ Figure 5.8

Floor plan of ward.
Source: Stefan Lundin, partner
at White Arkitekter

5.6.2.1 Specific Attributes Applied in Östra Hospital

- Nature connection and daylight: All patient rooms and communal spaces look out onto gardens in the enclosed courtyard or other natural elements. All communal and patient rooms have operable windows for accessing fresh air and nature sounds. The "core" of each of the four residential units (wards) is a small atrium with plants and benches that is fully accessible to patients and staff.
- Nature connection and access to outdoors: The secure outdoor courtyard gardens for each ward are accessible to patients (without an escort) year-round from communal areas. Each garden has seating choices and beds with flowers. Staff can easily observe the garden while inside.
- Noise control: Sound-absorbing environmental surfaces were used to reduce echoing and the spread of noise throughout the hospital. The high proportion of single rooms with walls and doors lessens patient exposure to noise.
- Flexible therapy spaces: Adjacent to each ward are various types of rooms for therapy, including group therapy, art therapy, and recreational therapy, as well as private offices for one-on-one consults.
- Nurse station observation: The floor plan was designed to afford good visibility and observation. Patient rooms are organized around a central space,

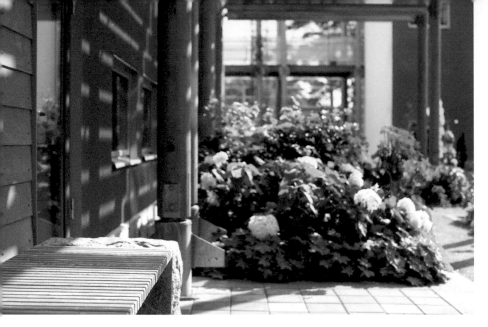

◀ Figure 5.9

One of the secure outdoor courtyard gardens.
Source: Stefan Lundin, partner at White Arkitekter; Photo by Hans Wretling

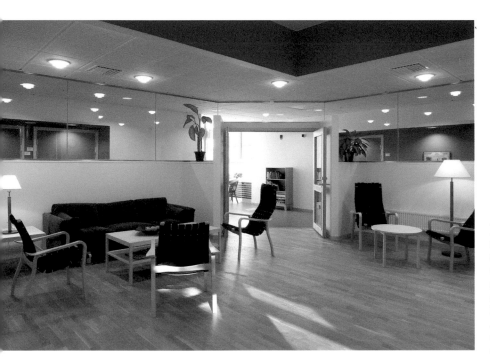

◀ Figure 5.10

One of the communal areas in the ward at Östra. Note the groupings of moveable and semi-moveable seating and half-wall partitions of break-resistant glass.
Source: Stefan Lundin, partner at White Arkitekter; Photo by Christoffer Hallgren

and staff can easily observe all seating areas, activity spaces, and bedroom doors.

- Private patient rooms: Seventy percent of beds at Östra are in single rooms with private bathrooms (toilet and shower). The other 30% of beds are in double (two-person) rooms. Each room is designed with multiple places to sit, including on the bed, in an armchair in a "reading corner", or in the recessed window nook.

Mardelle McCuskey Shepley and Naomi A. Sachs

5.6.2.2 Research With Östra Hospital's Acute Psychiatry Ward

A post-occupancy evaluation (POE) was conducted in this facility by Ulrich and colleagues (2018) to investigate the influence of design on stress which can trigger aggression and violent incidents across three Swedish psychiatric wards. Ulrich and colleagues tested a conceptual model they developed that includes four goals intended to reduce stress with ten design features outlined ahead. Many of these goals and design features align with the MBH EBD framework discussed earlier. In their empirical study, they investigated:

1. Crowding stress in relation to single patient rooms with private bathrooms, common areas with movable seating and enough space for patients to regulate social relationships, and a low-density design.
2. Environmental stress in relation to noise reduction design features and providing control of the environment, especially in the patient rooms.
3. Positive distractions in relation to accessible gardens, preferably without needing staff escort; nature views from windows; nature-inspired art, and exposure to daylight from indoors.
4. Ease in staff observation in relation to communal spaces and bedroom doors that can be observed from a central location.

For their study, Ulrich and colleagues (2018) compared data on two known clinical markers for aggressive behavior (compulsory injections and physical restraints) across three general psychiatric inpatient care wards for people with schizophrenia and affective disorders (but not addiction). Östra had nine of the ten recommended design features, whereas the other two hospitals had only one of the ten features. The authors found a statistically significant decrease in the proportion of patients receiving compulsory injections and a 50% decrease in physical restraints. Findings suggest that the inclusion of the ten design features can reduce stress and aggressive behaviors.

5.6.3 *The Next Door, Nashville, Tennessee, USA*

Client: The Next Door, Inc.
Architect: Earl Swensson Associates (ESA)
Square footage: 42,600
Site: 1.05 acres

The Next Door provides a continuum of care for women and their families who are impacted by mental illness, trauma, addiction, and/or incarceration as they transition from rehabilitation centers, domestic violence shelters, or correctional facilities. The 82-bed facility, completed in 2014, embodies the organization's human-centered mission that conveys a sense of community and well-being. The L-shaped building has three stories. The ground floor houses common areas, like the main kitchen, dining, children's space, chapel, administrative offices, and an in-house clinic. There is also a computer lab, library, and boutique, all of which are equipped for employment training. The second floor contains six medically monitored detox beds and 36 residential treatment

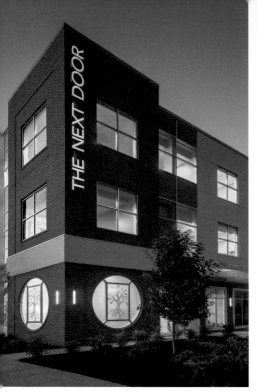

▲ Figure 5.11

Arrival view of The Next Door.
Source: Earl Swensson Associates; Photo by Michael Peck

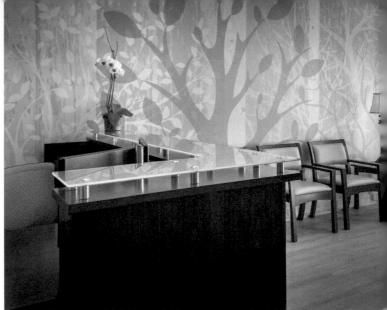

▲ Figure 5.12

Entrance lobby.
Source: Earl Swensson Associates; Photo by Michael Peck

beds with dedicated kitchenettes, lounge spaces, classrooms, and rehabilitation services. The third floor is dedicated to halfway house accommodations (40 beds) and related amenities.

5.6.3.1 Specific Attributes Applied in The Next Door

- Nature connection and daylight: Large windows are throughout the facility, including in resident rooms, living rooms, classrooms, dining areas, and staff offices. Rooms have at least one window for natural light and views. Windows afford views of the courtyard and the surrounding neighborhood.
- Nature connection and access to outdoors: The L-shaped building wraps around a landscaped courtyard adjacent to the dining area that is easily accessed, providing respite for residents and staff.
- Noise control: Most spaces are relatively small or can be divided by acoustical walls. Acoustical ceilings were used in the corridors and classrooms. Durable, sound-absorbent, low-maintenance flooring includes vinyl flooring with a wood-plank look in most of the spaces, and carpet in the chapel, classrooms, and offices.
- Flexible therapy spaces: Resident rooms on the two upper floors are grouped into small "communities" for 10–12 women supported by a lounge for informal meetings, and classroom spaces for counseling and other educational activities. Furniture in the chapel can be easily moved and repositioned to enable group meetings. The large, linear dining area is equipped with moveable partitions with whiteboard surfaces to accommodate smaller groups.

Mardelle McCuskey Shepley and Naomi A. Sachs

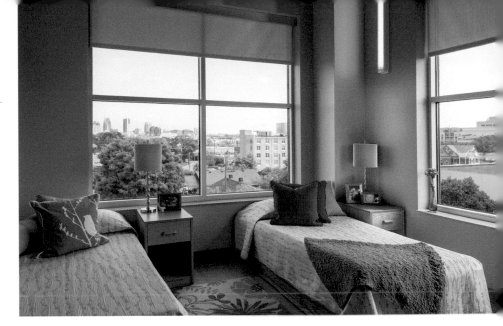

▶ Figure 5.13

Client bedroom.
Source: Earl Swensson
Associates; Photo by Michael
Peck

- Nurse station observation: In order to feel more like a home than a rehab facility, there are small staff offices rather than a true nurse's station. These offices are centrally located to each community of women. There is a central monitoring space for the detox unit and a small nurse desk at the clinic on the first floor.
- Private patient rooms: The Next Door felt strongly that residents should share semiprivate rooms because social support is crucial for treatment. Each room has two beds, except for the detox area, which has six beds, in one L-shaped, monitored room. Residents can bring in personal items to decorate their space.

5.7 Conclusions

The physical environment plays a significant role in the health and well-being of mental and behavioral health patients and the staff who care for them. Poorly designed environments can exacerbate patients' anxiety, aggression, and other negative emotions and behaviors. More recent research and EBD practices are working to change the story, to create places that embody holistic care and respect.

There have been a handful of ardent crusaders in the design of MBH facilities for many years. Fortunately, we are beginning to see broader interest among EBD design practitioners and researchers. Motivated by increased awareness of the number of individuals suffering from mental health challenges and the impact of the physical environment on health outcomes, the provision of adequate mental and behavioral health facilities appears to be the next frontier in healthcare design.

Acknowledgments

We are grateful for the contributions and help of Dina Battisto, Clemson University; Ellen Montiel and Francis Pitts, architecture+; Roger Ulrich, Chalmers University of Technology; Heather Bazille, Andrea Fronsman, Mio Jia, and Janhawi Kelkar, Cornell University; Sandra Dickerson, Tara Myers, and Shali Nelson, Earl Swensson Associates; Brian Giebink, HDR; Anne Garrity, Elizabeth Spelman, and Angela Watson, Shepley Bulfinch; Mary Therese Hankinson, Department of Veteran's Affairs New Jersey Health System; and Stefan Lundin, White Arkitekter.

Bibliography

Bailey, Keith A. "The Role of the Physical Environment for Children in Residential Care." *Residential Treatment for Children & Youth* 20, no. 1 (2002): 15–27.

Balan, Silviu, Arthur Leibovitz, Laurence Freedman, Boris Blagman, Mishiev Ruth, Shapira Ady, and Beni Habot. "Seasonal Variation in the Incidence of Delirium Among the Patients of a Geriatric Hospital." *Archives of Gerontology and Geriatrics* 33, no. 3 (2001): 287–293.

Benedetti, Francesco, Cristina Colombo, Barbara Barbini, Euridice Campori, and Enrico Smeraldi. "Morning Sunlight Reduces Length of Hospitalization in Bipolar Depression." *Journal of Affective Disorders* 62, no. 3 (2001): 221–223.

Boubekri, Mohamed, Ivy N. Cheung, Kathryn J. Reid, Chia-Hui Wang, and Phyllis C. Zee. "Impact of Windows and Daylight Exposure on Overall Health and Sleep Quality of Office Workers: A Case-Control Pilot Study." *Journal of Clinical Sleep Medicine* 10, no. 6 (2014): 603–611.

Brown, Juliette, Waleed Fawzi, Amar Shah, Margaret Joyce, Genevieve Holt, Cathy McCarthy, Carmel Stevenson, Rosca Marange, Joy Shakes, and Kwesi Solomon-Ayeh. "Low Stimulus Environments: Reducing Noise Levels in Continuing Care." *BMJ Open Quality* 5, no. 1 (2016): u207447–w4214.

Bryan, Craig J., M. David Rudd, and Evelyn Wertenberger. "Reasons for Suicide Attempts in A Clinical Sample of Active Duty Soldiers". *Journal of Affective Disorders* 144, no. 1–2 (2013): 148–152.

Capland, Ruth B. *Psychiatry and The Community in the Nineteenth Century America*. New York: Basic Books, 1969.

Carr, Robert F. "Psychiatric Facility." *WBDG Whole Building Design Guide*, 2011. www.wbdg.org/building-types/health-care-facilities/psychiatric-facility.

Christenfeld, Roger, James Wagner, Wagner Gary Pastva, and Wendy P. Acrish. "How Physical Settings Affect Chronic Mental Patients." *Psychiatric Quarterly* 60, no. 3 (1989): 253–264.

Cooper Marcus, Clare, and Naomi A. Sachs. *Therapeutic Landscapes: An Evidence-Based Approach to Designing Healing Gardens and Restorative Outdoor Spaces*. Hoboken: John Wiley & Sons, 2014.

Davis, Charles, Ira D. Guck, and Irving Rosow. "The Architectural Design of a Psychotherapeutic Milieu." *Psychiatric Services* 30, no. 7 (1979): 453–460.

Davis, Matthew C., Desmond J. Leach, and Chris W. Clegg. "The Physical Environment of the Office: Contemporary and Emerging Issues." *International Review of Industrial and Organizational Psychology* 26, no. 1 (2011).

Devlin, Ann Sloan. "Psychiatric Ward Renovation: Staff Perception and Patient Behavior." *Environment and Behavior* 24, no. 1 (1992): 66–84.

Diette, Gregory B., Noah Lechtzin, Edward Haponik, Aline Devrotes, and Haya R. Rubin. "Distraction Therapy with Nature Sights and Sounds Reduces Pain During Flexible Bronchoscopya: A Complementary Approach to Routine Analgesia." *Chest* 123, no. 3 (2003): 941–948.

Forster, Peter L., Cleve Cavness, and Molly A. Phelps. "Staff Training Decreases Use of Seclusion and Restraint in an Acute Psychiatric Hospital." *Archives of Psychiatric Nursing* 13, no. 5 (1999): 269–271.

Gjerden, Pål. "A Survey of Patient Satisfaction as a Means of Evaluating Quality of Care in an Open Psychiatric Ward." *Nordic Journal of Psychiatry* 51, no. 4 (1991): 235–242.

Grosenick, Judith K, and Claudia M. Hatmaker. "Perceptions of the Importance of Physical Setting in Substance Abuse Treatment." *Journal of Substance Abuse Treatment* 18, no. 1 (2000): 29–39.

Gutkowski, Silvio, Yigal Ginath, and Flor Guttmann. "Improving Psychiatric Environments Through Minimal Architectural Change." *Psychiatric Services* 43, no. 9 (1992): 920–923.

Ingham, B, and C. Spencer. "Do Comfortable Chairs and Soft Lights in the Waiting Area Really Help Reduce Anxiety and Improve the Practice's Image?" *Health Psychology Update* (1997): 17–20.

Kaiser Family Foundation Analysis of Data from SAMHSA 2015 NSDUH. www.healthsystemtracker.org/chart-collection/current-costs-outcomes-related-mental-health-substance-abuse-disorders/#item-30-percent-adults-serious-mental-illness-not-receiving-mental-health-treatment.

Kamal, Rabahm. "Mental Health and Musculoskeletal Disorders Are the Leading Causes of Years Lost to Disability in the U.S." *Health Systems Tracker*, Peterson-Kaiser. May 10, 2016.

Kirkbride, Thomas Story. *On the Construction, Organization, and General Arrangements of Hospitals for the Insane: With Some Remarks on Insanity and Its Treatment*. New York, NY: Arno Press, 1854.

Lynch Jr., Martin F., Robert W. Plant, and Richard M. Ryan. "Psychological Needs and Threat to Safety: Implications for Staff and Patients in a Psychiatric Hospital for Youth." *Professional Psychology: Research and Practice* 36, no. 4 (2005): 415.

Martin, Kimberly H. "Improving Staff Safety Through an Aggression Management Program." *Archives of Psychiatric Nursing* 9, no. 4 (1995): 211–215.

Maslow, Abraham H., and Norbett L. Mintz. "Effects of Esthetic Surroundings: I. Initial Effects of Three Esthetic Conditions Upon Perceiving 'Energy' and 'Well-Being' in Faces." *The Journal of Psychology* 41, no. 2 (1956): 247–254.

McMinn, Bryan G., and Lorraine Hinton. "Confined to Barracks: The Effects of Indoor Confinement on Aggressive Behavior Among Inpatients of an Acute Psychogeriatric Unit." *American Journal of Alzheimer's Disease* 15, no. 1 (2000): 36–41.

Nanda, Upali, S. Eisen, R. S. Zadeh, and D. Owen. "Effect of Visual Art on Patient Anxiety and Agitation in a Mental Health Facility and Implications for the Business Case." *Journal of Psychiatric and Mental Health Nursing* 18, no. 5 (2011): 386–393.

Nejati, Adeleh, Susan Rodiek, and Mardelle Shepley. "The Implications of High-Quality Staff Break Areas for Nurses' Health, Performance, Job Satisfaction and Retention." *Journal of Nursing Management* 24, no. 4 (2016): 512–523.

Nejati, Adeleh, Mardelle Shepley, Susan Rodiek, Chanam Lee, and James Varni. "Restorative Design Features for Hospital Staff Break Areas: A Multi-Method Study." *HERD: Health Environments Research & Design Journal* 9, 2 (2016): 16–35.

NIMH (National Institute of Mental Health). "Mental Health Information." n.d. www.nimh.nih.gov/health/topics/index.shtml.

Partonen, Timo, and Jouko Lonnqvist. "Bright Light Improves Vitality and Alleviates Distress in Healthy People." *Journal of Affective Disorders* 57, no. 1–3 (2000): 55–61.

Perkins, Elizabeth, Helen Prosser, David Riley, and Richard Whittington. "Physical Restraint in a Therapeutic Setting; A Necessary Evil?" *International Journal of Law and Psychiatry* 35, no. 1 (2012): 43–49.

Salerno, Silvana, Laura Forcella, Ursala Di Fabio, Talamanca I. Figà, and Pablo Boscolo. "Ergonomics in the Psychiatric Ward Towards Workers or Patients?" *Work* 41 (2012): 1832–1835.

SAMHSA (Substance Abuse and Mental Health Services Administration). "Behavioral Health Treatment Services Locator." n.d. https://findtreatment.samhsa.gov/. Accessed November 22, 2018.

Shepley, Mardelle McCuskey. "The Role of Positive Distraction in Neonatal Intensive Care Unit Settings." *Journal of Perinatology* 26, no. S3 (2006): S34.

Shepley, Mardelle McCuskey, and Samira Pasha. *Design for Mental and Behavioral Health*. Oxon: Routledge, 2017.

Shepley, Mardelle McCuskey, Samira Pasha, Pamela Ferguson, Jamie C. Huffcut, Guy Kiyokawa, and Joe Martere. *Design Research and Behavioral Health Facilities*. Concord, CA: The Center for Health Design, 2013.

Shepley, Mardelle McCuskey, Angela Watson, Francis Pitts, Anne Garrity, Elizabeth Spelman, Andrea Fronsman, and Janhawi Kelkar. "Mental and Behavioral Health Settings: Importance & Effectiveness of Environmental Qualities & Features as Perceived by Staff." *Journal of Environmental Psychology* 50 (2017): 37–50.

Shepley, Mardelle McCuskey, Angela Watson, Francis Pitts, Anne Garrity, Elizabeth Spelman, Janhawi Kelkar, and Andrea Fronsman. "Mental and Behavioral Health Environments: Critical Considerations for Facility Design." *General Hospital Psychiatry* 42 (2016): 15–21.

Shepley, Mardelle McCuskey, and Peni Wilson. "Designing for Persons With AIDS: A Post-Occupancy Study at the Bailey-Boushay House." *Journal of Architectural and Planning Research* (1999): 17–32.

Shorter, Edward. *A History of Psychiatry: From the Era of the Asylum to the Age of Prozac.* New York, NY: Wiley, 1997.

Sidman, Jack, and Rudolf Moos. "On the Relation Between Psychiatric Ward Atmosphere and Helping Behavior." *Journal of Clinical Psychology* 29, 1 (1973): 74–78.

Sørlie, Tore, Alexander Parniakov, Grigory Rezvy, and Oleg Ponomarev. "Psychometric Evaluation of the Ward Atmosphere Scale in a Russian Psychiatric Hospital." *Nordic Journal of Psychiatry* 64, no. 6 (2010): 377–383.

Stansfeld, S. A., M. M. Haines, M. Burr, B. Berry, and P. Lercher. "A Review of Environmental Noise and Mental Health." *Noise and Health* 2, 8 (2000): 1.

Talbott, John A. *The Death of the Asylum: A Critical Study of State Hospital Management, Services, and Care.* New York, NY: Grune & Stratton, 1978.

Tomes, Nancy. "Kirkbride, Thomas Story (1809–1883), Psychiatrist." *American National Biography* (2000). https://doi.org/10.1093/anb/9780198606697.article.1200493.

Torres, Denise, and Steven Estrine. *Behavioral Health.* Oxford: Oxford University Press, 2013.

Tuke, Samuel. *Practical Hints on the Construction and Economy of Pauper Lunatic Asylums; Including Instructions to the Architects Who Offered Plans for the Wakefield Asylum, and a Sketch of the Most Approved Design.* New York, NY: W. Alexander, 1815.

Turlington, Richard. "Creating a Planetree Inpatient Psychiatric Unit." *Health Facilities Management Magazine* 17, no. 6 (2004): 12–13.

Tyson, Graham A., Gordon Lambert, and Lyn Beattie. "The Impact of Ward Design on the Behaviour, Occupational Satisfaction and Well-Being of Psychiatric Nurses." *International Journal of Mental Health Nursing* 11, no. 2 (2002): 94–102.

Ulrich, Roger S., Lennart Bogren, Stuart K. Gardiner, and Stefan Lundin. "Psychiatric Ward Design Can Reduce Aggressive Behavior." *Journal of Environmental Psychology* 57 (2018): 53–66.

Ulrich, Roger S., Lennart Bogren, and Stefan Lundin. "Towards a Design Theory for Reducing Aggression in Psychiatric Facilities." *ARCH 12: Architecture / Research / Care / Health.* Gothenburg: Chalmers Institute of Technology, 2012.

Ulrich, Roger S., Robert F. Simons, and Mark A. Miles. "Effects of Environmental Simulations and Television on Blood Donor Stress." *Journal of Architectural and Planning Research* (2003): 38–47.

US Department of Health and Human Services. "Mental Health and Mental Health Disorders." 2019. www.healthypeople.gov/2020/topics-objectives/topic/mental-health-and-mental-disorders.

Warm, Joel S., William N. Dember, and Raja Parasuraman. "Effects of Olfactory Stimulation on Performance and Stress." *Journal of the Society Cosmetic Chemists* 42, no. 3 (1991): 199–210.

Watts, Bradley V., Yinong Young-Xu, Peter D. Mills, Joseph M. DeRosier, Jan Kemp, Brian Shiner, and William E. Duncan. "Examination of the Effectiveness of the Mental

Mardelle McCuskey Shepley and Naomi A. Sachs

Health Environment of Care Checklist in Reducing Suicide on Inpatient Mental Health Units." *Archives of General Psychiatry* 69, no. 6 (2012): 588–592.

Whitehead, Clay C., Richard H. Polsky, Carol Crookshank, and Edward Fik. "Objective and Subjective Evaluation of Psychiatric Ward Redesign." *The American Journal of Psychiatry* 82 (1984): 454–462.

Chapter 6

Renewing the Human Spirit Through Design
Celebrating Maggie's Centres

Jamie Mitchell

6.1 Introduction

In May 1993, Maggie Keswick Jencks was told that her breast cancer had returned and that she had two to three months to live. Maggie went on to live with this advanced cancer for two years, and during that time she created a blueprint for a new approach to cancer care that would help people to "live well with cancer". Her vision was for a center that would provide information to people with cancer so they could become informed participants in their medical treatment, and included stress-reducing strategies, psychological support, and opportunities to meet other people going through similar experiences. Maggie, a garden designer and author, was married to the architectural theorist Charles Jencks. Given their backgrounds, it is not surprising that an important part of her vision for a new kind of cancer care involved the creation of a community around well-designed and tranquil places.

Since the first Maggie's Centre opened in 1996, these ideas of supporting people with cancer as well as their families and friends in a nonclinical way, and in a nonclinical environment, have grown beyond the experience of Maggie herself. There are now 22 Maggie's Centres across the UK and abroad, and more are being planned. Even as the number of Maggie's Centres continues to grow, they have stayed true to her vision.

6.2 Genesis of the Idea for a Maggie's Centre: Philosophy and Approach

Before there was even an idea of a "Maggie's Centre", Maggie Keswick Jencks wrote about her experience with cancer, and about her struggles coming to terms with living on "borrowed time". In a 1995 essay called "A View From the Front Line", she observed,

> A diagnosis of cancer hits you like a punch in the stomach. Other diseases may be just as life-threatening, but most patients know nothing about them. Everyone, however, knows that cancer means pain, horrible treatments and—though no longer quite the unmentionable "Big C" of twenty-five years ago—early death.
>
> (Keswick 2007, p. 9)

Even so, Maggie became determined that she would not "lose the joy of living in the fear of dying", and she wanted this for other people facing cancer too (Keswick 2007, p. 23). During her treatment and the inevitable hours of waiting between appointments at Edinburgh's Western General Hospital in the United Kingdom, Maggie often wished she could find respite from the clinical environment. This wish was the catalyst for a new kind of cancer support center that could work alongside the hospital.

Over the course of seven years, Maggie experienced cancer diagnosis, treatment, remission, and recurrence. During that time, she took the insight and experience she had gained and transformed it into a pioneering approach to cancer care. Maggie noticed several key things that were to lead to the formulation of the first Centre. She saw, despite her initial fears, how much better she felt when she began to take an active role in her own treatment. She came to believe that this quite deliberate move from passive to active participant was the single most important step she took in grappling with her illness.

In a conversation with Laura Lee, who was at that time Maggie's oncology nurse, Maggie and Laura discussed the need for both practical and emotional support in addition to necessary medical treatment. Both women knew that many other people were in the same predicament. Maggie felt that her needs could not be met exclusively by medical treatment in the hospital. The fear, anxiety, and loneliness were as difficult to tolerate as the illness itself. Maggie died in 1995, but her ideas became a blueprint for the first Maggie's Centre, which opened in 1996, in a converted stable block at Edinburgh's Western General Hospital.

6.3 The First Maggie's Centre

To understand how Maggie's Centres developed into what they are today, it is helpful to look back to the first Maggie's Centre, in Edinburgh. Maggie's Edinburgh was designed by architect Richard Murphy, who transformed what had been an abandoned stable block into a place of warmth, comfort, and daylight. People being treated at the hospital could wander in and would immediately feel welcome. There is no reception desk, but a large dining table is the focal point in the open kitchen. This welcoming, informal convivial space became the inspiration for every Maggie's Centre that has followed.

Murphy's design is a modest, modern intervention woven into the fabric of the existing historic stables. "The idea was clearly domesticity", Murphy says. But, as he also says, designing the first Maggie's Centre was not without its challenges:

> There were problems with the brief—the wooliness of it. What exactly was the building for? We knew it wasn't going to be a clinical building, but Maggie was going on about all kinds of things: relaxation, a library, meetings, yoga, beauty care. How would we fit all this in?
>
> (Jencks 2015, p.112)

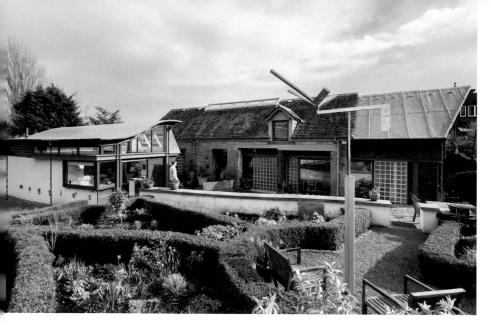

◀ Figure 6.1

Maggie's Edinburgh,
1996, designed by Richard
Murphy Architects.
Source: Philip Durrant

Maggie wanted the Centre to be special, not for some luxury add-on value but because it needed to do so much for the people who would use it. The building would set the scene and tone for everything that would happen inside it. The architect's task was not to answer a functional brief but to create the right kind of atmosphere to allow the Centre's professional staff to do their jobs most effectively—to help people live well with cancer.

At first glance Maggie's Edinburgh looks reassuringly familiar, a small rectangular stone block with a pitched roof (Figure 6.1). The small scale and shape of the building give visitors a taste of what they will find when they venture in. The building was designed to be anti-institutional, with no corridors, big windows, bright colors, and lots of niches and intimate spaces. Within the domesticity is the idea of the kitchen as the pivot around which the building revolves, creating a space where people instantly feel at home. The interior space is flexible, with dividing sliding doors. From the large entrance it is possible to understand what is going on in all other areas of the building. There are no intimidating closed doors with specific labels. As one visitor noted, "The bright modern building is as informal as a private home", continuing: "Nobody is obviously in charge, nor is anyone too busy to greet a recent arrival or hear the latest news. The atmosphere is hard to pin down, but it is far more 'coffee morning' than 'cancer ward'" (Blakenham 2007, p. 27–28).

6.4 Architecture for Elevating the Human Spirit: Design Goals and Strategies

Though designed to be practical, British National Health Service (NHS) hospitals are often not very pleasant places. Illness shrinks the patient's confidence, and arriving for the first time at a huge hospital is often a time of high anxiety. Simply finding your destination can be exhausting. Although much is done to improve the interior environments of these hospitals—such as adding plants and hanging art—limited fiscal resources often inhibit the ability to make significant architectural renovations. Consequently, most people spend time waiting for treatment in uncomfortable seating under harsh lights—both of which increase, rather than decrease, feelings of stress. The original concept of a Maggie's Centre was a direct reaction to this environment. The concept of a Maggie's Centre is based on five overarching design goals, discussed ahead, that shape the character of these distinct places.

6.4.1 Create a Hopeful and Healing Environment

A Maggie's Centre is intended to elevate the human spirit through the integration of architecture and landscape design. To subvert the hierarchies inherent in traditional waiting rooms that consist of rows of chairs under harsh lighting, waiting areas at Maggie's Centres are conceived of as places where time waiting can be used positively. Lounge seating arranged in various groupings, thoughtful lighting, and a view to the outdoors are simple design provisions that are less commonly seen in typical hospital environments, but better allow for relaxation and talking among others going through similar difficulties. Bathrooms also reflect this residential approach to space: Rather than a partitioned row of toilets, bathrooms are designed to give privacy for crying, water for washing the face, and a mirror for getting ready to deal with the world again. There could be a tea and coffee machine to use while waiting, and a small cancer library for those who want to learn more about their disease. These individual touchpoints along a cancer patient's journey had to be thought out in detail to be as familiar and navigable as possible, to counteract the disorientation a patient may feel post-diagnosis.

As a garden designer herself, Maggie believed in the power of gardens to renew the human spirit. Part of the Maggie's Centre brief is recognizing that

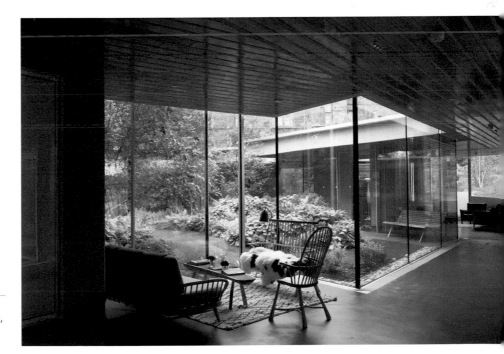

▶ Figure 6.2

Maggie's Glasgow, 2011, designed by Rem Koolhaas, OMA.
Source: Nick Turner

gardens are essential for promoting well-being, improving mindfulness, and reducing stress. During her illness, Maggie spent as much time as she could in her own garden. She wanted gardens to be visible through the windows of the Centres, so that there would always be a connection to nature. For those who were able, tending to the garden could also be therapeutic.

All Centres are designed to embrace nature in some way, as shown in Maggie's Glasgow. Designed by Rem Koolhaas from OMA, the Maggie's Centre is a single-story building framed as a ring around a landscaped internal garden, creating a private oasis on the hospital grounds (Figure 6.2). Huge windows afford views from all rooms in the Centre. Rooms flow into one another while remaining separate, where an atmosphere of domesticity is framed by the kitchen, dining room, and library. This makes the Centre feel welcoming, in direct contrast to the institutional atmosphere of most hospitals.

Similar in the organization of spaces among landscape is Norman Foster's design of Maggie's Manchester, set in a peaceful garden and inspired by natural themes that engage the outdoors (Figure 6.3). Foster noted, "Our aim in Manchester, the city of my youth, was to create a building that is welcoming, friendly and without any of the institutional references of a hospital or health centre—a light-filled, homely space where people can gather, talk or simply reflect". He added, "That is why throughout the building there is a focus on natural light, greenery and views; with a greenhouse to provide fresh flowers, and an emphasis on the therapeutic qualities of nature and the outdoors" (Frearson 2016). A timber frame structure that is envisioned to be partially planted with vines was used to connect the building with the surrounding greenery and help the Centre blend in with the gardens. The greenhouse, a signature element of this Centre, is located on the south-facing end of the building, inviting patients to grow flowers and other produce (Figure 6.4). Following this idea that the garden is a therapeutic vehicle to help reduce stress, treatment and counseling rooms along the eastern façade each face their own private garden designed by landscape architect Dan

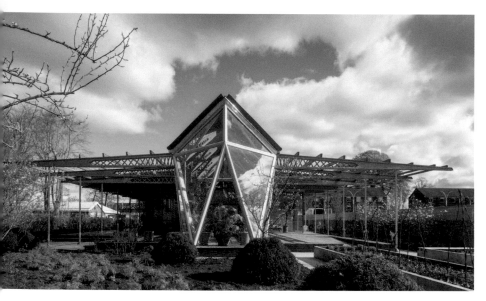

◀ Figure 6.3

Maggie's Manchester, 2016, designed by Foster+Partners. A view looking toward the greenhouse, a place to grow flowers and produce. *Source*: Nigel Young/ Foster+Partners

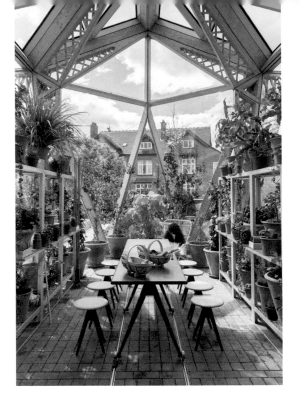

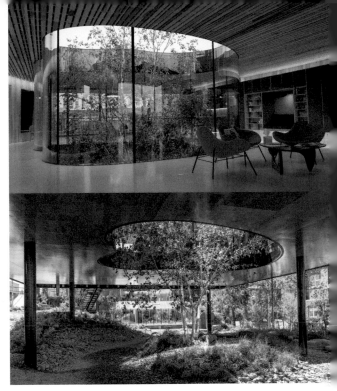

▲ Figure 6.4

Maggie's Manchester, 2016, designed by Foster+Partners.
A view looking outside from the greenhouse.
Source: Nigel Young/Foster+Partners

▲ Figure 6.5

Maggie's Oldham, 2017, designed by Alex de Rijke of dRMM.
Source: Nick Turner

Pearson. Foster wrote, "Seen from the outside, I hope the building looks spectacular, but it's what's inside that matters most. The palette of materials we have used combines warm, natural wood, tactile fabrics, and natural clay tiles for the floor" (Frearson 2014).

The gardens at each Centre are designed to create a unique and authentic setting. They are also tended to by Centre visitors, who take part in therapeutic gardening groups. The sunken garden at Maggie's Oldham offers another example of the seamless connection between building and landscape (Figure 6.5). Designed by Alex de Rijke of dRMM, Maggie's Oldham combines "elements of a modernist villa, an industrial shed and a wooden cabin". Underneath the building is a modest, contemporary garden offering a quiet, somewhat austere place for contemplation. There is also a birch tree growing up into the glazed lightwell, which is a symbolic reminder of both the fragility and persistence of life (Smisek 2017).

Everything in a Maggie's Centre, from the fact that the building gives you a choice of whether to sit in the open with other people or find your own quite space to the materials of the interior design—such as wood and stone chosen for their natural and tactile qualities—to the uniqueness of the building itself, combines to create a first impression of openness and welcome. Each Centre provides a sense of comfort and familiarity and, eventually, of ownership and belonging.

Just as kitchens are the center of most homes, the kitchen—and particularly the kitchen table—is the heart of every Maggie's Centre. A fairly large "island" with additional seating for two or three people is essential for nutrition workshops and provides extra space for setting up food or drinks during large gatherings or events. As exemplified by the Maggie's Centre in West London as shown in Figure 6.8, the kitchen table is more than just a design requirement: It's a central concept in the way a Maggie's Centre functions. When people first enter, they are usually offered a cup of tea, but they are also told that they are welcome to go and help themselves if they prefer. The kitchen table serves as a space where visitors can participate in conversations.

6.4.2 Stimulate Curiosity and Imagination

Many healthcare facilities are institutional, uninspiring places that feel drab and lifeless. Instead, Maggie's Centres are designed to be striking, unforgettable, and unique. The Centre footprints are small in relation to the hospital yet intended to shine out like a beacon of hope. A snapshot of a handful of Maggie's Centres shows a wide range of architectural styles, creating an idiosyncratic collection of wonderfully vivid and inspiring buildings. Place and location affect and influence the design of Maggie's Centres in ways that are both obvious and surprising: in both scale and design.

The first newly built Maggie's Centre after Edinburgh was Maggie's Dundee, designed by world-famous architect Frank Gehry and built in 2003 (Figure 6.6). Maggie's Dundee is a white, cottage-like building with a wavy silver roof modeled on a traditional Scottish dwelling, with a tower that extends from the building's roof. In addition, the garden, landscaped by Arabella Lennox-Boyd, contains a labyrinth design based on Chartres Cathedral in France. The Centre conveys a welcoming sense of calm and feels like a sanctuary.

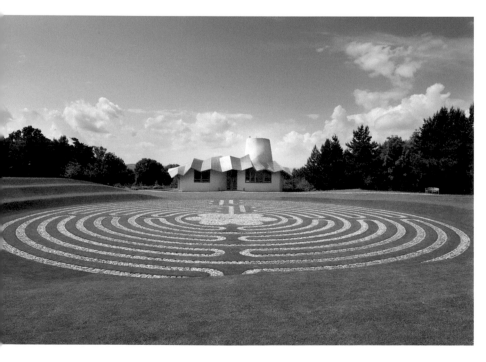

◀ Figure 6.6

Maggie's Dundee, 2003, designed by Frank Gehry.
Source: Maggie's Centre

Jamie Mitchell

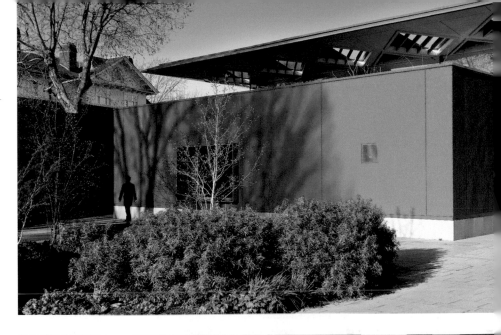

► Figure 6.7

Maggie's West London, 2008, designed by Rogers Stirk Harbour + Partners.
Source: Nick Turner

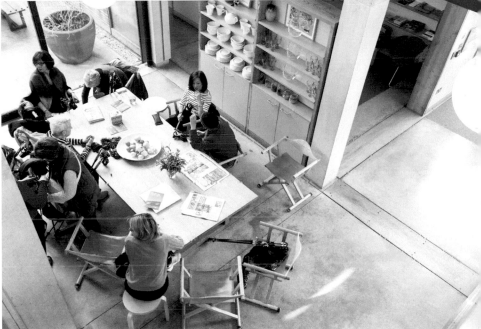

► Figure 6.8

Maggie's West London dining area, 2008, designed by Rogers Stirk Harbour + Partners.
Source: Philip Durrant

Another example to illustrate this design goal is Maggie's West London. Designed by Rogers Stirk Harbour + Partners, Maggie's West London was inspired by Richard Rogers's concept of a heart nestled in the protective wrap of a building's four walls (Figure 6.7). Rogers said, "The idea was to try to minimize the overbearing impact of Charing Cross Hospital. The roof, the landscaping, the hearth inside, the views out, each was to take you away from the hospital and the bustle of the road" (Maggie's Centre, https://www.maggiescentres.org/our-centres/maggies-west-london/architecture-and-design/).

The bright orange walls carry visitors into an equally uplifting interior with cozy rooms, bright open spaces, and transitional walls that provide the flexible space needed to host everything from intimate chats to lively exercise classes (Figure 6.8).

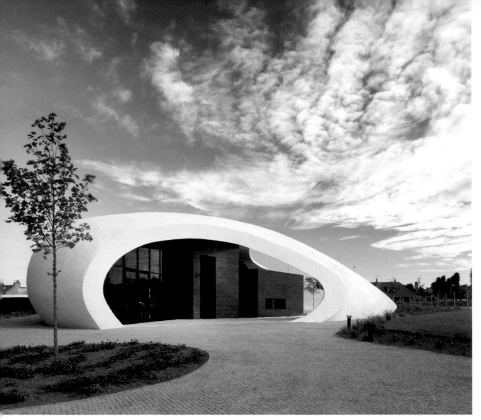

◀ Figure 6.9

Maggie's Aberdeen, 2013, designed by Snøhetta. *Source*: Philip Vile

Maggie's Aberdeen was also designed with the goal of evoking a sense of safety and curiosity. The shell-shape building sits among sculpted green lawns, like a pebble on the grass, with a group of beech trees marking the main entrance (Figure 6.9). The architect, Snøhetta's Kjetil Thorsen, expressed gratitude for the opportunity to design the Centre. He said, "In a world of architectural commercialism, it has been the most meaningful task to seek employment with spaces, materials and landscapes in the service of psychological and emotional healing processes" (Davis 2013).

To evoke emotion, thought, and curiosity, art is incorporated into every Centre. Art that challenges as well as delights is featured, such as Anthony Gormley's *Another Time X*, which stands on a hillock overlooking the Maggie's Centre in Dundee. The art critic and historian Richard Cork, who has helped arrange works of art displayed in Maggie's Centres, has said,

> Artists working in hospitals should never feel tempted to settle for bland decoration. They must opt instead for images that are centrally involved with their own uncompromising visions of the world. The imaginative nourishment provided by such work in a hospital context is incalculable.
>
> (Jencks 2015, p. 87)

6.4.3 Foster a Sense of Self-Reliance and Empowerment

Put simply, the job of those who work at Maggie's Centres is to help people work out how to live with cancer. Each person needs to find the way that is right for him or her, but most people will need some help, at some stage, in finding out

Jamie Mitchell

what that way is. Maggie's Centres have a carefully worked-out series of options, or "set of tools" to choose from: from individual to group support, workshops on different aspects of living with cancer, relaxation strategies, and help with information.

Everything in a Maggie's Centre, from the way it is furnished to the art on its walls or in its gardens, is designed to help people draw on their strengths even and especially when they think they have lost them. Distress can make a person feel paralyzed. There can be a temptation, when things are tough, to curl up and withdraw. To counteract these natural tendencies, landscape designers and architects work together from the beginning of all Maggie's Centre projects with a focus on the important role of the environment in empowering individuals. Sheltered inside, it helps to be reminded, by a seasonal and changing scene outside, that you are still part of a living world. This helps soothe people's fears and start the journey to actively participate in their therapy (Figure 6.10). The architects of Maggie's Oxford, Chris Wilkinson and Jim Eyre, explain,

> Our design encapsulates the philosophy and principles on which the Maggie's Centres are based—the tree house concept maximises the relationship between the internal space and the external landscape offering discreet spaces for relaxation, information and therapy. It will provide a sympathetic and caring retreat, in tune with its surroundings.
> https://www.maggiescentres.org/our-centres/maggies-oxford/architecture-and-design/

There are no clocks in Maggie's Centres because it is important for people to feel that they can do things in their own time and that they aren't going to be rushed out of the door or held to appointments—cancer patients get

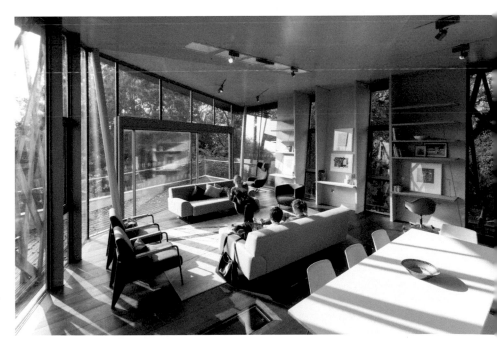

▶ Figure 6.10

Maggie's Oxford, 2014, designed by Wilkinson Eyre. *Source*: Hasselblad H5D

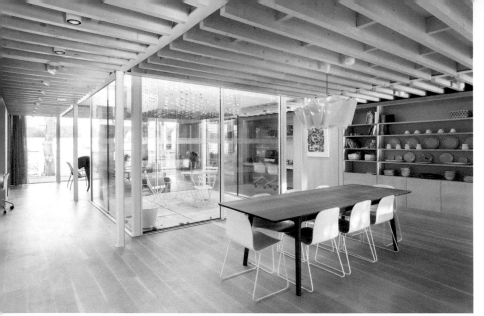

◀ Figure 6.11

Maggie's Lanarkshire, 2014, designed by Reiach and Hall.
Source: Philip Durrant

enough of that at the hospital. Maggie's Centres are open only during the day, but while they are open, they are flexible and welcoming. While exercise groups, cancer-specific support groups, and nutrition workshops take place at particular times, there is never a time when someone who needs support is turned away. Many people use Maggie's Centres as a place to come before or after their hospital appointments, finding that having a cup of tea and sharing their experiences can make the experience of chemotherapy feel a bit more normal. In a way, these are small things, but can make a huge difference to someone who is struggling after a cancer diagnosis.

If a person is in acute distress, all that the person can bear sometimes is to look out of the window from a sheltered place. At Maggie's Lanarkshire, the essence of the design was to create a matrix of courtyards that result in a porous building, an extension of the landscape that offers moments of visibility and outlook with places of privacy and solitude (Figure 6.11).

6.4.4 Design for a Diverse Array of Programs

Maggie's has been pioneering in its approach toward providing a comprehensive program of nonclinical cancer support activities—from yoga and exercise classes to art groups, and from group therapy to information about treatment and side effects. Some of the programs target the need for practical, emotional, and social support for people living with cancer. Some of the practical programs help visitors learn how about eating well, coping with hair loss, advice on benefits and entitlements, and what to expect when starting treatment, to name a few. Some of the emotional support programs offered include managing stress, professional counseling, expressive art, creative writing, and talking to children about cancer. A host of other programs to help with social support include group support on various topics, gardening groups, and how to care for a person with cancer. In addition to scheduled events and structured programs, the Centres provide a place to meet others in a relaxed domestic environment, with the kitchen table providing a place where people can talk openly about cancer. It's a place to sit and read; a place to talk to other people; a place to find support from

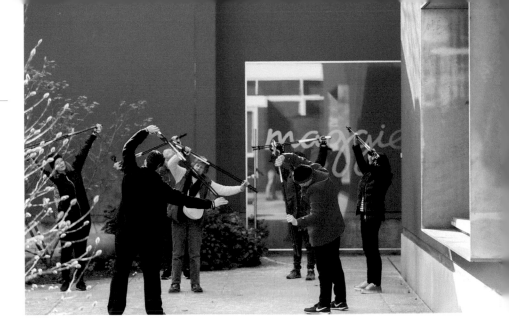

► Figure 6.12

Maggie's West London, 2008, designed by Rogers Stirk Harbour + Partners. *Source*: Philip Durrant

professional experts. The spaces in the Maggie's Centres are integral to supporting the programs. Some of core spaces are the welcoming kitchen, sitting areas, a library, an office with access to computers, consultation rooms, larger rooms for group activities, and quiet away spaces for people to retreat.

It is all too common for people with cancer to feel vulnerable and painfully alone. So, Maggie's provides psychological support both individually and in weekly support groups, which are led by a clinical psychologist. Meeting other people in the same predicament helps people who are feeling isolated to see that they have hopes and fears and experiences in common. Centres also have space and programs for relaxation therapies and stress-reducing strategies (Figure 6.12). These go a long way toward greatly improving quality of life.

Visitors also have access to useful information related to cancer support, such as information on nutrition, supplements for boosting the immune system, medical insurance, exercise, and self-care. The open kitchen offers a vibrant backdrop to the social gathering to discuss shared experiences and education workshops on nutrition. Cancer can fuel fear and helplessness, especially when considering the misconceptions that often exist around a disease as challenging as cancer. Knowledge helps individuals regain both dignity and autonomy.

6.4.5 Be Inclusive and Accessible

The Centre is a place for anybody who wants help in dealing with cancer: friends and family as well as those who just want to visit. Hospitals generally focus on clinical diagnosis and treatments, yet do not offer the other support services that are vital to recovery.

While the Centres welcome all people, some Centres are tailored to specific populations. For Maggie's Newcastle, the architect, Ted Cullinan, adopted the challenge of appealing to a more male "Geordie" constituency, for whom the Maggie's idea of opening up about problems and illness might seem less attractive. Design elements were chosen to make the Centre appeal to men, who tend to feel that a cancer support center isn't for them. Some of these

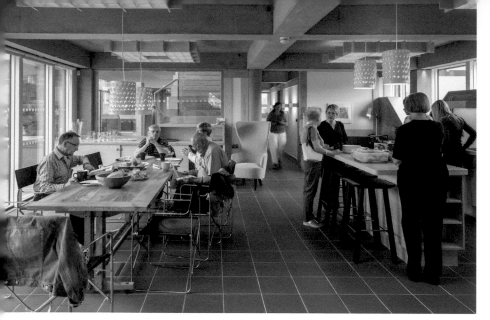

◀ Figure 6.13

Maggie's Newcastle, 2013, designed by Ted Cullinan. *Source*: Paul Raftery

design elements include the use of Corten cladding (referring to the industrial and ship building history of the North East), the building form itself, the roof terraces, and the location of the partly enclosed courtyard. In addition, there are exercise bikes perched in the highest point of the Centre beneath the circular roof. The interior features lots of wood and clay tiles, materials chosen for their warm and calming properties (Figure 6.13). As with all Maggie's Centres, there is a large library, which here forms the central section of the Centre, and the rest of the building is divided into two wings—one contains counseling rooms and a large living room space, the other leads to a kitchen table. There is built-in furniture, such as banquettes and bookshelves, that help to partition the interior into smaller, more intimate spaces surrounded by books instead of bare walls.

While the buildings should look friendly and welcoming, they should not belittle what people are going through by being too "cozy". Having cancer is not "alright" . . . facing the brutal possibility that you could die and what that means for you and your family is not something you can fix with some comfy armchairs and cheerful paint on the walls. These places should look as if they are acknowledging what people are going through, saluting the magnitude of the challenge they are facing and themselves rising to the challenge of trying to help.

As Maggie had wanted, each Centre was—and still is—open to all, regardless of age, gender, or cancer type. It is for anybody who wants help to live well with cancer: friends and family as well as those with cancer themselves. Maggie knew how hard it was to be close to, and look after, someone with cancer. She was determined that financial restraints would not stop people from using the Centre who need it. From the very beginning, all the support offered by Maggie's has been free of charge.

6.5 Conclusions

Maggie's Centres have become examples of how great architecture and design can be used to improve well-being for people who are going through a traumatic experience. Twenty years after the genesis of an idea, Maggie's is now an established charity that has grown into a network of cancer caring centers across the UK, each located on the grounds of a major NHS hospital. There are currently two Centres abroad, one in Hong Kong and another in Tokyo, with more in development.

Maggie's Centres are consistently lauded and awarded for their architecture, but these are not simply status buildings. Every element of design for each Centre is meticulously thought through and tested for how it will be experienced by those who use it. Designing a "Maggie's" has become something of a badge of honor in the architecture world, following in the illustrious footsteps of Frank Gehry, Zaha Hadid, and Richard Rogers, among many others. Designing a Maggie's has also had a profound impact on the architects as well, forming the exact culture of positivity Maggie sought to foster. Norman Foster said, "This project has a particular personal significance, as I was born in the city and have first-hand experience of the distress of a cancer diagnosis. I believe in the power of architecture to lift the spirits and help in the process of therapy" (Frearson 2014).

Bibliography

"A Design Competition for a New Maggie's Centre." Maggie's Centre. www.maggiescentres.org/media/uploads/file_upload_plugin/competition-resource-pack/Maggies resource pack-3.pdf. Accessed June 20, 2019.

"Annual Review 2015." Maggie's Centre, 2015. www.maggiescentres.org/media/uploads/publications/annualreviews/annual_review2015_16.pdf.

Blakenham, Marcia. "Maggie's Centres: Marching On" In *A View from the Front Line*: Edinburgh: Maggie's Cancer Caring Centre, 2007, 27–36 https://www.maggiescentres.org/media/uploads/file_upload_plugin/view-from-the-front-line/view-from-the-front-line_1.pdf.

Campbell, Denis. "NHS England Hospitals Overspend by up to £141m a Year." *The Guardian*, January 17, 2019. www.theguardian.com/society/2019/jan/18/nhs-hospitals-overspend-by-up-to-141m-a-year.

Davis, Ashleigh. "Maggie's Aberdeen by Snøhetta." *Deezen*, September 13, 2013. https://www.dezeen.com/2013/09/13/maggies-centre-aberdeen-by-snøhetta/.

Frearson, Amy. "Norman Foster's Maggie's Centre Opens in Manchester." *Dezeen*, April 27, 2016. www.dezeen.com/2016/04/27/norman-foster-partners-maggies-centre-cancer-care-manchester-england/.

Frearson, Amy. "Norman Foster Unveils Maggie's Centre for Home Town of Manchester." *Deezen*, February 12, 2014. https://www.dezeen.com/2014/02/12/norman-foster-maggies-centre-manchester/.

Jencks, Charles, and Edwin Heathcote. *The Architecture of Hope: Maggie's Cancer Caring Centres*. London: Frances Lincoln, 2015.

Keswick, Maggie. *A View from the Front Line*. Edinburgh: Maggie's Cancer Caring Centre, 2007. https://www.maggiescentres.org/media/uploads/file_upload_plugin/view-from-the-front-line/view-from-the-front-line_1.pdf.

"Maggie's Architecture and Landscape Brief." Maggie's Centre, 2015. www.maggiescentres.org/media/uploads/publications/otherpublications/Maggies_architecturalbrief_2015.pdf.

"Maggie's 2018 Key Facts." Maggie's Centre, 2018. www.maggiescentres.org/media/uploads/publications/otherpublications/PR_Fact_Sheet_v27.pdf.

Quddus, Sadia. "Design with Empathy: An Exhibit Honoring Maggie's Architecture of Cancer Care." *ArchDaily*, September 12, 2014. www.archdaily.com/547453/design-with-empathy-an-exhibit-honoring-maggie-s-architecture-of-cancer-care.

Smisek, Peter. "Maggie's Centre, Oldham: 'Alex De Rijke Is Right to Be Proud of This Project'—Icon Magazine." Maggie's Centre, Oldham: 'Alex De Rijke Is Right to Be Proud of This Project'—*Icon Magazine*, 2017. www.iconeye.com/architecture/news/item/12773-maggie-s-centre-oldham-alex-de-rijke-is-right-to-be-proud-of-this-project.

"The Architecture and Design of Maggie's West London." Maggie's Centre. https://www.maggiescentres.org/our-centres/maggies-west-london/architecture-and-design/. Accessed June 18, 2019.

The Architecture and Design of Maggie's Oxford Centre. Maggie's Centre. https://www.maggiescentres.org/our-centres/maggies-oxford/architecture-and-design/. Accessed June 18, 2019.

YouTube. "Building Hope: The Maggie's Centres Full BBC Documentary 2016." www.youtube.com/watch?v=QkVcZuAikrl. Accessed May 14, 2019.

Part 2 | Community Health

This domain is based on the belief that the design of architectural settings should promote the health of organizations and communities. At this scale, design promotes a healthier future for different social groups across multiple populations. Architectural responses are guided by a shared vision, purpose, and set of goals to improve the health of all members in the community.

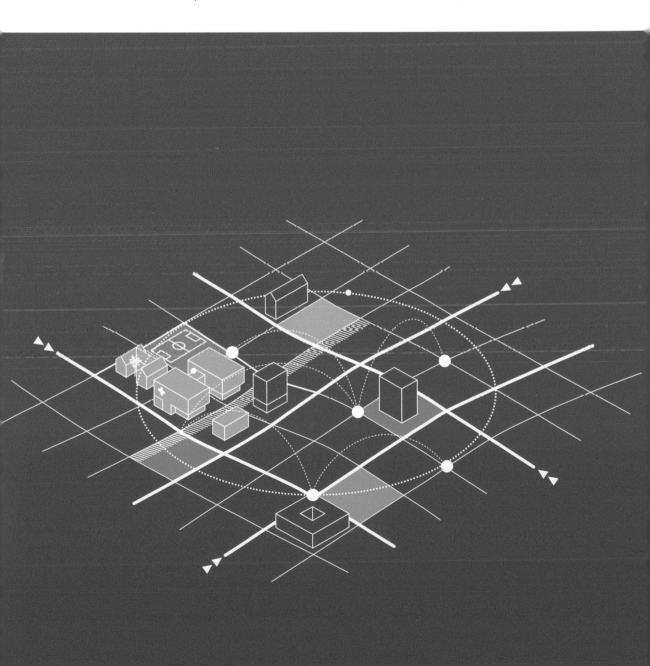

Chapter 7

Creating Healthy Communities Through Wellness Districts and Health Campuses

Shannon Kraus, Kate Renner, Dina Battisto and Brett Jacobs

7.1 Introduction

By most indicators, people in the United States should be happy. We are in an unprecedented era of peace and prosperity. As a nation, we have a strong economy, low unemployment rates, stable wages, plentiful food, and clean water. While these traditional metrics might suggest Americans are happy, the reality is that our global happiness ranking has been declining since 2002. According to a 2019 survey of the state of global happiness, the United States currently ranks nineteenth (Helliwell, Layard, and Sachs 2019). Perhaps the traditional metrics we use to measure happiness do not give a complete picture. Can this decline in ranking be linked to contemporary approaches to community and neighborhood design?

Some reports would say yes. According to a 2013 Robert Wood Johnson Foundation study, life expectancy of most Americans is largely predicted by zip code. When you parlay this finding with the fact that almost 90% of our health is directly related to individual behaviors, socioeconomic factors, and the physical environment (Choi et al. 2018), it becomes apparent that the planning and design of our communities are essential for achieving a high quality of life. It is becoming widely recognized that neighborhood and community design creates affordances that can collectively promote, maintain, and/or improve the health of members of the community (McKenzie, Pinger, and Seabert 2018).

Community health has focused historically on reducing risk factors, decreasing acute and chronic disease burdens and injury occurrence, and promoting health (Goodman, Bunnell, and Posner 2014). Today, however, health is viewed from a broader perspective. There is increasing awareness that to elevate the health of individuals, we need to think beyond access to healthcare services. We need to think about how to create healthy communities.

7.2 Defining a Healthy Community

In the United States, we have built our community infrastructure around the automobile, and it is becoming more apparent that this organizational scheme chokes the life from communities. Planning principles have focused on cultivating "central business districts", which often result in separations between residential and business areas, with neither benefitting from full-time activity and livelihood. These planning principles have also created programmatic divisions as well as social inequalities in many urban areas.

By contrast, a well-designed neighborhood should be a microcosm of society, with active street life, communal areas that promote strong social relationships and support, and healthy codependencies among neighbors. Auto-centric sprawling developments pose a striking parallel to Jane Jacobs's criticism of mid-century neighborhoods redevelopments. They are frequently devoid of urban density, mixed-use neighborhoods, public infrastructure, and shared communal space. Jane Jacobs claimed that people are drawn to the human activity found on a healthy street. It is through opportunities for serendipitous encounters that people build "social capital" to be used in times of need. Furthermore, lively street life give rise to "eyes on the street", helpful for promoting safety, but essential for creating convivial communities (Jacobs 1961).

Communities designed to draw people in are generally planned with a mix of diverse programs (e.g., retail, residential, the arts, entertainment, and health and wellness programs), and include civic amenities, public parks and plazas, and what Smart Growth America calls "complete streets". These are streets that have wide sidewalks for pedestrian life (areas on sidewalks that can be occupied and pathways for pedestrian movement) as well as bike lanes, lanes for public transportation, and dedicated areas for on-street parking and vehicular traffic. These are the fundamental elements of a healthy community.

A healthy community is "one that continuously creates and improves both its physical and social environments, helping people to support one another in aspects of daily life and to develop to their fullest potential" (Center for Disease Control 2006). Healthy communities are places that are designed to offer a range of programs that promote healthy lifestyles and behaviors. They offer programs and features that advance ideas ranging from active transportation to equity to healthy food access. When defining how the design of communities promotes health, a report by Health Resources in Action states that "healthy community design encourages mixed land uses to bring people closer to the places where they live, work, worship, and play. Doing so reduces dependence on cars and provides affordable housing, good bicycle and pedestrian infrastructure, space for social gathering, and access to transit, parks, and healthy foods (Health Resources in Action 2013, p. 6)".

Ideally, communities utilize data to measure and track health outcomes and can leverage this information to address concerns through the implementation of specific programmatic and design strategies. Findings from emerging data sources irrefutably demonstrate the links between many diverse factors, such as the impact that access to healthy food has on diabetes or the relationship between neighborhood walkability with safety and stress. This builds the case for a more integrated design approach toward the composition of healthy communities as shown in the guidelines in Table 7.1.

Shannon Kraus et al.

Table 7.1 Guidelines for creating healthy communities

The design of campuses, neighborhoods, districts, and/or communities should promote public health and the welfare of multiple populations. Community design should promote healthy behaviors and lifestyles, a high quality of life and health-promoting building practices. Healthy communities should reflect the shared vision by multiple constituencies, utilize local assets, and embrace a broad view of health.

Design goals	Design strategies
Multi-sector partnerships	Use collaborative partnerships across multiple sectors to identify a shared vision and set of principles that are rooted in community values and based on a broad definition of health.
Physical activity	Design environments conducive to active transit modes (walking and biking) through the provision of safe routes, conveniences between destinations, and public infrastructure, such as bike racks, shaded pathways, and seating opportunities. The design should encourage active living by supporting recreational physical activity.
Public transportation and infrastructure	Provide accessible and affordable public transportation options, such as bus, train, or trolley, and encourage connectivity through public amenities, local assets, and resources.
Housing and neighborhood quality	Encourage density, mixed land-use (commercial, residential, civic, etc.), and shared infrastructure (i.e., sidewalks). Also, plan around wildlife and ecological features, such as waterways, wetlands, green spaces parks, trees, and gardens.
Social interaction and social cohesion	Encourage incidental social interactions, civic engagement, and a welcoming atmosphere. Common areas, building facades (porches, outdoor seating, and large-sized sidewalks), parks, and public spaces should be designed to foster social relationships.
Engagement	Promote community participation, ownership, and ongoing commitments to maintain public areas. Include health-related activities in the community and support educational initiatives.
Community safety and security	Design for crime prevention and incorporate social infrastructure (or common areas) to reduce actual or perceived threats.
Healthcare and preventative health services	Provide a continuum of healthcare services that are high-quality, accessible, and affordable for all people. Structure public policies and laws to promote public health and monitor health outcomes in the community. Encourage academic medical institutions and community-based healthcare programs.
Access to healthy food and water	Support local food production by preserving agricultural lands and shared/co-op farming. Provide sites for healthy food options that are fresh, nutritional, and affordable. Ensure strong water infrastructure.
Avoid environmental hazards	Minimize man-made activities that negatively impact the surrounding natural environment and public health (e.g., the transfer of toxic chemicals to air, water, and soil, greenhouse gases, noise and air pollution from neighboring highways, and exposure to harmful chemicals).
Educational opportunities	Invest in educational institutions, both K-12 and higher education. Provide opportunities for lifelong learning as well as training community residents to expand employment opportunities and be secure financially.
Strong economy	Provide a range of employment opportunities as well as other opportunities for economic growth, and business retention and vitality. Ensure access to mainstream financial services. Invest in clean, renewable energy.
Equity	Support social equity and quality of life for all people (accommodating for different age groups, socioeconomic groups, family arrangements, gender, cultures, etc.).
Sustainable ecosystems	Utilize renewable energy, such as solar, geothermal, and wind power. Protect local assets and resources, and protect natural resources. Seek harmony between the community of living organisms and man-made environments and artifacts.

Source: Dina Battisto and Brett Jacobs. Adapted from various references in the bibliography

Healthcare systems have opportunities to provide state-of-the-art healthcare services as well as community-enriching services, such as education and community centers, and public infrastructure, like bike paths, public parks, and farmers markets. Additionally, these organizations may support local building activities, such as public housing and business development, to further improve the economic status of their community. In all of this, the healthcare planner/designer must encourage thinking beyond the initial ideas of the client and must advocate for how a hospital project may have an impact beyond its defined walls. Healthy community design may influence the following:

- Urban density
- Dependence on vehicles
- Opportunities for physical activity and social engagement for people as a part of their typical routine
- Ability for people to age in place
- Access to healthy, affordable food, including fresh produce

Programs and key design features that yield outcomes like those listed earlier are necessary to support healthy behavior change, leading to healthier lifestyles and communities. Best practice healthcare systems are now studying the broader health determinants of the communities they serve, so that facilities can be located, sized, programmed, and designed accordingly (Health Resources in Action 2013).

Designing for community health does not happen in a vacuum. It is most effective when community organizations and design professionals collaborate to maximize impact across the many determinants of health (Figure 7.1). Collaboration among healthcare systems, government departments, and philanthropic groups can bring health-focused programs and design elements into care facilities and campuses.

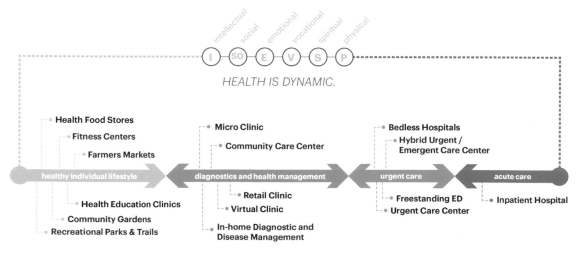

▲ Figure 7.1

Community health spectrum.
Source: HKS 2015

Shannon Kraus et al.

7.3 Creating a Healthy Community

Three steps are essential to the creation of healthy communities. First, it is necessary to assess the community's assets and shortcomings. A variety of community assessment tools and methodologies exist for this purpose. Designers, planners, healthcare systems, and policy organizations can utilize these tools to assess health disparities and gaps in the community, survey assets for current and future projects, and understand how interventions can be leveraged to improve health. Once needs have been identified in a community, a plan needs to be developed based on these findings that includes the scope and scale of the intervention. Will it encompass multiple sites and infrastructure across the community, or will it focus on a specific site? Finally, a coalition of committed stakeholders must be established. They must work together to define health priorities in relation to budget, develop a strategic vision, set short-term and long-term goals, and identify strategies for implementation.

To create a healthy community, two planning typologies are essential and manifest differently based on the needs of the community as shown in Figures 7.2 and 7.3:

- A health campus is a planning typology that aims to promote health through the design of healthcare facilities and campuses that include nonmedical programs that address the diverse nature of health determinants. Health campuses focus on providing the latest advancements of medical science on a campus to treat disease as well as deliver services related to health prevention and promotion.
- A wellness district is a planning typology that aims to promote health through the design of mixed-use developments at a community-wide scale. These neighborhood and community-scale developments span multiple sites and target improvements to population health and the promotion of healthy behaviors through community design.

The development of health campuses and wellness districts (also referred to as health districts or medical districts) is starting to take shape around the

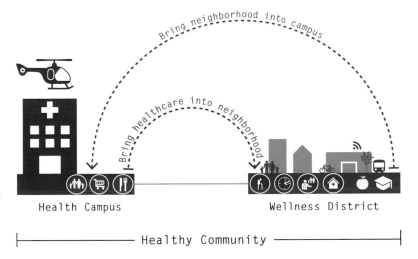

► Figure 7.2

Two planning typologies for healthy communities.
Source: Dina Battisto and Eva Henrich

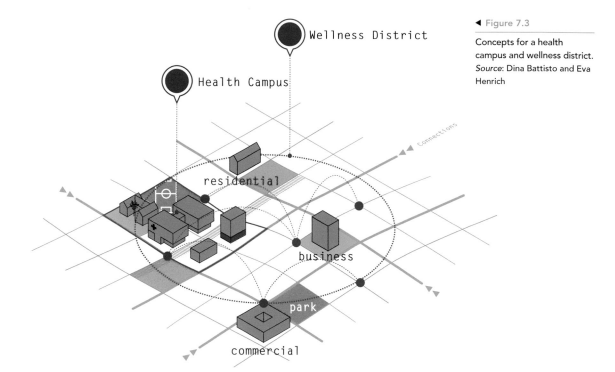

◀ Figure 7.3

Concepts for a health
campus and wellness district.
Source: Dina Battisto and Eva
Henrich

world. Although early in their implementation, these typologies are expected to
improve individuals and community health by better addressing the entire range
of health determinants, many of which have often been overlooked. In the next
two sections, case studies are introduced to show how these two typologies are
being implemented in practice. The first two projects are health campuses and
the last two projects are larger-scale wellness districts. To provide an overview
of the four case studies, Figure 7.4 summarizes the main programs for each case
study organized by the two typologies.

7.4 From Isolated Healthcare Facilities to Integrated Health Campuses

The first essential typology for creating a healthy community begins with the
transformation of established healthcare facilities into health campuses that
address specific community health needs. Healthcare systems are doing this
in several ways, including renovating and replacing old facilities and pairing
campus investments with infrastructure to seed preferred development. Further,
the integration of diverse programs into these campuses, such as education
spaces, libraries, retail, healthy dining options, farmers markets, community gardens, and fitness centers, provides opportunities for healthcare organizations
to curate a community centered on wellness. At the same time, these developments assemble the most advanced healthcare technologies, equipment,

TWO TYPOLOGIES:	HEALTH CAMPUS		WELLNESS DISTRICT	
Goal	Promote health through the design of neighborhoods and communities		Promote health through the design of health care system facilities and campuses	
Four Case Studies:	Metro Health Master Plan	Focal Point	Las Vegas Medical District	Baton Rouge
Programming Components				
Housing	●	●	●	●
Healthcare	●	●	●	●
Pharmacy	●	●	●	●
Civic functions (i.e. bank, post office, police, etc.)	●	●	●	●
Social services (i.e. childcare, shelters, foodbanks, etc.)		●	●	●
Entertainment (i.e. theater events programming, etc.)	●		●	

Food
  a. farmer's market
  b. grocery store
  c. restaurants
	●
	
	●
		●
		●
		●
			
			●
			●
				
				●

Education
  a. community space
  b. K-12 school
  c. higher education
	●
	●
	●
		●
		●
		●
			●
			
			●
				●
				
				●

Community amenities
  a. public event space
  b. fitness center
  c. library
	●
	●
	●
		●
		●
			●
			●
			●
				●
				●

Recreation / greenspace
  a. community garden
  b. parks / green space
  c. playground
  d. sports fields
  e. bike paths
  f. walking trails
	●
	●
	●
	●
	●
	●
		●
		●
		●
		●
		●
		●
			
			●
			●
			●
			●
			●
				
				●
				●
				●
				●
				●

Public transportation	●	●	●	●
Source:	Metro Health Master Plan 2016	HDR website www.hdrinc.com	Las Vegas Medical District Master Plan Executive Summary, 2015 Smith Group	A Master Plan for Baton Rouge Health District, 2015, Perkins and Will

▲ Figure 7.4

Overview of case studies for two planning typologies.
Source: Authors

and specialists. While wellness districts involve multiple sites, a health campus is on a specific site, yet the boundaries are permeable and bleed out into the surrounding community. Two case studies are presented ahead to convey the health campus concept.

7.4.1 MetroHealth

MetroHealth is undergoing a transformation, focused on community health and the creation of a health campus through physical building changes, programming, and amenities. MetroHealth serves both the city of Cleveland and greater Cuyahoga County in Ohio, both areas with severe health challenges. According to some common health metrics, Cleveland is 20% or more below the national average (Cleveland & Cuyahoga County Health Resource 2017).

Reflecting the challenges faced by Cleveland and Cuyahoga County, the neighborhoods surrounding MetroHealth have a Walk Score of 64, a Transit Score of 44, and a Bike Score of 52, which represent values in the fair to poor range of the scoring system (Walk Score 2017). The site has been identified as a food desert, and the only green space near the campus is a cemetery. Cuyahoga County, in partnership with MetroHealth and a coalition of neighborhood stakeholders, has been focused on addressing many of these identified shortcomings, including limited food access, unhealthy eating habits, poor air quality, and physical inactivity. MetroHealth's Main Campus has been identified as an opportunity to engage the community and act as a catalyst for change to stimulate growth through the development of housing, retail, and commercial properties on their health campus. Additionally, these planning initiatives have outlined

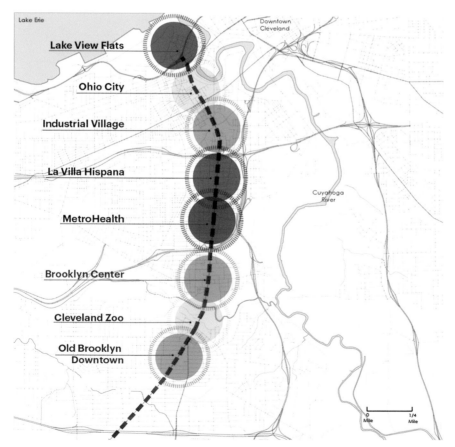

◀ Figure 7.5

MetroHealth Main Campus to encourage growth across multiple neighborhood nodes.
Source: HKS

plans for street improvements with bike lanes and pedestrian safety features to increase walkability, public transit access, and walkable environments, all with a unified branding strategy to link the nodes together (Figure 7.5).

The MetroHealth system has taken a mindful, responsive approach to serving the community. In 2013, the system began by re-envisioning its mission statement into one that is more community-focused, with the primary aim of "leading the way to a healthier you and a healthier community". MetroHealth's transformation is centered on flipping the health delivery paradigm from focusing on the hospital as the first line of defense to seeing it as the last stop.

The MetroHealth transformation design and planning process began with strategic assessments of both the health system and the neighborhoods surrounding the main campus. Economic and residential potential was established, and MetroHealth formed partnerships with more than 25 local organizations, including the Cuyahoga County Library, community development corporations, the Cleveland Sustainability Office, Enterprise, Bike Cleveland, and the Greater Cleveland Regional Transit Authority. These connections have exponentially expanded the impact the system has within Cuyahoga County.

MetroHealth engaged more than 275 community residents, 70 Metro-Health staff members, 29 patients/family members, and more than 30 community groups in a series of engagement meetings, including visioning sessions and a Community Health Design Assessment. Feedback from residents on how a future campus could support the goals and vision of the surrounding neighborhood uncovered the need for affordable housing, healthy food access, safe parks and sidewalks, bike paths, health education, and better access to transportation. A resulting key design driver for the project became connecting the campus with the surrounding community (Figure 7.6).

In addition to physically transforming the campus, MetroHealth's partnerships with local community groups have already begun to address this feedback through more than 100 community programs. For example, MetroHealth Farm Stand provides fresh, affordable produce weekly during the Ohio growing season. Additionally, the Cuyahoga County Library has a branch in the main hospital, allowing patients, staff members, visitors, and community members to have convenient access to reading materials. The new health campus is expected to stimulate neighborhood revitalization and economic development along Cleveland's urban corridor (Figure 7.7). Furthermore, the campus transformation project is expected to support 5,618 permanent jobs, provide $837 million in economic benefit to Cuyahoga County, and generate more than $95 million in new local, state, and federal tax revenue (Cleveland Urban Design Collaborative 2012).

7.4.2 Focal Point Community Campus

Yet another project in early phases of development is the Focal Point Community Campus in southwestern Chicago (Figure 7.8). Planned by HDR, and in partnership with Saint Anthony Hospital, the Chicago Southwest Development Corporation, and Jones Lang LaSalle, the Focal Point project aspires to become the most comprehensive healthcare campus in America.

It is sited on a 32-acre campus, much of which is contaminated by the chemical manufacturing companies who previously occupied the site. Owing to

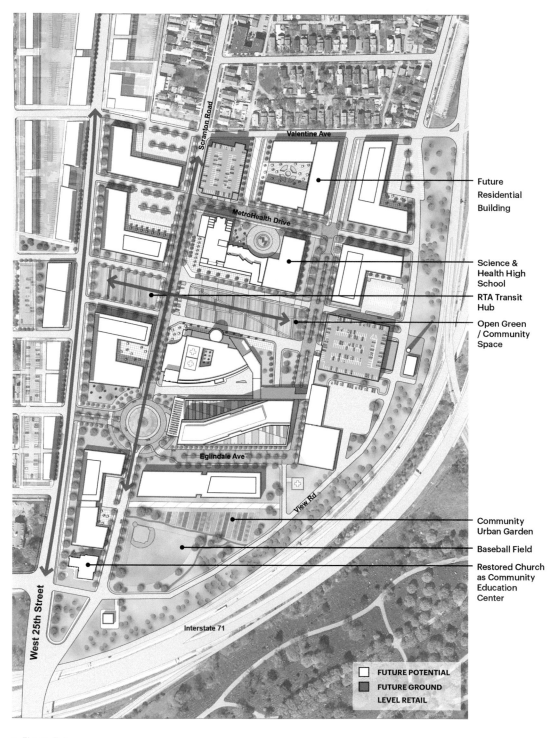

Future
Residential
Building

Science &
Health High
School

RTA Transit
Hub

Open Green
/ Community
Space

Community
Urban Garden

Baseball Field

Restored Church
as Community
Education
Center

FUTURE POTENTIAL

FUTURE GROUND
LEVEL RETAIL

▲ Figure 7.6

MetroHealth master plan.
Source: HKS

Shannon Kraus et al.

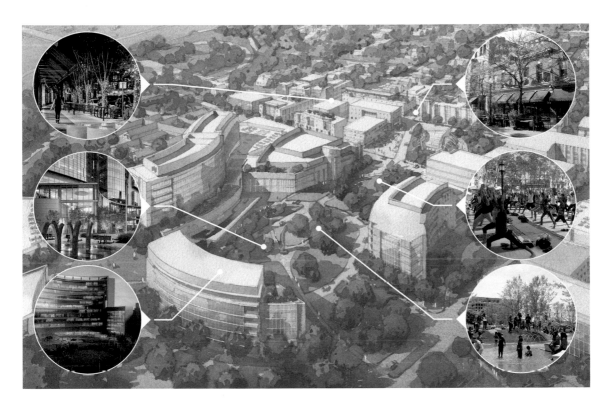

▲ Figure 7.7

MetroHealth master plan detail.
Source: HKS

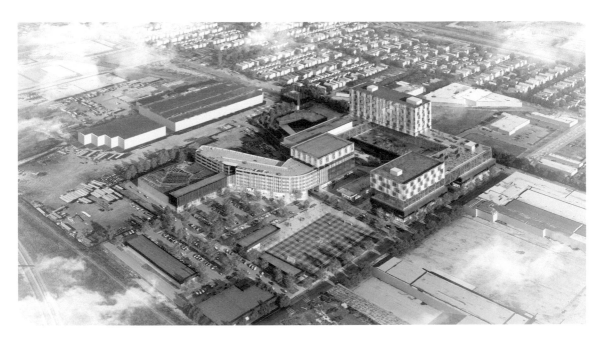

▲ Figure 7.8

Focal Point master plan.
Source: HDR

this state, one of the initial project goals has been site remediation. The stakeholders and designers intend to transform unused space into a vibrant, active, and holistic community asset.

The site is also located in an economically challenged district. On top of remediating the land, the stakeholders and designers have had to devise a self-sustaining business plan for development. To this end, it was determined that a portion of the rental income from the campus's diverse range of programs will be used to subsidize community amenities, including education spaces, wellness classes, a creativity center, parks, a recreation center, and subsidized housing. The campus truly intends to be self-reliant, almost as if a microcosm of the greater city.

The design team and Saint Anthony Hospital worked together, developing plans for the campus. Programs were selected in accordance with the needs of the surrounding community as verified by research and quantifiable metrics. All things considered, the primary goals of the campus are centered around creating a true "one-stop-shop", where all the various programs associated with healthy living can be collocated into a dense, mixed-use community as well as spur development outward across the community (Figure 7.9).

In addition to providing a full spectrum of healthcare services, the Focal Point team established five additional goals for the development. The first of these goals is to increase access to early childhood education, daycare, and family services to ensure developmental success for children. Ultimately, Focal Point aspires to lift the community out of poverty by providing for the needs of children, adequately preparing them to become healthy, productive citizens. To accomplish this, a daycare and early childhood development center are currently being planned for, as are numerous preschool educational programs. Building upon the idea of enabling "upward mobility", the second major goal of the Focal Point Community Campus is to partner with K-12 programs to increase the percentage of college-bound teens. To this end, plans are in the works for extracurricular activity centers, a high school, and a vocational school.

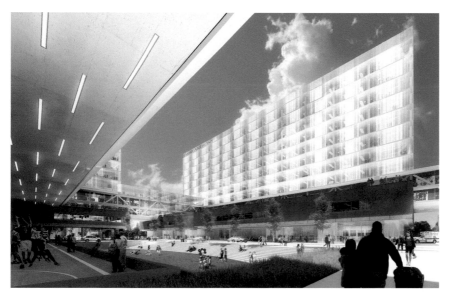

◀ Figure 7.9

Focal Point courtyard.
Source: HDR

Following a Community Health Needs Assessment, the stakeholders and design team identified diabetes, mental health, nutrition, physical activity, obesity, and access to care as areas significantly in need. Thus, a third major goal of the campus is to facilitate a true, comprehensive sense of holistic wellness for the local community. To achieve this, plans are in the works for a myriad of parks, gardens, athletic fields, and a fitness center. To tackle the concept of "access", alternative modes of transportation are being designed for, most notably through the incorporation of bike lanes into the road network.

The fourth major goal of the campus is to provide for the basic housing needs of over 100 families in the area. This will be accomplished through the inclusion of Veterans Associate (VA) housing and other subsidized family housing on-site. Additionally, other VA facilities will be located on the campus to reduce the occurrence of homeless veterans.

The final goal of the Focal Point Community Campus is to create a self-sustaining network of jobs for the area to serve as a boon for the local economy. With over 1.2 million square feet of construction to be completed, and a variety of retail businesses and medical services in need of staff, the campus is expected to create 1,400 new, permanent jobs, in addition to hundreds, if not thousands, of temporary construction jobs. Also, as has been stated earlier, vocational and job training programs are being planned to increase the skilled local workforce. Rather than viewing their mission through the lens of providing medical care exclusively, the Saint Anthony Hospital aspires to be truly transformational. There are plans underway not only for state-of-the-art clinics and a general hospital, but also for affordable housing, parks, outdoor and public community spaces, childcare, other educational programs, and retail (Figure 7.10). The Focal Point Community Campus aspires to be the path forward not only for southwestern Chicago but also as an example of how a hospital can serve as a catalyst for urban renewal through comprehensive, holistic campus programming and design.

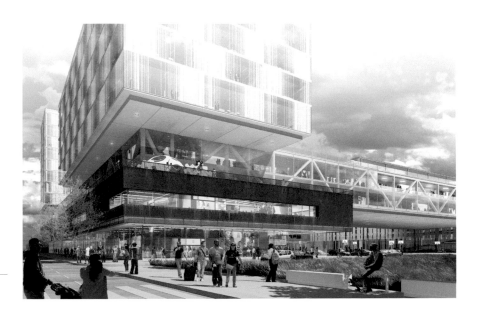

▶ Figure 7.10

Focal Point summer retail.
Source: HDR

7.5 The Rise of Wellness Districts

The second essential typology for creating healthy communities is the cultivation of wellness districts. Wellness districts are mixed-use developments that support a combination of zoning practices and land uses rather than developing an area for a single purpose. These developments aim at improving population health outcomes and encourage healthy behaviors for the community. Wellness districts have demonstrated many positive outcomes, including increased physical activity, active transportation, and reduced vehicle miles traveled (Mixed-Use Development 2017). These neighborhood developments prioritize wellness at their core, creating synergies between healthcare, whole-life living concepts, fitness, retail, dining, and entertainment through careful planning of the user experience.

7.5.1 Las Vegas Medical District (LVMD)

One such master plan is the Las Vegas Medical District (LVMD) in Clark County, Nevada. This 674-acre district, located near downtown Las Vegas, is the nexus of several health-focused partners. These include Valley Hospital, the University Medical Center, and the Cleveland Clinic's Lou Ruvo Center for Brain Health, to name a few.

Though the district was established back in 1997, it has been badly neglected. When the county performed a Community Health Needs Assessment in 2015, the depths of the neglect were revealed. Routine health metrics in Las Vegas were found to be far below national averages. The percentage of medically uninsured or underinsured was one of the worst cases in the United States, and a severe shortage of hospital beds per person was uncovered. The availability of affordable housing was insufficient, commutes were shown to be plagued by severe congestion, and air pollution was extreme. To top it off, the unemployment rate peaked at 14% in 2010, nearly 50% higher than the United States national average that year. The district and its residents were not healthy. Following the results of the report, the LVMD engaged more than 20 stakeholder organizations, surveyed over 800 residents, held numerous town hall meetings, and conducted extensive polling through both online portals and engagement booths stationed throughout the district.

The results of this extensive outreach and research effort revealed impressive opportunities. Reports indicate that with carefully considered district-wide interventions, an additional $3.6 billion can be generated by the year 2030, contributing 24,000 permanent jobs and $181 million in additional government tax revenue. Preliminary analysis revealed two key considerations: (1) plentiful opportunities exist for collaboration among the key stakeholders (especially pertaining to security and parking services, and district-wide amenities), and (2) the creation of a new four-year accredited medical school would be essential for achieving the district's goals. Not only would it attract young, talented professionals to the area (which has long suffered from healthcare worker shortages), but also it would bring much-needed fiscal resources through the development of mixed-use communities and with the money brought in by research dollars, grants, and technological advancements.

Shannon Kraus et al.

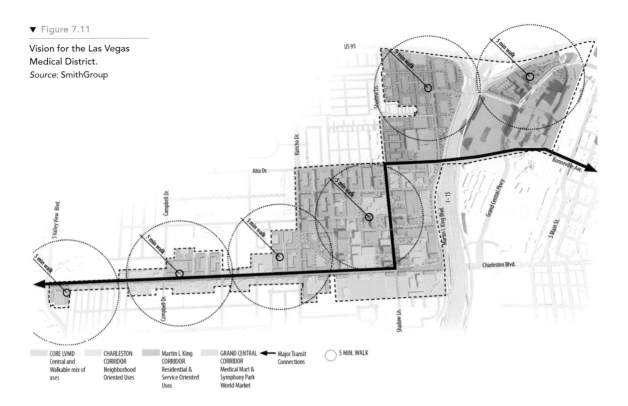

| CORE LVMD Central and Walkable mix of uses | CHARLESTON CORRIDOR Neighborhood Oriented Uses | Martin L King CORRIDOR Residential & Service Oriented Uses | GRAND CENTRAL CORRIDOR Medical Mart & Symphony Park World Market | ← Major Transit Connections | 5 MIN. WALK |

Visioning sessions with the stakeholders and planning/design team revealed the "live, learn, work and play" concept, which has since become the district's mantra. Three primary goals were identified to move closer to this vision. These include: (1) creating a series of connected and walkable neighborhoods throughout the district with individual character and identity, (2) encouraging collaborative efforts between the stakeholders, and (3) promoting and developing a diversity of mixed uses throughout the district (Figure 7.11).

With vision and goals set, numerous strategies were then created to bring them to fruition (Figures 7.12 and 7.13). Pertaining to the creation of small, interconnected communities, the design team realized they will need to activate the street by increasing the urban density of the "core" zone. This necessitates street renovations in accordance with the "Complete Streets" approach and revealed the need for a district-wide transit shuttle service, as well as new parking structures. Relating to the goal of collaboration between major entities, it was determined that the creation of a joint 501(c)(3) nonprofit would be essential. This cooperative entity will organize and administer collective services for the district, including parking, security, and various concierge and amenity services. Finally, relating to the goal of promoting mixed-use development, the design team and stakeholders have committed to working together with the local jurisdiction's planning, zoning, and design-review boards.

The largest and most important "neighborhood" to the new LVMD will be the revitalized district known as the "Core". With densification as the top

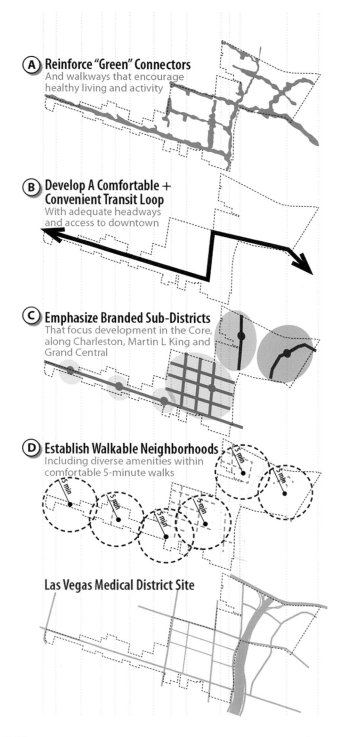

A **Reinforce "Green" Connectors**
And walkways that encourage
healthy living and activity

B **Develop A Comfortable +**
Convenient Transit Loop
With adequate headways
and access to downtown

C **Emphasize Branded Sub-Districts**
That focus development in the Core,
along Charleston, Martin L King and
Grand Central

D **Establish Walkable Neighborhoods**
Including diverse amenities within
comfortable 5-minute walks

Las Vegas Medical District Site

▲ Figure 7.12

Las Vegas Medical District—four primary systems.
Source: SmithGroup

Shannon Kraus et al.

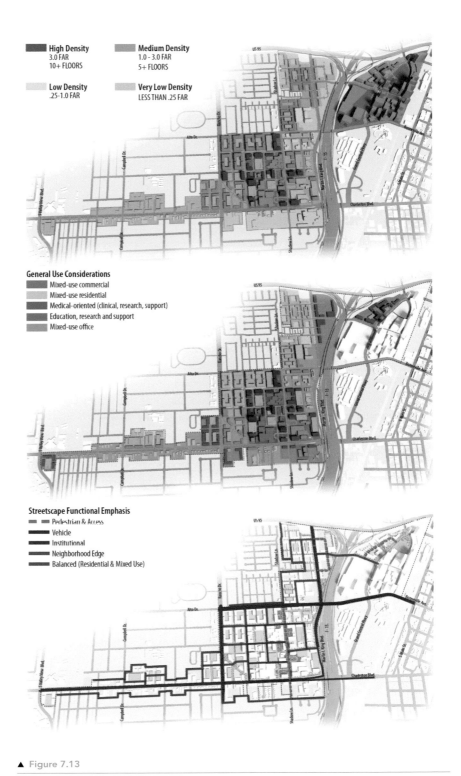

High Density
3.0 FAR
10+ FLOORS

Medium Density
1.0 - 3.0 FAR
5+ FLOORS

Low Density
.25-1.0 FAR

Very Low Density
LESS THAN .25 FAR

General Use Considerations
Mixed-use commercial
Mixed-use residential
Medical-oriented (clinical, research, support)
Education, research and support
Mixed-use office

Streetscape Functional Emphasis
Pedestrian & Access
Vehicle
Institutional
Neighborhood Edge
Balanced (Residential & Mixed Use)

▲ Figure 7.13

Las Vegas Medical District—urban design strategies.
Source: SmithGroup

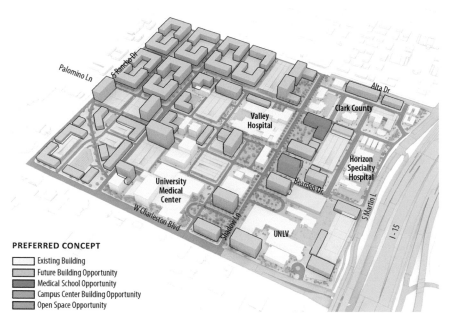

◄ Figure 7.14

Las Vegas Medical District—
mixed use and walkable core.
Source: SmithGroup

PREFERRED CONCEPT

- Existing Building
- Future Building Opportunity
- Medical School Opportunity
- Campus Center Building Opportunity
- Open Space Opportunity

concern, the design team established another set of goals now more narrowly focused on the Core (Figure 7.14). This zone will be home to the new UNLV medical school and will require enough parking to handle the new load. To address this, multiple parking structures are currently part of the master plan. However, a parallel series of considerations at the legislative level is pivotal to the success of Core redevelopment initiatives. The design team and stakeholders are working alongside relevant community boards to consolidate small adjacent parcels to enable larger-scale development. Efforts are underway to lobby for increased allowable floor-to-area ratios. Negotiations to re-designate random, interspersed, single-use parcels for mixed-use development and negotiate for reduced building setbacks are in various stages of progress.

From the efforts to improve and redevelop the Las Vegas Medical District we can see the importance of process. Comprehensive preliminary analysis was conducted. An overarching vision was established with clear-cut goals, as well as strategies to realize those goals. Finally, narrower goals and strategies were developed to achieve urban densification of the Core, from both design and legislative points of view. Clearly, for large-scale projects the use of scalar thinking, whereby goals and strategies are broken down into ever more specific interventions, seems to be a useful way to deal with complexity. Additionally, the scale and scope of the interventions made it necessary to employ a comprehensive approach, where design efforts run in tandem with legislative efforts.

7.5.2 Baton Rouge Health District

The Baton Rouge Health District in Louisiana is one of the largest wellness districts currently being planned in the United States. In an innovative pre-design analysis study, the project planners and stakeholders imagined the entire district as if

Baton Rouge Health District intervention methodology.
Source: Perkins and Will

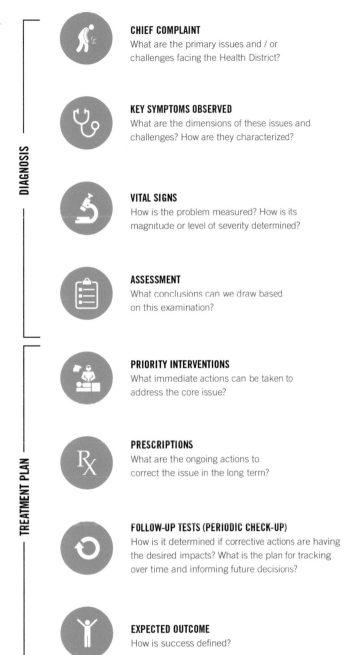

DIAGNOSIS

CHIEF COMPLAINT
What are the primary issues and / or challenges facing the Health District?

KEY SYMPTOMS OBSERVED
What are the dimensions of these issues and challenges? How are they characterized?

VITAL SIGNS
How is the problem measured? How is its magnitude or level of severity determined?

ASSESSMENT
What conclusions can we draw based on this examination?

TREATMENT PLAN

PRIORITY INTERVENTIONS
What immediate actions can be taken to address the core issue?

PRESCRIPTIONS
What are the ongoing actions to correct the issue in the long term?

FOLLOW-UP TESTS (PERIODIC CHECK-UP)
How is it determined if corrective actions are having the desired impacts? What is the plan for tracking over time and informing future decisions?

EXPECTED OUTCOME
How is success defined?

it were a "patient", developing a "diagnosis" and "treatment plan" to address the overarching project vision, as defined in collaborative visioning sessions (Figure 7.15). The four topical areas addressed are the following: (1) healthy place, (2) health education and research, (3) healthcare innovation, and (4) resiliency and disaster preparedness. Each of these four areas received its own independent diagnosis and treatment plan according to the district intervention methodology. This analysis structure was essential for clarifying the programming, planning, and design interventions that will ultimately be included in the district.

Downtown Baton Rouge was identified as a "sick patient" for a myriad of reasons. It suffers from acute vehicular congestion on major thoroughfares, has extremely limited access to alternative means of transportation, and is the very embodiment of sprawl. Regarding access to medical care, there are few incentives for medical professionals to choose to practice in the region as it currently exists. Consequently, there are not enough medical professionals to serve the needs of the community, and the medical services that do exist are not well suited to it. These services tend to focus on acute care, rather than on preventative treatments or the management of chronic diseases.

Using the methodology previously described, the project planners and stakeholders identified numerous goals and strategies to improve the district. One of the primary goals was to build up the district's network of streets, to both create hierarchy and mitigate congestion (Figure 7.16). To accomplish this goal, they determined that constructing Midway Boulevard, extending Dijon Drive, and rerouting Picardy Drive would be essential interventions.

Another goal identified for the district was to enable walking, biking, and the use of mass transit. To this end, the designers developed a set of street guidelines that include features such as widened sidewalks, bike lanes, medians, plazas, and bus stops, in conjunction with bike and car share programs, an intra-district shuttle, and a new transit center (Figure 7.17). Yet another separate (but related)

The Health District will be the hub of a well-connected and efficient transportation network that supports the daily operations of the district and serves the region.

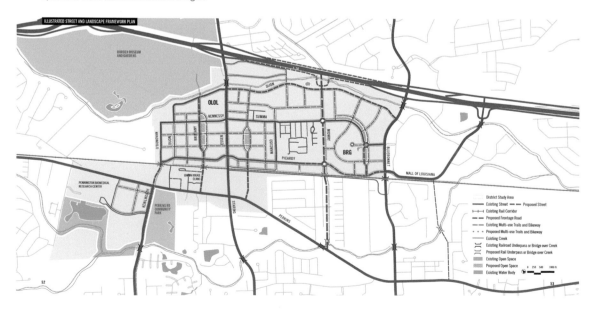

▲ Figure 7.16

Baton Rouge Health District street framework.
Source: Perkins and Will

Shannon Kraus et al.

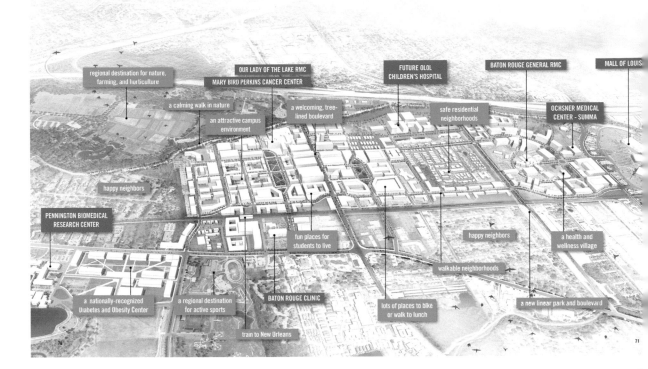

▲ Figure 7.17

Baton Rouge Health District master plan.
Source: Perkins and Will

▼ Figure 7.18

Baton Rouge mixed-use zoning creates vibrant street life.
Source: Perkins and Will

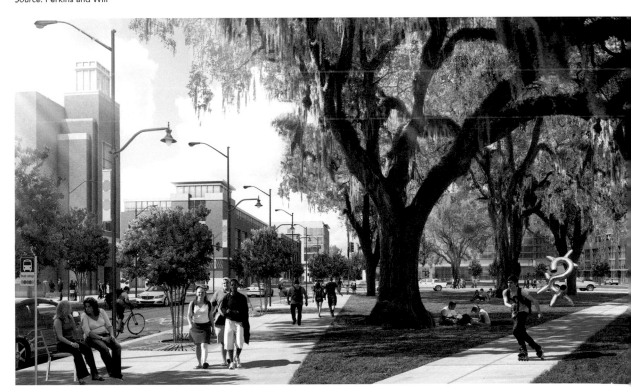

goal was for the district to connect to parks and open spaces. To this end, the designers developed a landscape framework plan to connect the site with existing green spaces as well as construct new signature parks. To promote balanced, diverse, and orderly development, the planners decided that all buildings must contribute in some way to the public domain (Figure 7.18). One recommendation to ensure this possibility was for the district to be designated as a mixed-use institutional zone. After all, programs ranging from housing, healthcare, and childcare to education and recreation spaces, just to name a few, are all included in the program.

To tackle the primary health needs of the community served, the stakeholders have drafted plans for the creation of a Diabetes and Obesity Center. This facility will collocate the following services: nutrition, exercise, clinics, healthy meals for purchase, a demonstration kitchen, medical education classes, and research. In line with the research aspirations of the center, plans are also being drafted to extend LSU's School of Medicine (in New Orleans) into the district.

A bold and diverse coalition of foundations and care providers has been instrumental in advancing this project. A partial list of stakeholders includes the following: The Baton Rouge Area Foundation, Baton Rouge General Medical Center, Blue Cross and Blue Shield of Louisiana, the Mary Bird Perkins Cancer Center, the Ochsner Medical Center, Our Lady of the Lake Regional Medical Center, the Pennington Biomedical Research Center, and the Woman's Hospital. The complexity and capital required to develop a project as extensive as the Baton Rouge Health District necessitate strategic partnerships and wouldn't be possible without these planners.

7.6 Conclusions

Health systems in the United States, and around the world, are working to address the many health disparities facing communities today. From access to care to access to wellness programs, initiatives that impact the built environment are being undertaken by designers and providers. The most successful initiatives look beyond the walls and property lines of traditional healthcare facilities and consider health in its full complexity. Wellness districts, health campuses, and healthy buildings are the fundamental building blocks of a healthy community.

Healthy communities are often the result of cross-disciplinary stakeholders coming together to identify needs and design features to improve opportunities for safety, physical activity, nutrition, and healthy lifestyles. To this end, we offer the following healthy community planning and design guidelines:

1. Evaluate—Assess the broader picture around any project or engagement:

   • Understand the healthcare system's current efforts with community outreach and programming
   • Understand the healthcare system's current priorities for infrastructure and development
   • Assess community needs and conduct a community health gap analysis utilizing the tools

2. Expand—Move beyond a siloed approach:

- Identify ongoing or already funded community, local, and regional initiatives
- Seek traditional and non-traditional community, stakeholder, and agency partnerships and alliances
- Identify strategies and scopes for projects that advance community goals, including health campuses and wellness districts

3. Explore—Think beyond the property lines:

- Evaluate opportunities for campus, neighborhood, and community design interventions
- Consider how any project must be designed to maximize community impact
- Assess success and failures of strategies, and share results

Following these guidelines will help every development, healthcare-focused or otherwise, positively address all determinants of health. Designing for health is not just an opportunity but also a responsibility that architects and designers must embrace. They must embark on initiatives to raise local economies, increase quality of life, and improve health outcomes. The key to impacting community health rests in breaking down the silos between civic, community, private, and public stakeholders. It is about designers leveraging stakeholders' combined interests in creating healthy communities for us to live, work, play, and heal.

Acknowledgments

The authors would like to thank the following people for helping to develop the case studies in the chapter: James J. Atkinson from HDR on the Focal Point Community Campus project; Michael Johnson from SmithGroup on the Las Vegas Medical District master plan; and David Green and Basak Alkan from Perkins and Will on the Baton Rouge Health District master plan. In addition, we would like to thank the countless other people and organizations who contributed to the development and realization of the case studies included in this chapter.

Bibliography

Alberta Health Services. *Built Environment Indicators Review: Summary Report*. www.albertahealthservices.ca/ps-4131-be-indicators-report.pdf.

Baton Rouge Area Foundation. *Health District Master Plan*, December 11, 2015. www.braf.org/braf-research/2016/2/29/health-district-master-plan.

Center for Disease Control. *Healthy Community Design Fact Sheet*, November 2006. https://www.cdc.gov/healthyplaces/factsheets/Designing_and_Building_Healthy_Places_factsheet_Final.pdf.

Center for Disease Control. *Healthy Places*, January 23, 2014. www.cdc.gov/healthyplaces/about.htm.

Choi, Edwin, Juhan Sonin, Giknvo Hrothgar, and Kelsey Kittelsen. *Determinants of Health*. GoInvo, October, 2018. www.goinvo.com/features/determinants-of-health/.

Cleveland & Cuyahoga County Health Resource. *What Determines Our Health*, 2017. www.healthdatamatters.org/health-overview.

Cleveland Neighborhood Progress, Parsons Brinckerhoff, Baker, 4ward Planning, Kent State University CUDC. *W. 25 Transit Development Strategy. Community Planning Process Final Report*. Cleveland, Ohio, 2015.

Cleveland Urban Design Collaborative. *W. 25th Street Corridor Initiative*, 1–82, Rep. Cleveland, Ohio: Kent State University, 2012.

Coupland, Kerry, S. Rikhy, Kaitlyn Hill, and Deborah McNeil. *State of Evidence: The Built Environment and Health 2011–2015*. Edmonton: Public Health Innovation and Decision Support, Population & Public Health, Alberta Health Services, November 2011.

Downtown Cleveland Alliance. *Downtown Cleveland Fast Facts 2014* (2017). http://rethinkcleveland.org/Data-Reports/fast-facts-2014_list.aspx?ext=.pdf.

Goodman, Richard A., Rebecca Bunnell, and Samuel F. Posner. "What Is 'Community Health?' Examining the Meaning of an Evolving Field in Public Health." *Preventive Medicine* 67 (2014): S58–S61.

HDR website. www.hdrinc.com/portfolio/focal-point-community-campus.

Health Resources in Action: Advancing Public Health and Medical Research. *Defining Healthy Communities*. Boston, MA: Health Resources in Action, July 25, 2013. https://hria.org/wp-content/uploads/2016/10/defininghealthycommunities.original.pdf.

Helliwell, John F., Peter R. G. Layard, and Jeffrey Sachs, eds. *World Happiness Report 2019 Update*. New York: Sustainable Development Solutions Network, 2019. https://worldhappiness.report/ed/2019/.

Institute of Medicine Committee on Post-Disaster Recovery of a Community's Public Health, Medical, and Social Services. *Healthy, Resilient, and Sustainable Communities after Disasters: Strategies, Opportunities, and Planning for Recovery*. Washington, DC: The National Academies Press, 2015. www.ncbi.nlm.nih.gov/books/NBK316532/pdf/Bookshelf_NBK316532.pdf.

Jacobs, Jane. *The Death and Life of Great American Cities*. New York: Random House, 1961.

Key Stats & Figures. http://rethinkcleveland.org/Data-Reports/Key-Stats-Figures-(1).aspx.

Kraus, Sigma, and Renner, Kraus. "How Architecture Can Help Progress Population Health." *Health Facilities*, October 5, 2016. www.hfmmagazine.com/articles/2434-how-architecture-can-help-progress-population-health.

Las Vegas Medical District. *Las Vegas Medical District Facilities Master Plan Executive Summary*, December, 2015. https://lasvegasmedicaldistrict.com/wp-content/uploads/2016/01/LVMD-Executive-Summary-Dec-2015.pdf.

Levi, Jeffrey, Laura M. Segal, Amanda Fuchs Miller, and Albert Lang. *A Healthier America 2013*. Trust for America's Health and Robert Wood Johnson, January 2013.

McKenzie, James F., Robert R. Pinger, and Denise M. Seabert. *An Introduction to Community & Public Health*. 9th ed. Burlington, MA: Jones & Bartlett Learning, 2018.

MetroHealth. *MetroHealth Annual Report 2016* (2016). http://mhannualreport.org/.

"Mixed-Use Development." *What Works for Health: Policies and Programs to Improve Wisconsin's Health*. Madison: The Board of Regents of the University of Wisconsin System, 2017. http://whatworksforhealth.wisc.edu/program.php?t1=109&t2=126&t3=45&id=298.

NSW Department of Health. *Healthy Urban Development Checklist: A Guide for Health Services When Commenting on Development Policies, Plans and Proposals*. North Sydney, NSW: Better Health Centre—Publications Warehouse, 2009.

Paine, Gregory, and Susan Thompson. *Healthy Built Environment Indicators*. City Wellbeing Program, CFRC, UNSW, Australia (2016).

Schneider, Eric C., Dana O. Sarnak, David Squires, and Arnav Shah. *Mirror, Mirror 2017: International Comparison Reflects Flaws and Opportunities for Better U.S.*

Health Care. The Commonwealth Fund, July 2017. www.commonwealthfund.org/interactives/2017/july/mirror-mirror/.

U.S. Centers for Disease Control and Prevention. *Community Health Assessment for Population Health Improvement: Resource of Most Frequently Recommended Health Outcomes and Determinants*. Atlanta, GA: Office of Surveillance, Epidemiology, and Laboratory Services, 2013. https://wwwn.cdc.gov/CommunityHealth/PDF/Final_CHAforPHI_508.pdf.

U.S. Department of Housing and Urban Development (HUD) and Healthy Homes. "Healthy Communities Assessment Tool (HCAT)." Adapted for use by San Diego, CA. http://hci-sandiego.sandag.org/indicators.

Walk Score. *Raw data*, 2017. https://www.walkscore.com/.

Chapter 8

Superhospitals
The Next Generation of Public Hospitals in Scandinavia

Klavs Hyttel

8.1 Introduction

This chapter will focus on a Scandinavian approach to achieving healing architecture. The recent building boom within the healthcare sector has demanded an evidence-based approach to designing hospitals that are not only state-of-the-art from a contemporary perspective but also robust in relation to future developments. The solution builds on humanistic and democratic values that are characteristic of Scandinavian design traditions, and especially embraces nature and daylight as primary therapeutic elements. With the intent of pioneering a new benchmark for a highly specialized health service, a framework is proposed to ensure healing and patient-centered design. This holistic approach is exemplified in a C.F. Møller–designed "superhospital".

8.2 Scandinavian Healthcare Design

8.2.1 Transforming the Healthcare Sector

In Denmark, hospitals were previously run by either counties or municipalities and offered the same services within the same geographic area. This put them in mutual competition in terms of attracting staff and being the best within the clinical fields. In 2007, counties were abolished in favor of five large regions, which now run the entire hospital service. The restructuring of the health sector aimed to create a more centralized, specialized, and efficient hospital service, as well as foster better conditions for the patients. These extensive structural changes were the catalyst for a major rebuilding of the hospital. Approved and co-financed by the government, the various proposals crafted by each region have resulted in the construction or rebuilding of 16 hospitals. The hospital buildings are a massive economic investment with a lot of political and public awareness, and through public hearings, the structural changes and building projects have been heavily debated with the citizens. The projects have all been offered through prequalification for an international architectural competition, and all constructions are now well underway, with an expected finish date within the year 2025 (Regeringens Ekspertpanel 2008). Because of this massive redistribution and expansion of health services, and in order to set the standard for the future of healthcare in Denmark, a new typology of hospital was deemed necessary. Superhospitals, defined here as an evolution of the traditional hospital, elevate the role of healthcare in modern Scandinavia. Cathedrals of the Nordic welfare societies, here all are on equal footing and receive the same service and treatment. Similarly, the public hospitals hereby become an image of the state's social capacity and priorities. Inherently large in scale due to the wide range of patients and treatments they need to provide for, the mixing of programs they offer, and the financial efficiencies required in state services, superhospitals act as a campus of uses. Recognizing the social capital they create, a superhospital provides value to its service area by offering a wider range of care beyond the immediate treatment of illness. A focus on wellness, disease prevention, research, and technology is common in a superhospital, along with the ability to adapt to the rapidly changing field of medicine. All of these aspects and more contributed to what the twenty-first-century hospital should give back to patients in Denmark for future growth.

Part of this inventory of care centers is six new superhospitals, which will each have a joint emergency department with the capability of supporting doctors from several specialties around the clock. These new centers will each cover an area of at least 200,000 citizens. With the theories behind evidence-based design, it has become evident that the buildings should not only provide a framework for medical treatment but also by virtue of themselves contribute to the healing process. To create what is known as healing architecture, the evidence-based approach is inevitable, and has been adopted not only by architects but also by the politicians, who have commissioned the buildings.

8.2.2 Established Requirements for Healing Architecture

According to published evidence within the field of healthcare design, there are multiple factors that contribute to a healing environment. Daylight, views of nature, private patient rooms, a flexible floorplan, better safety, noise reduction, legible wayfinding, lighting, comfortable and aesthetic furnishings, and so forth all contribute to user experience, many strategies of which are featured throughout this book. There is an obligation to embrace all of the relevant evidence, but it still leaves a certain artistic freedom in the implementation (Ulrich et al. 2004; Hamilton 2010; Kroll 2005).

In Denmark, strict laws have been formulated regarding the work environment, enshrining aspects of an architecture for health into written law. Specifically, regulation around access to daylight in workspaces demonstrates the articulation of social priorities in the built environment. The requirements that concern daylight and views, dictated by the Danish labor inspectorate, can be summarized as follows (Arbejdstilsynet 2007):

- There must be sufficient access to daylight in workrooms. Under certain circumstances, access to daylight may be indirect. Exemption may be given for work that does not allow daylight.
- From the workrooms, there must be a view of the outside environment. Under certain circumstances, this view may be indirect or to a large glass-covered area.

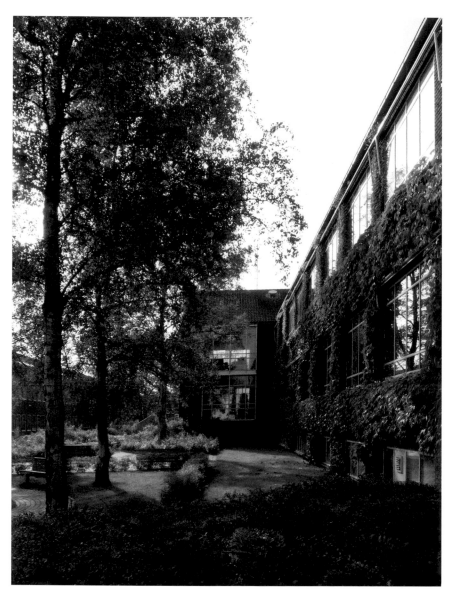

◀ Figure 8.1

Aarhus Kommunehospital.
Source: Julian Weyer

142

Klavs Hyttel

Securing the health, overall well-being, and safety for all personnel in both the physical and mental senses is part of the Danish heritage. This is particularly evident in the incorporation of multiple large window sections—windows are even provided in the most dense or subdivided sections of the hospital, such as operating theaters—and large work areas. These laws are secured in a symbiosis with the principles of healing architecture and are characteristic of healthcare projects in Denmark.

A previously completed C.F. Møller project of the Akershus University Hospital, Oslo, also helps set required standards for large-scale healthcare facilities. This hospital, designed and built from 2000 to 2008, has been awarded for its design, which eminently integrates humanistic principles while ensuring the highest level of clinical functionality. Serving as a benchmark project, the evidence-based approach it followed quickly became politically acknowledged in Scandinavia and is now required for all new hospital buildings (International Academy Award 2015 Report, by The Design & Health International Academy Awards, winner of International Health Project Over 40,000 m²). These standards lay the foundation for what any future superhospital should contain in terms of program, spatial relationships, finishes, technological adaptability, and more.

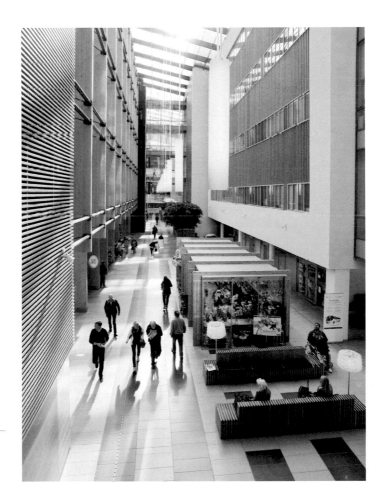

▶ Figure 8.2

Akershus University Hospital, Oslo. The glass-covered main street.
Source: Jørgen True

8.2.3 A Democratic Process

In the evidence-based process, all relevant information is gathered and used in the most effective way. This means combining theories, data, previous experience, and the expertise of technical and clinical professionals, thereby creating unique and adapted solutions on a solid knowledge base (Hamilton 2009).

In Scandinavia, there is a tendency toward flat and democratic organizational structures, which emphasize the importance of bottom-up influences. It is important that all employees are thriving and have a say about their workplace. In the case of designing healthcare buildings, a democratic approach calls for a comprehensive user involvement process. Employees from all organizational layers are involved from the initial conceptual phases and throughout the design phases. Representatives participate in work groups, facilitated by C.F. Møller's consultants, and their clinical insights about an ideal workplace influence the finalized project. Furthermore, the state has issued efficiency standards for logical and functional flows that further necessitate collaboration with clinicians to achieve performance goals. Representatives from patient associations also participate in work groups, to make sure all perspectives are incorporated in the design.

Besides securing a flow of relevant data and information to the project, user involvement ensures that the users take ownership of the project, thereby easing the transformation to a new physical and cultural work environment. This degree of user involvement is unique to the Scandinavian approach to design, thereby displaying humanistic and democratic values not only in the final design but also in the process.

8.2.4 Building for the Future

Until the twenty-first century, much of the hospital inventory of Denmark was scattered around the country, landing in smaller cities and random urban locales. Each hospital was composed of several autonomous buildings as a result of a rapid increase in building stock without overall master planning, making the layouts intricate and the wayfinding cryptic. In contrast, the new hospital stock is being gathered in large urban centers with a defined structural layout that optimizes functionality for easier, more intuitive wayfinding. Whereas the old hospitals were centered on the building mass, the new hospitals center around the landscape, allowing for a wealth of daylight, views, and access to nature. Another important lesson learned over years of hospital operations is that hospitals get outdated quicker than other types of buildings due to the rapid nature of technology and research developments. Consequently, new hospitals are being designed to accommodate these expected future changes. Building hospitals that can maintain their timeliness requires a flexible design, where rooms and sections can be diminished, enlarged, or otherwise transformed within the existing framework. Furthermore, the anticipated future technological solutions have been taken into account, so that they can be easily implemented when applicable. This adaptability extends to the whole building complex, where future extensions have been accounted for from the beginning (Heslet 2007).

8.2.5 Aarhus University Hospital

At approximately 400,000 m², which includes an existing C.F. Møller design from the 1980s of 150,000 m², the Aarhus University Hospital is proposed as the largest Danish hospital to date. Construction in its entirety is expected to be completed in 2019, making this the first superhospital in the country. The massive scale sets high demands on the design, where the resemblance between the hospital complex and a small city really becomes clear.

▶ Figure 8.3

Aarhus University Hospital, nearing completion.
Source: Projektafdelingen DNU

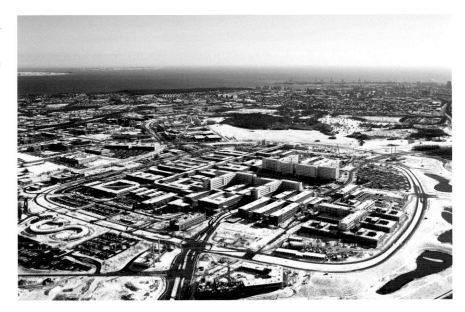

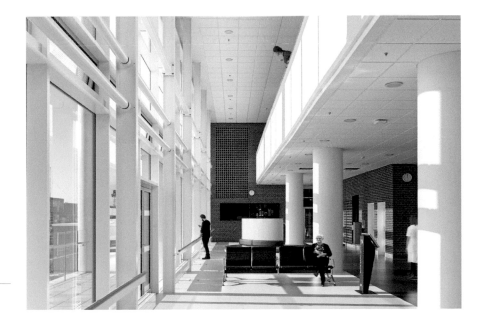

▶ Figure 8.4

View of a gallery.
Source: Thomas Mølvig

8.3 Implementing Healing Design Principles

8.3.1 Urban Layouts as a Means of Organization

As a publicly funded resource for the surrounding community, superhospitals become more accessible through mirroring their urban contexts. By creating neighborhoods, each with a unique visual identity, the large structure is scaled down and broken into recognizable parts, which makes it navigable and comprehensible. This urban approach guides circulation and creates a logic infrastructure. The facility is furthermore well connected to the larger urban context, and by placing activities that attract healthy citizens, such as health talks, self-check workshops, and children's learning facilities, the facility is able to provide care in ways not restricted to the treatment of illness. Public programs and a centralized location position the superhospital as an approachable activity hub for promoting health.

Much like the network of parks that take on an elevated role because of their contrast to the cityscape in urban centers, landscape is an important part of the overall structure in superhospitals. By varying the landscape across different zones, it can become another element to aid in wayfinding. The outdoor season is short in Nordic countries, but can be extended by providing shelter from the wind and rain. By blurring the border between the inside and outside, it is possible to maintain physical and visual contact with nature during the winter months. Views of the surroundings are accommodated in every patient room by large window sections, which also allow for maximum ingress of daylight. The healing powers of landscape and daylight are reckoned as one of the most important features in superhospitals, combined with the layout and a legible wayfinding strategy. These design aspects create a soothing and friendly environment that focuses on the patients' well-being.

8.3.2 Functional Zoning of Blocks

The complex is structured in blocks, each of which has been assigned a color that is repeated on the exterior as well as in the interior for easy visual navigation. The blocks are connected by a thoroughfare containing larger squares that branch out into byroads and enclosed courtyards. In the heart of the complex is a large park, and surrounding the entire facility is an outer ring road, allowing for direct access to the blocks regardless of where you have arrived. Upon arrival, visitors are met with large galleries at ground level that connect the inside with the outside and bring daylight to the work spaces placed internally. Each courtyard and park area at the Aarhus University Hospital is landscaped with its own theme and plant palette, and thus becomes a recognizable landmark. The landscape is made easily accessible and visible from all parts of the facility, and offers patients, relatives, and staff respite in a calm and soothing environment. Diverse landscapes will develop over time, and once established, will only further strengthen views and navigation throughout the facility.

Klavs Hyttel

▶ Figure 8.5

View of an arcade.
Source: Tonny Foghmar

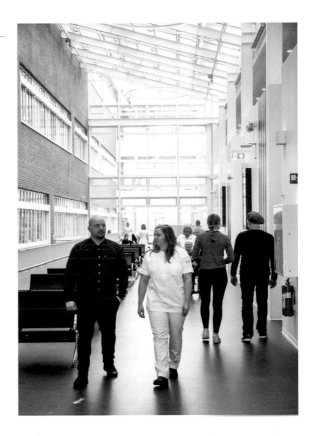

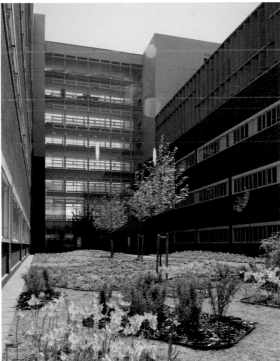

▶ Figure 8.6

View of a courtyard.
Source: Schønherr

Vertically the hospital is structured in functional layers:

Level 1: Wardrobes, archives, mechanical, and university facilities. Admittance for staff only.
Level 2: (Ground level) Arrival area and outpatient clinics.
Level 3: Surgery, intensive care, and diagnostic imaging.
Level 4: Mechanical logistics, clinical support functions, and canteens. Admittance for staff only.
Levels 5–8: Patient wards and office space.

This structure ensures an elasticity at each level, opening up the opportunity to easily extend or shorten sections within the building frame, and allows for the future possibility of expanding functions between levels with minor construction efforts. Future extensions are possible both vertically and horizontally (as shown by the dotted buildings in Figure 8.7). By establishing identical rooms that can be used by many different medical specialties, a cross-sectional elasticity is ensured. This is especially evident in the office facilities, which are shared across professional and specialist fields, outpatient clinics, and operating theaters. Standardization across functions and staff groups is reflective of the democratic and flat organization structures in Scandinavia.

Each ward consists of 24 single patient rooms, divided into three equally large units that emerge from a central square. An arrival point and natural gathering place for patients and staff, the central squares provide views of all three units. Furthermore, this structure secures short distances for minimized traffic. Other amenities include private bathrooms, noise-reducing ceiling tiles, varied lighting, accommodation for one relative per patient room, and a homelike environment through choice of materials and residential furnishings.

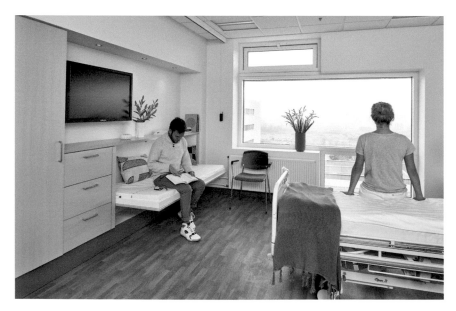

◀ Figure 8.7

The patient room.
Source: Kirstine Mengel

These aspects give the patients empowerment and a sense of control, in that they can find their way around the complex, be private, take part in the community, seek nature and other positive distractions, or be with relatives. Not only does this reduce stress and increase well-being, but also the empowerment allows the staff to spend their time on the actual care. The caregiving is furthermore supported by efficient workflows and the creation of a work environment that focuses on safety and comfort.

8.3.3 Healing Wayfinding

Large hospital facilities are complicated to navigate, requiring staff to use a certain amount of time showing people around—time that is better used on patient care. To lose orientation is stressful and can cause frustration and a feeling of helplessness. Therefore, it is not enough to focus on good signage for wayfinding. Wayfinding must instead be the result of an overall system that incorporates multiple factors (Ulrich et al. 2004). Large-scale hospital projects, inherently difficult to relate to because of their size, can improve patient, staff, and visitor experience by following a two-step plan for wayfinding. Step 1 focused on the programming and organizational planning of a building. Step 2 introduces added features, typically scalable, soft infrastructure, like artwork, furnishings, and signage to help contribute to a section's overall identity. The strategies that fall under each step are presented here as a starting point for implementation on projects of any size.

Step 1

- Compose a logical and intuitive structural layout—the organizational layout should follow a simple pattern that is easy to comprehend and easy to extend without breaking the pattern.
- Place the main circulation flows both inside and outside in connection with the main entrances.
- Secure daylight and views from all parts of the building—to be able to orientate in relation to the surrounding environment helps navigation.

Step 2

- Create different themes in the surrounding landscape and courtyards to establish identifying features and recognizable waypoints.
- Create an art strategy that divides the hospital in different themes—art will serve as orientation marks and can be used as such both inside and outside.
- Divide the hospital into color themes—the themes can be continuous from the exterior to the interior.
- Develop a signage strategy that covers the inside and outside. The signage should be logical, simple, systematic, legible, and flexible—for example, by using numbers instead of department names.
- Design different pavements that lead from the parking area to the entrances.
- Prepare for organizational wayfinding initiatives, such as volunteer guides and interactive information screens with directions.

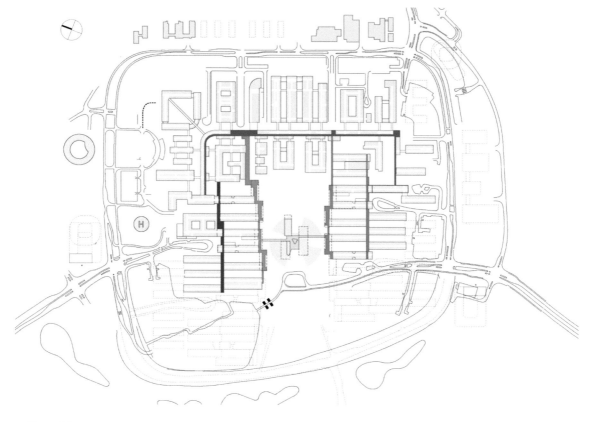

▲ Figure 8.8

The main circulation flows each have their own visual theme.
Source: C.F. Møller Architects

Wayfinding that considers these two steps at the onset of a project can avoid complicated navigation that only further alienates patients and staff from their surroundings. It is in this sense that wayfinding can be considered healing, or a necessary part of any healing environment.

8.4 Conclusions

The healthcare sector in Scandinavia is undergoing a transformation toward centralized and optimized patient care, which requires the hospital mass to meet a new standard of functionality. With this great investment comes a great opportunity, as well as a great responsibility, to create a new generation of superhospitals vetted through and designed with an evidence-based approach. Other countries outside of Scandinavia, whether currently providing healthcare through the government or just aiming to make services more efficient, can learn from the democratic principles and features of realizing the superhospital. They can insert their own goals, values, and contexts for more tailored approaches across cultures.

Today it is not a question of either-or in the Scandinavian approach to healthcare design, but rather a holistic vision where all voices are heard. Attention to scale, organization, healing principles, and wayfinding forms part of a mutualism, each enhancing the other's effect, thereby increasing the overall effectiveness of a hospital. Humanistic and democratic values permeate the hospital projects in process and therefore product, and create healthcare buildings that promote the healing of patients, staff, and visitors alike. The healing principles build upon the humanist tradition, a natural progression for healthcare buildings in Scandinavia. It is this humanistic vision that not only ensures the continued functionality of a country-wide healthcare system but also guides all future growth to stay on course for improved health outcomes.

Bibliography

Arbejdstilsynet. "At-vejledning." In *Grænseværdier for stoffer og materialer.* Danish Working Environment Authority. Copenhagen, Denmark 2007.

Aslaksen, R., B. Brismar, H. Kirk, K. Møller Pedersen, and E. Juhl. "Regionernes Investerings-Og Sygehusplaner: Screening Og Vurdering." In *Afgivet af regeringens ekspertpanel november, København, Ministeriet for Sundhed og Forebyggelse, København.* Denmark: Ministry of the Interior and Health, 2008.

Hamilton, D. Kirk, and Mardelle McCuskey Shepley. *Design for Critical Care: An Evidence-Based Approach.* New York: Routledge, 2010.

Hamilton, D. Kirk, and David H. Watkins. *Evidence-Based Design for Multiple Building Types.* Hoboken, NJ: John Wiley & Sons, 2009.

Heslet, Lars, and Kim Dirckinck-Holmfeld. "Sansernes Hospital." *Bibliotek for Læger,* 280–309. Copenhagen: Saxo, 2007.

Kroll, Karen. "Evidence-Based Design in Healthcare Facilities." *Building Operating Management,* Trade Press, 2005.

Ulrich, Roger, Craig Zimring, Anjali Joseph, and Ruchi Choudhary. *The Role of the Physical Environment in the Hospital of the 21st Century: A Once-in-a-Lifetime Opportunity.* Concord, CA: The Center for Health Design, 2004.

Chapter 9

A Rebirth of the Consolidated Health Campus
The New Parkland Hospital

Matthew Suarez and James J. Atkinson

9.1 Introduction

The embattled frontier of the American hospital has experienced a tumultuous evolution in recent decades. Rapid changes in the healthcare landscape have created an unstable environment for health organizations and the facilities they inhabit. The resulting effect has been nothing short of an explosion, scattering service lines traditionally found in the hospital broadly across the urban landscape and the communities they serve. Large regional hospitals of the past have been deconstructed and redistributed as multiple small, local, specialized facilities. Though much has contributed to the decentralization of hospital-based programs, the main drivers are cost containment, new forms of payment, technological developments, consumer preferences, and national health reform efforts (Shortell, Gillies, and Devers 1995).

The innumerable problems of large hospitals of the past proved an important catalyst toward decentralization efforts. Given the complications that oversized hospitals have in coordinating large numbers of patients, staff, materials, supplies, and technologies, the care continuum was frequently overshadowed by organizational needs, resulting in diminished patient experiences. Additionally, the growth of these facilities over many decades created wayfinding challenges and excessive walking distances between care destinations. The choreography of several thousand employees across large campuses created logistical nightmares.

Large-scale "safety-net" hospitals are the most challenged. An estimated 1,300 hospitals nationwide accept protected patient populations (the uninsured or underinsured) that lack mobility and choice (Legnini et al. 1999). While these patients have been a mainstay of urban hospitals for years, the Affordable Care Act (ACA) has allowed underprivileged people to experience choice for the first time (Sommers et al. 2015). As protected patient populations become more empowered regarding their care choices, larger facilities have suffered.

Street view of New Parkland
Hospital.
Source: Dan Schwalm/HDR

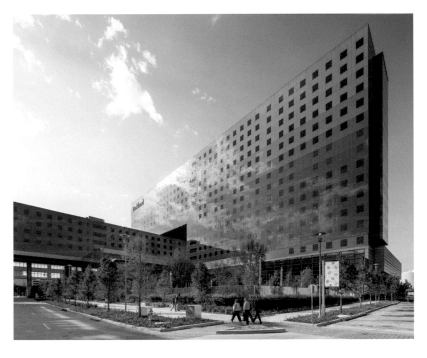

Exterior view of NPH.
Source: Dan Schwalm/HDR

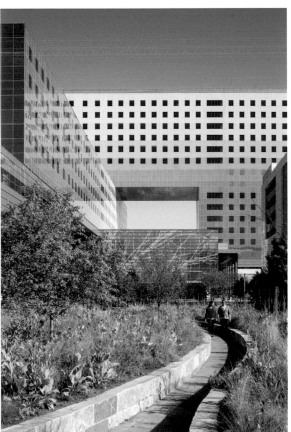

Safety-net hospitals are additionally burdened by untenable reimbursement policies that emphasize efficiency over quality (Institute of Medicine [US] 2002). Looking to avoid these regulatory demands, many physicians have sought new venues in the outpatient setting. The shift of physicians to multiple, distributed locations has further reduced aggregate procedure volumes in large hospitals (Grube, Kaufman, and York 2013). In response to these pressures, large health systems have resorted to a decentralized community care model in which services are distributed into the community across multiple locations.

As the "decentralized" paradigm ages, unforeseen problems have raised inquiry into the reliability of dispersed community care. In modern population health-based systems, the unraveling of this care model has already begun. The allure of the decentralized care model has slowly eroded, as evidenced by rising staffing complexities, inconvenient access to services, and social inequalities (Franz et al. 2019).

To curtail these issues, health systems are shifting back to large-scale replacement hospital projects. Healthcare systems are consolidating services on health campuses to support a high level of integrated care delivery unmatched in dispersed care settings. The concept of the hospital as a "one-stop shop" is the new mission of many health systems attempting to re-engage the community. This became the rationale for the New Parkland Hospital (NPH).

9.2 A Vision for a Patient- and Family-Centered, Consolidated Health Campus

Population growth in Parkland's home, Dallas County, Texas, has given rise to social inequalities and healthcare disparities in the area's major urban center. When compared to the 2017 national average of 8.8%, a considerably higher 27.3% of Dallas residents did not have health insurance at any point during the year. During this same year, 21.8% of the people living in the Dallas area lived in poverty, significantly above the national average of 12.3% (Fontenot et al. 2018). For this disadvantaged population, the dispersion of services across multiple locations has resulted in difficulties accessing these services, particularly for those who lack reliable transportation.

Service line chiefs have also experienced adverse results as they have been saddled with new and unforeseen staffing irregularities. By moving specialties to a split service line model between the hospital and outpatient settings, an increased need for full-time employees across multiple locations increased. This issue challenged an already overburdened regional workforce that often suffers from health provider shortages.

Given these forces, three key driving questions became central to Parkland:

1. Can a hospital maintain the traditional form of a "mega-hospital" but adapt its programs to encompass the amenities of smaller, integrated community facilities?
2. Can a hospital be accessible and provide affordable care while also supporting the demands of a massive medical teaching facility?

3. Can a hospital maximize its outreach to the larger population but still deliver a quality care experience to individual patients?

Many points of alignment exist between a health system's desire to return to a consolidated model of care and to shift away from primarily decentralized care models. It became increasingly important during the planning process for NPH to tackle the stigmas associated with large, aging hospitals: they disproportionately focus too much on the needs of the institution rather than the patient experience.

9.3 Aligning the Client Vision With Health Improvement Goals

Today, comprehensive care initiatives must be holistic, including both medical and nonmedical health programs. The Institute for Health Improvement (IHI) highlights three common goals dubbed the "triple aim": (1) improve the individual experience of care, (2) improve the health of populations, and (3) reduce per capita costs of care for populations (Berwick, Nolan, and Whittington 2008). The design team used these key principles to establish a framework to guide decisions for the new mega-hospital, ensuring that results were patient-centered and convenient for the community serviced.

Prior to commencing the programming and planning process, the design team engaged hospital leadership to establish the project vision. Intended to be free of normal restrictions, such as budget, facilities, and staffing, visioning sessions explored the core objectives of the project, identified critical client expectations, and established a design vision statement. As shown in Table 9.1, the design team used the framework of the "triple aim" objectives to guide client expectations.

9.4 The Immersive Planning Process

The overarching theme for a hospital master plan should grow from addressing core requisites of exceptional care delivery from the perspectives of patients, employees, and the public. At Parkland, three "Communities" were formed to help the design team gain insight into the unique needs of each group. The "Communities" provided a forum and vehicle to test new ideas, seek innovative ways of delivering care, and explore best practices. The Patient, Staff, and Public Communities had ample opportunities to participate in a variety of activities. Each group was given a similar starting point—start with the smallest unit—the bedside—and work outward. This approach led to organizational ideas that addressed transportation, navigation of the site and facilities, the patient and family experience, and affordable care delivery. Feedback from the Communities ultimately helped the designers align design goals with the perspectives of these vital stakeholders.

Table 9.1 Client expectations and design goals aligned with Triple Aim objectives

Triple Aim Objectives	Client Expectations	Provide Easy Access to the Hospital	Create Intuitive Wayfinding and a Pleasant Arrival Sequence	Consolidate Service Lines on One Campus	Streamline the Patient-Centered Care Delivery Process	Separate Traffic Flows	Promote Therapeutic Experiences	Increase Patient Empowerment and Family Involvement in Care	Accommodate Change Over the Lifespan of the Hospital
Improve the individual experience of care	Create a "Hospital in the park"		●				●	●	
	Promote a strong campus identity	●	●	●			●		
	Clear hierarchy of pathways and inter-campus connections	●	●	●	●	●	●		
	Provide on-stage/off-stage circulation throughout the campus		●		●	●	●		●
Improving the health of populations	Design park-like outdoor spaces		●				●	●	
	Embrace the multi-cultural aspect of the Dallas community				●			●	
	Create an acute care hub with direct access to the Medical District	●	●	●	●			●	
	Provide places for community outreach initiatives				●		●	●	●
Reducing per capita costs of care for populations	Provide flexibility and adaptability for future changes in healthcare delivery								●
	Co-locate similar services for cross-training and sharing of staff	●	●	●	●				
	Design separate building structures to decrease first cost		●		●				●

9.4.1 Capturing the Patient Perspective

Patients who experience the full breadth of care services typically offer the best insight. To harness their perspective, a Patient and Family Advisory Council (PFAC) was established consisting of frequent Parkland guests. The PFAC helped the team focus design energy on the areas that most influence patient experience and wellness. Engagement with the design team occurred at strategic intervals throughout programming, planning, and schematic design phases. This ensured that feedback was applied to operational planning at pivotal moments in the decision-making process.

9.4.2 Capturing the Staff Perspective

Staff perspective is the most comprehensive, covering the full gamut of operations, from materials management to patient care. To solicit these viewpoints, a nurse liaison team was formed to study a patient-centered care delivery process. This team was also instrumental in studying culture and change-management and removing operational bottlenecks. Parkland staff also studied different patient care scenarios with HDR's design team through schematic visioning sessions. Each group was given a scenario to explore patient experiences. Various empathetic scenarios were studied across different clinical areas and different user groups. For example, a patient in the emergency room, a physician in an exam room, and a family member with a child in the Neonatal Intensive Care Unit (NICU) were examined. The groups studied humanistic considerations in relation to functional requirements. Once input was integrated from all groups into the final design of patient care spaces (e.g., patient rooms, operating rooms, and exam rooms), nursing staff practiced medical codes and procedures in physical mock-up rooms to confirm the functionality of the design. This process reassured Parkland nurses and clinical staff that the design team satisfied patient care needs.

9.4.3 Capturing the Public Perspective

For many publicly funded hospital projects, taxpayers represent the larger community and provide the main source of funding. Aligning a project's design initiatives with the surrounding community's priorities must be a top concern. At the time of its inception, the Parkland project was the largest publicly funded construction project in the U.S. It was essential to engage the neighboring residents, build consensus, and encourage a sense of ownership over the process and results. This Community group helped the design team focus on a human-centered approach to the patient experience. Community members collaborated with nurse liaison teams, attended town hall meetings, and participated in mock-up room reviews and walking distance studies.

9.5 The New Parkland Hospital Master Plan and Program

Parkland serves as the public hospital for Dallas County (population 2.4 million). It operates a system of 11 community-oriented primary care clinics, is a Level I Trauma Center, and has the only burn unit in North Texas. Parkland also operates the area's only Level III Neonatal Intensive Care Unit (NICU).

Like many great institutions, the Parkland Health System is seen as the foundation for health leadership in its community. As suggested by the IHI Triple Aim objectives, community-based programs are to be the new cornerstone of the modern hospital's mission. Thus, Parkland set out to become a civic anchor for the community alongside three cornerstone institutions that create the medical district:

UT Southwestern (UTSW) Medical Center, a premier academic medical center; the Children's Medical Center, a leading institution for comprehensive care; and Parkland Hospital, a world-renowned teaching hospital. The master plan demonstrates the intent of creating connections across institutions in the medical district, the surrounding urban context, the community, and the new light rail transit system. The master plan aimed to stimulate a thriving medical or wellness district.

The Parkland program was designed to move patients and their families beyond individual site-specific care and consolidate multiple care destinations and community amenities on one site. A "health campus" concept served as the backdrop to merge three state-of-the-art medical services at Parkland: Adult Inpatient Medical Care, Women's and Infants' Care, and Outpatient Clinical Care. Each of these centers is duly represented in the program requirements

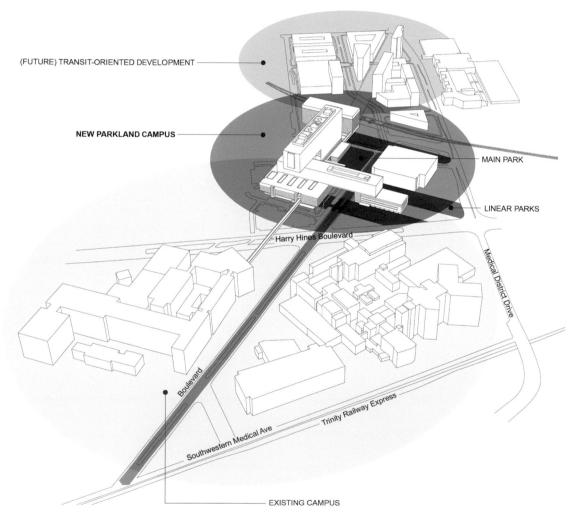

▲ Figure 9.3

Creating a new medical district.
Source: Joshua Domingo/HDR

Matthew Suarez and James J. Atkinson

and the final expression of building form. The following is an overview of the centers and key programs:

- Adult Inpatient Medical Care Center—1,342,000 square feet

  - 579 private adult beds shared across six specialties (Medical, Surgical, Neurology, Orthopedics, Burn, and Psychiatry)
  - Emergency Department—140 exam, 10 trauma, and 4 resuscitation rooms
  - Diagnostic and Treatment—27 operating rooms

- Women's and Infants' Care Center—560,000 square feet

  - 48 Labor Delivery Recovery beds
  - 96 Neonatal Intensive Care Unit (NICU) beds
  - 216 Post-Partum/Ante-Partum beds
  - 64 Gynecological beds

- Outpatient Clinical Care Center—387,000 square feet

  - 650 clinic exam rooms

- Shared services across the three centers

  - Administrative areas of 269,000 square feet
  - Healthcare retail areas (pharmacy and gift shop)
  - Nonmedical public areas (museum, dining, community wellness park, and chapel)
  - Parking for 1,800 staff and 2,000 patients/visitors
  - Logistics building—123,000 square feet
  - Central utility plant

9.6 Design Goals and Strategies

In this section, eight key design goals for the New Parkland Hospital are presented followed by design strategies aimed at achieving these goals. These goals align with the IHI Triple Aim objectives and client expectations as shown in Table 9.1.

9.6.1 Provide Easy Access to the Hospital

Guests arrive at the hospital through a variety of transportation methods other than private cars, so easy access to the hospital was essential. It was necessary to create a hospital that could accommodate all forms of transportation in a single location, including the existing elevated light rail stop incorporated on the new hospital site. This approach helped the project team imagine the hospital and surrounding grounds as a community center for people from many different socioeconomic backgrounds and geographic locations.

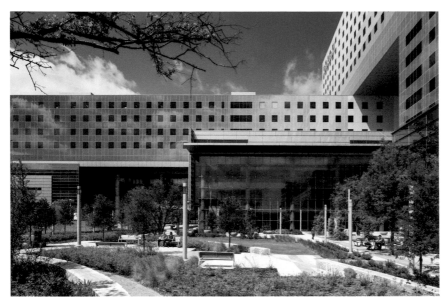

To facilitate access, the design team used an "onstage offstage" concept, commonly used in hospital interiors, to assist with transportation management. Parking structures were positioned to welcome guests from different directions. Patients and visitors access parking from the interior of the site while staff access parking from the perimeter—essentially keeping out cars that do not need to be in the interior of the campus. Additionally, ambulances have dedicated access to the emergency department, and service vehicles are relegated to the back-of-house, effectively leaving public circulation free of congestion and creating a stress-free first impression.

As with any urban hospital, finding a "backyard" can be difficult. Every face of the hospital is on display and may be used for pedestrian and vehicular access. Removing logistic support from the main hospital and connecting through a basement tunnel promotes a friendlier face to the community and creates opportunities for a more inviting multimodal arrival experience. This approach had two primary benefits: it eliminated service traffic at public points of entry and it obscured the less attractive everyday operations.

Another concept developed early in the master plan was the idea of putting the "park" back in Parkland. At the center of the new campus is a "wellness park", a two-acre garden space accessible from the hospital. Within the new park is a meditation area opening directly into the hospital chapel. The combination of this relationship to public transportation and linear parks established a robust navigational framework for the overall master plan (Moore 2012).

9.6.2 Create Intuitive Wayfinding and a Pleasant Arrival Sequence

In order to create a mega-hospital that is responsive to the complete patient experience, it is important to break down the scale of the buildings so they feel inviting and user-friendly. This can be accomplished through intuitive wayfinding

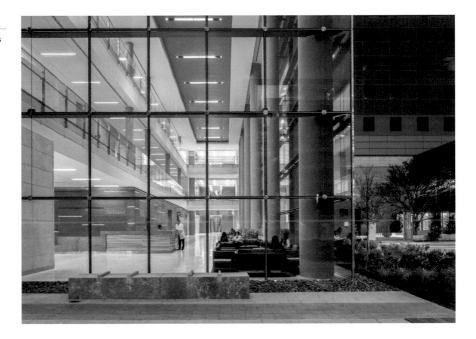

cues that encourage movement and accessibility. By pushing public spaces and circulation to the edges of the buildings, exterior points of reference were used to establish a pleasant arrival sequence. Whether visitors use the park, the garage, or the Dallas Skyline, each of these is visible from all public spaces and act as a continuous orientation device to inform circulation.

Furthering the concept of a pleasant arrival sequence, all public elevators were placed on axis with the main lobby. Aided by simple geometries of the overall building design, each care portal is visually separate but equally accessible from the multistory main entry lobby. This space was condensed and then vaulted to create a sense of spatial hierarchy that helps activate the entry and encourage movement to each care destination. Programs like the park, the cafeteria, and the chapel are accessed via the main onstage concourse, whereas connections to the medical office buildings and the old hospital were raised a level to separate through-traffic from the mass transit station and other buildings. These simple moves created a clear hierarchy of staff, care pathways, and inter-campus connections that help with self-directed navigation in an otherwise complex mega-hospital landscape.

9.6.3 Consolidate Service Lines on One Campus

Hospitals like Parkland that were originally built at the heart of population centers are repeatedly challenged by urban development pressures and land restrictions. Urban hospitals considering a "one-stop shop" model are weighing the trade-offs and feasibility of building a single large building versus multiple specialized care centers on one campus.

For the new hospital, the project team approached the urban challenge in three significant ways: create a health hub with available land adjacent to the

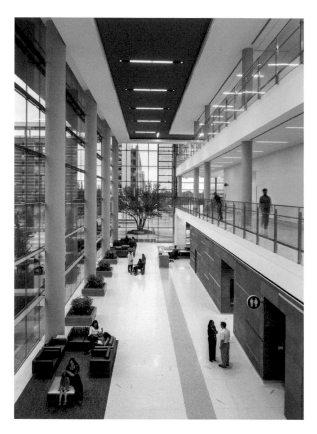

Hospital atrium.
Source: Dan Schwalm/HDR

medical district, accommodate the three centers of care on one site for accessibility, and place ambulatory care centers at the periphery of the building massing so they can be built at lower construction costs. To facilitate access between centers, main circulation pathways were added to connect the centers with the existing campus. In so doing, service line connections between inpatient and outpatient specialties have alleviated many staffing redundancies through combined care platforms. Also, by separating the outpatient care center from the main hospital via a connector, the clinic could be built to a lower building code, thus reducing first costs and promoting budget consciousness.

9.6.4 Streamline the Patient-Centered Care Delivery Process

Creating a health campus has two significant benefits: convenient access to many different service lines for high-risk patients and a reduction in staffing inefficiencies that occur when staff cover multiple sites. To improve the effective delivery of care services, complementary service lines were strategically co-located. For example, Labor/Delivery and Surgery were programmed on the same level to form the footprint of the diagnostic and treatment base and to allow for the co-location of procedural services to share code team staff for high-risk patients. In addition, a vertical relationship was established between the emergency department on the ground level and Imaging, located directly above, to facilitate easy access.

To help streamline the care process at the department level, standardized care spaces were created so physicians and nurses could benefit from spatial familiarity. Research suggests that if care zones are easily accessible, care providers can respond more effectively to stressful patient care needs and complete standard tasks faster and with fewer errors (Chaudhury, Chaudhury, and Mahmood 2007). Therefore, the design team organized the program into strategic groupings based on the frequency of nurse access during a typical shift. Patient units were sized to ensure that staff would not have to walk further than five patient rooms for frequently accessed support spaces, such as care team-work areas, medication areas, nourishment, clean utility, and soiled utility rooms. Additionally, staff would not have to walk by more than nine patient rooms to get to less frequently accessed spaces, such as team workrooms, the business center, and personal lockers. These approaches, along with decentralizing care team stations to the bedside, resulted in increased bedside care time.

9.6.5 Separate Traffic Flows

In a consolidated health campus model, the massive scale can often overshadow the patient experience. To counteract this pitfall, the flows of different user groups should be separate and streamlined with definitive arrival and discharge points. In addition, staff and materials should be sequestered in offstage areas to eliminate patient exposure. To separate traffic flow, a series of front-of-house and back-of-house interventions was planned across multiple departments. This distinction prevents high volumes of visitors and public from inadvertently accessing inpatient spaces and reduces adverse traffic flows, which can impede stretcher mobility and diminish patient privacy.

To provide a calming environment for inpatient care, eight elevators were dedicated in the transportation core to separate vertical movements of staff

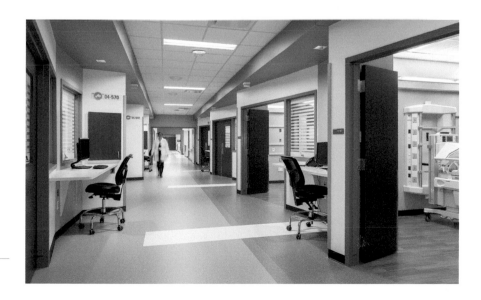

► Figure 9.7

Nursing unit.
Source: Dan Schwalm/HDR

and patients, clean material, and waste removal. To maintain a quiet patient environment, supplies and patients do not move horizontally between units. Instead, horizontal movement was relegated to the lower diagnostic and treatment podium. In offstage areas of patient care departments, patients are moved by staff utilizing restricted patient transport elevators, which helps to maintain dignity and patient privacy. Supplies travel horizontally at the basement level from cart staging points, and then vertically in strategically located supply elevator cores. Once the supplies reach their intended floor, they are distributed offstage to storage spaces. This eliminates the visibility of logistics from the patient's point of view.

9.6.6 Promote Therapeutic Experiences

Creating a therapeutic environment that merges a patient's emotional needs with the practical needs of a hospital is about addressing the holistic care of the patient, as well as acknowledging the impact that the built environment can have on clinical outcomes and staff effectiveness. At a time when patients are unsure of their health outlook and are separated from their normal social relationships, visiting the hospital can be a particularly stressful experience (Smith and Watkins 2016). At Parkland, attention was paid to creating environments that promote healing and reduce stress.

From the patient's experience, waiting and care spaces were strategically located at the perimeter of the building to take advantage of daylight and views of the park and city skyline. Finishes promoted personalization and order so patients can feel ownership over their care spaces, and artwork was selectively located to create positive distractions. Additionally, patient units were designed to reduce cart traffic and alarms and increase staff bedside time.

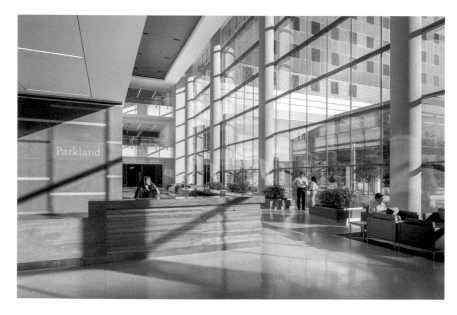

◀ Figure 9.8

Waiting areas.
Source: Dan Schwalm/HDR

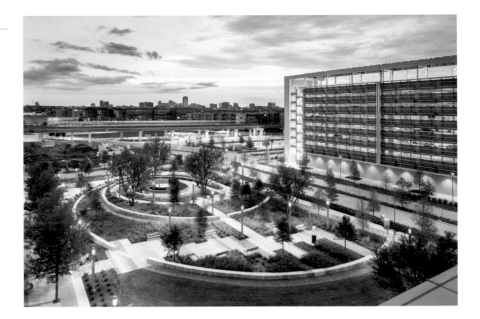

For the staff, mental fatigue was addressed through a variety of staff amenity spaces and noise reduction strategies. Special attention was paid to lowering staff stress and raising employee retention rates by providing staff lounges and administrative workrooms with exterior views to gardens, parks, and the city. Respite spaces are provided in each department, and parks and gardens are readily available.

9.6.7 Increase Patient Empowerment and Family Involvement in Care

In a patient- and family-centered environment, institutional resources and personnel are organized around the patient rather than around clinical departments. Whenever possible, care is brought to the patient rather than moving the patient to receive care. Patient- and family-centered care considers patients' cultural traditions, personal preferences and values, family situations, and lifestyles. Responsibility for aspects of self-care and monitoring is put in the patient's and family's hands (Institute for Healthcare Improvement 2019).

In an environment where semiprivate rooms are the norm, patient incompatibility issues are unavoidable. These issues lead to transfers and rework as well as dissatisfied patients, families, and caregivers. The move to private rooms has eliminated these inconveniences, contributed to the reduction in hospital-acquired infections, improved staff, patient, and family satisfaction, and resulted in fewer medical errors. Private patient rooms are designed to include space for a family member to spend the night and include a desk and Internet access. Providing dedicated family space encourages participation in care and often leads to better patient outcomes. Other amenities that encourage patient empowerment include a large-screen television, room temperature control, different lighting settings, outside views, and secure storage.

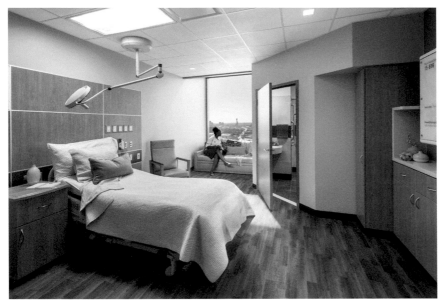

Patient room.
Source: Dan Schwalm/HDR

9.6.8 Accommodate Change Over the Life Span of the Hospital

Patient needs, healthcare delivery methods, treatment modalities, and technologies frequently change over time, requiring buildings, building systems, and infrastructure to respond to these changing factors. A new hospital's ability to efficiently accommodate these inevitable changes contributes to the hospital's overall operational and financial well-being. To accommodate unforeseen changes over time, Parkland was designed to be flexible. This was accomplished through internal conversion–ready spaces and strategic expansion plans. Internal conversion required preplanning "soft" spaces in areas of planned expansion. Expansion required consideration during the planning phase for building systems and components to be right-sized for simple horizontal additions. This includes structural, mechanical, electrical, and IT systems along with circulation components, such as corridors, elevators, and stairs.

To be flexible, the major structural grid was standardized to modular units of 30' x 30'. This grid size has proven to be highly flexible when reconfiguring clinical departments. The immovable vertical elements, such as HVAC chases, stairs, and major structural elements, were located at or near the building perimeters or in designated zones within the building; this leaves most of the floor plate free of obstacles, allowing it to be easily adapted over time. To complement the interchangeable chassis, a designated flex space was planned on each inpatient unit. These flex areas vary based on specialty, from rehab gyms and procedure spaces to newborn nurseries, allowing the units to be redesigned without major renovations. The patient rooms were designed to adapt easily to higher acuities with light rework. The IT and electrical infrastructure backbones were amply sized to support future devices and the growing dependence on wireless and mesh networks.

9.7 Conclusions

Paradoxically, the focus on population health has led to a deconstruction of the modern hospital to make way for a decentralized, community care approach to healthcare delivery. However, many problems have emerged, such as staffing complexities, compromised access, and social inequalities. Squaring the impact that population health has on current approaches to healthcare has led many health systems to reconsider the merits of the decentralized model. This has spurred a rebirth of the consolidated health campus.

The main objective of the Parkland Hospital design was to co-locate services on a site while simultaneously de-emphasizing the institutional image of the healthcare facility by increasing regional and community elements. These strategies were designed to reduce spatial disorientation, improve the patient experience, and enhance the care of the whole person. Furthermore, incorporating strong planning and design strategies can help health systems create a hospital that merges community needs with the practical needs of a hospital.

The viability of the consolidated health campus begins and ends with addressing the needs of the community. When a replacement hospital project begins, architects are uniquely positioned to build a bridge of communication between the healthcare system and the population it serves. By engaging local residents early in the design process, patients were given equal footing in establishing design interventions in the continuum of care. The inclusion of community-based amenities makes the public feel invested in the hospital that serves them, and finally, for the sake of the hospital, it creates a facility that exists for the community and not for itself.

Bibliography

Berchick, Edward R., Emily Hood, and Jessica C. Barnett. "Health Insurance Coverage in the United States: 2017." In *Current Population Reports. U.S. Department of Commerce Economics and Statistics Administration*, 60–264. Washington, DC: U.S. Census Bureau, 2018. www.census.gov/library/publications/2018/demo/p60-264.html.

Berwick, Donald M., Thomas W. Nolan, and John Whittington. "The Triple Aim: Care, Health, and Cost." *Health Affairs* 27, no. 3 (2008): 759–769.

Bureau of Labor Statistics. "Occupational Outlook Handbook." *United States Department of Labor*, 2018. www.bls.gov/oco/.

Chaudhury, Habib and Atiya Mahmood. *The Effect of Environmental Design on Reducing Nursing and Medication Errors in Acute Care Settings*. Concord, CA: The Center for Health Design, 2007.

Fontenot, Kayla, Jessica Semega, and Melissa Kollar. *Income and Poverty in the United States: 2017*. Washington, DC: US Government Printing Office, 2018.

Franz, Berkeley, Daniel Skinner, Jonathan Wynn, and Kelly Kelleher. "Urban Hospitals as Anchor Institutions: Frameworks for Medical Sociology." *Socius* 5 (2019): 2378023118817981.

Grube, Mark, Kenneth Kaufman, and Robert York. "Decline in Utilization Rates Signals a Change in the Inpatient Business Model." *Health Affairs Blog*, 2013. http://healthaffairs. org/blog/2013/03/08/decline-in-utilization-rates-signals-a-change-in-the-inpatient-business-model.

Institute for Healthcare Improvement. *Patient-Centered Care on Medical/Surgical Units*. Boston, MA: Institute for Healthcare Improvement, 2019. www.ihi.org/resources/Pages/Changes/PatientCenteredCare.aspx.

Institute of Medicine (US). *The Future of the Public's Health in the 21st Century*. Washington, DC: National Academy Press, 2003.

Legnini, Mark, Stephanie Anthony, Elliot K. Wicks, Jack A. Meyer, Lise S. Rybowski, and Larry S. Stepnick. *Privatization of Public Hospitals*. Washington, DC: Economic and Social Research Institute, 1999.

Moore, Adam. "New Parkland Hospital by HDR + Corgan." *Commercial Interior Design & Architecture*. Last modified February 24, 2012. www.interiorsandsources.com/article-details/articleid/13590/title/new-parkland-hospital-by-hdr-corgan.

Shortell, Stephen M., Robin R. Gillies, and Kelly J. Devers. "Reinventing the American Hospital." *The Milbank Quarterly* 73, no. 2 (1995): 131–160.

Smith, Ren, and Watkins, Nicholas. "Therapeutic Environments." National Institute of Building Sciences. Last modified September 22, 2016. Whole Building Design Guide: www.wbdg.org/resources/therapeutic-environments.

Sommers, Benjamin D., Munira Z. Gunja, Kenneth Finegold, and Thomas Musco. "Changes in Self-Reported Insurance Coverage, Access to Care, and Health Under the Affordable Care Act." *JAMA* 314, no. 4 (2015): 366–374.

Valentin, Andreas, and Julian Bion. "How Safe Is My Intensive Care Unit? An Overview of Error Causation and Prevention." *Current Opinion in Critical Care* 13, no. 6 (2007): 697–702.

Chapter 10

Defining a Project Method
Ensuring Project Success with Pre-Design Planning

Harm Hollander

10.1 Introduction

A hospital is a stage set for the processes that run inside its walls. The positive, negative, or neutral effects a design can have on these processes are often experienced as side effects rather than the manifestation of clear design intent. At a basic level, those involved with the planning and design of a new hospital are charged with developing a vision and translating it into a real environment. If this vision clearly outlines objectives such as deinstitutionalization, safety for patients, enhanced clinical outcomes, and improved efficiency in building operations, then the design team can identify the strategies that best fit the given situation. For these strategies to then be successfully implemented, all participants in their execution need to know and believe in the overall objectives of the project, not defaulting to functional rationales.

This undertaking is surprisingly complex, one that can be derailed, through distraction, along several points throughout the journey. This complexity is only amplified when the project objectives need to consider specific populations. How a design is proposing to interact with the needs of children, for example, is necessary to establish early on, in order for opportunities to be maximized and sensitivities to be observed.

This chapter demonstrates the relevance of this concept—establishing an overall project vision—by unpacking the design process for the Queensland Children's Hospital (QCH), formerly the Lady Cilento Children's Hospital, in Brisbane, Australia. It does not outline all the design strategies of a healing environment for children, but exemplifies how replicable strategies can be identified and employed. Because of its complexity in terms of user, scale, and location, the QCH project showcases the several key ideas necessary as a footing for the design journey: ensuring the whole team has informed imagination, a passion to improve the lives of patients, and a collective, clear mind, free from preconceptions.

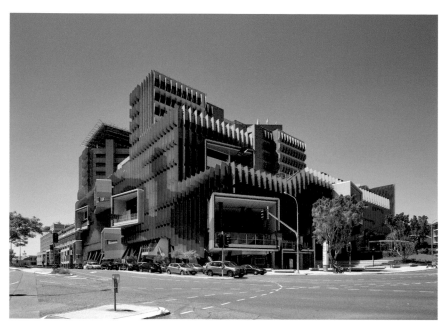

◄ Figure 10.1

Queensland Children's
Hospital as viewed from
the SouthBank Parklands,
Brisbane, Australia, 2015.
Source: Christopher Frederick
Jones

10.2 Identifying Project-Specific Principles

Defining who a building is serving reveals principles that expand on what is traditionally expected of hospitals for the general public. Population-specific care centers, for children, the elderly, a cultural group, or those receiving specialized treatment, will all have shared and unique principles. At the commencement of the QCH project briefing, the client and design teams co-observed and collated the principles underpinning children's hospitals (references associated with some of these principles show similar conclusions in parallel to other studies):

- The experience of the child: Since many hospitalized children and adolescents have serious illnesses, the whole experience can be scary, exhausting, and unpleasant. The design of a facility should do its best to mitigate these harsh aspects of their stay there.
- Carer support: Other than the capacity for healing and relief through clinical means, family access to resource support is one of the primary comforts that should be available to all carers and patients.
- Culture: A pleasant, genuine, caring, and competent environment is likely to win a carer and child's confidence. This will reflect on the feelings associated with working or lodging at the hospital.
- Continuation of life: Distraction, normalization of the environment, natural light, exposure to nature, rest, security, exploration, orientation and wayfinding, and fresh air provide comforts and respite to children, parents, and the care team.
- Community: A hospital is not an illness fixer or a fortress that is separated from the rest of the world. Its spaces need to be perceived as being interconnected

Harm Hollander

The experience of the child	A youth forum and a patient carer stakeholder group were enthusiastically supported by the executive throughout the design and construction phases.
Carer support	As the brief developed, there was continued reflection on further opportunity. This resulted in amenities such as Long-day Lounge (a place of retreat for long-distance families who undergo a series of appointments during a day).
Culture	Environment has an influence on culture if it activates relationships between staff, patients and carers. The continuing focus of the design process was to provide opportunistic and pleasant spaces where people may casually interact.
Continue with life	Sitting for a long time in an institution's waiting rooms does not produce a helpful atmosphere, especially if you are from out-of-town and have nowhere else to go for your stay in the city. Banking, laundry, entertainment, homework and other daily activity were given consideration. Exposure to continue-with-life activity was provided by the building's public spaces. Last-minute waiting systems, which allowed freedom to continue roaming for as long as possible, were developed.
Part of the community	The precinct is a pivotal connection within the city fabric. Urban links, a pedestrian flow through the building and activated street frontage ensured the hospital was not isolated from the community. Parts of the building were made identifiable and transparent, giving an inside/ outside relationship. Specific upper building areas were provided with views down to the streetscape and entrance in order to keep a relationship with daily life.
Universal values	International facilities revealed exemplars and provided inspiration. Values, such as the family's need to withdraw and be together, in grief, for a dying child, were an example of a universal theme. This research resulted in a special facility away from more bustling areas. Some parochial considerations also became evident through research. Indigenous culture, for instance, highlighted the need for outdoor areas for family gatherings.
Design innovation	Innovation can be activated if asking the right questions at the right time. Before defining accommodation, a series of sessions asked questions and proposed alternative operational models.

▲ Figure 10.2

Co-observed principles for planning, programming, and envisioning a children's hospital.
Source: Conrad Gargett Lyons

with the outside world to form important links to the healing environment. A hospital is more a place of life, where people interact, heal, play, confer, and access beneficial resources. A hospital relates to a city and the city responds to it.

- Universal ethics: Despite the cultural differences and variances in regulations, core values are international. In the West, and many other parts of the world, these priorities include considerations of transparency, dignity, access to healthcare, comfort of the child, and carer support. Although the levels of success may vary, a universal intent is evident in global exemplars.
- Design innovation: Any brief that is functionally centered in describing a definitive schedule of rooms will not achieve a healing environment despite any overarching vision statements. At best, a good result will be a cosmetic adjustment. Innovation in design will, however, emerge in a well-articulated, objective-based brief toward a people-centered building.

Since some of these principles go against other clinical priorities, a way to balance the design must be sought. The balance should never be perceived as a need to make a sacrifice of one over the other. These principles are often ignored, misidentified, or not acted on for a variety of reasons. These reasons are often budgetary, but are also frequently due to engaging primary stakeholders who focus only on what a hospital has been, rather than on a future of architecture for health. On larger projects, spanning several years, there are also inevitable changes to the management team, clinical organization, and project team personnel. Projects at this scale can become fractured into isolated components, where the overall vision can be difficult to maintain. Team members such as building contractors and various expert consultants can skew the viewpoints. The project can also be further complicated by political opposition or media headlines. QCH went down this rugged route and even had a Queensland state government election fought over the project advancing on the chosen site. It is not unusual for major hospital developments to have parallel disruptions that potentially distract from and place pressure on the realization of the overall objectives.

10.3 Building a Project Team

Apart from the many potential derailment points along the journey of a major development, there is also often a concern in the rigor associated with the commencement of the project. Without a team that involves key stakeholder and occupant groups, the vision to create a therapeutic environment for children will be overrun by the challenges noted earlier. Any resulting outcomes proposed by the design team would likely be a token gesture, explained but not necessarily experienced. At the commencement of the QCH as a project, the proposed organization of the new hospital board was an emerging one, amalgamating three existing children's health bodies: one nonprofit public health provider and two government bodies from diverse geographic parts of Brisbane. It had been recognized that collaboration between parties would provide clinical benefits, and the initiative was arranged by visionaries at top levels of government. The various organizational representatives were well informed, knowledgeable, and passionate about the project vision. The representatives understood the new hospital would have the eyes of the world on it. By the time the design consultants were engaged, the client team had already undertaken a global study tour and articulated why exemplars were considered worthy. The group also sourced reports from stakeholders of various, recently completed, international projects, and provided coordinated summaries of lessons learned. Most significantly, the client leaders were open in acknowledging that they "did not know what they did not know". The first all-day workshop session and associated bundle of reports articulated a wide range of issues but did not attempt solutions.

Because all members of the newly formed project team were solicited for their input and engaged in the workshopping sessions, illuminating discoveries were made. Not only was there passion and unity, but also there was a universal focus on the child being first and foremost in all considerations, including how any proposed environments would provide support, respite, and comfort to their families. There was an overall desire to do away with silo thinking, to provide smoother clinical pathways, and to create a place which was "not like a hospital". This became the overarching project vision. It recognized the child being in a place that was not exclusively clinical, but also where children experience a part of their lives; a place where the community interacts; where outside spaces are experienced; where life continues for the child and family. The project vision also acknowledged that the hospital's place in the community assumed a wider role than that of any one facility. A banner of the key findings, including the expression "not like a hospital", was included in the concluding summary, and became the defining culture for the project moving forward, being displayed on various personal pin boards for some years afterwards.

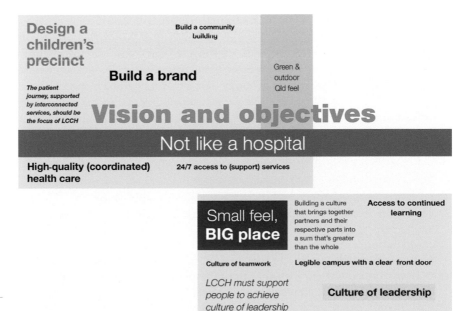

▶ Figure 10.3

Briefing banner.
Source: Conrad Gargett Lyons

10.4 Brief Development

A series of consultation sessions led to the development of the brief (program document). These sessions were significant exercises, each being a good portion of a day for the collaborative group exercises, in addition to the research, preparation, distribution of preparatory packs, and reporting. At an early session, there was a detailed briefing from the clients to the consultants on amalgamating findings to date. This included the ideals in culture, and further ideals illustrated by relevant exemplars. The information gained through the forum founded a series of further workshops. The basis of workshopping was to structure the profile of participants to represent all levels of the hospital hierarchy (i.e., not "executive-centric" nor "department-operational-staff-based"), and to ask a series of fundamental, patient-centered questions for subgroup discussions and then whole-of-session analysis. The results were a brief that was not budget-led but allowed a provisional target with staged definition of the final scope to comprehensively provide the emerging, best solution. The brief also recognized the developmental culture of the new organization and how design could work hand in hand to enhance the best ways forward. The briefing document continued with a context study, including analysis of permeability toward the community, goals of urban regeneration, and the relationship with three significant neighbors (two private schools and the neighboring private nonprofit partner of QCH). The briefing document also included future growth scenarios that capitalized on the link to the adjacent South Bank Parklands (which could be used as healing spaces for the hospital) and access to surrounding amenities, particularly public transport infrastructure. In other words, the brief was part of a living instruction, seeking further development by exploring opportunities.

10.5 Establishing a Vision: Expanding on the Brief

The first design solutions were proposed, stepping back from directly addressing hospital issues. They were undertaken in the design studio as well as interactive consultations with a "zoom-out" technique—that is, not just focusing on the knowledge that came from within the project stakeholder team but also asking these questions: "What can this project do for the whole of Brisbane and what can Brisbane do for the project?" A series of ideas that were outside the immediate brief emerged from this process:

1. A road realignment would simplify cross traffic flows between the new hospital, the adjacent schools, and collocated private hospital campuses.
2. An underpass with retail or other active spaces would link the hospital with South Bank Parklands without having the barrier of the major arterial road, which currently interrupts flow between the two landmarks.
3. A connection between the basement and the adjacent bus tunnel would allow emergency vehicle pathways to be virtually uncluttered from any point within the Brisbane road network at peak traffic times.

Harm Hollander

4. A partial land swap between the two adjacent private schools would allow more beneficial sites for both schools and extensive parking facilities to be created in conjunction with commercial initiatives.
5. A main entrance could be built on the back street, allowing a peaceful atmosphere in both the external forecourt and its transition to internal areas. The opportunity could extend to divert and minimize vehicular traffic at that zone and allow a mixed zone of light vehicles and pedestrians in the resulting entrance forecourt.

The ideal scenario of integrating these five recommendations is slightly "blue-sky" and a full execution is difficult to achieve; however, by thinking at this scale, the project vision is more likely to be completed. Aspects of a final design, like site arrival, public engagement, and traffic patterns, can always be exploited to decrease the burden a new development could pose to a city. The ideas of road realignment and the land swap with the inclusion of a multistory carpark were pursued, and are fully realized in the precinct as it is today. The idea of the quiet entrance with a pedestrianized streetscape was captured in

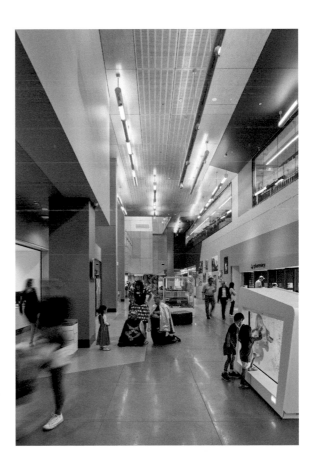

▶ Figure 10.4

Outpatient public space connections.
Source: Christopher Frederick Jones

the final solution as well, but only partially. The integration of these solutions formed the core of the success in the overall development. Written to accept opportunity, the brief was focused on best-outcome solutions, a fully defined scope prior to the issue of budget, and open enough to address emerging issues.

Because the project was part of a larger hospital capital works program by the Queensland state government, there was a parallel investigation of standards and further opportunity through strategic reference groups, covering four parallel major hospital developments. Clinical standards, developments, and expectations were discussed, and a series of recommendations emerged from these groups. This informed development of the Australasian Health Facility Guidelines, as well as providing project benchmarks. One beneficial conclusion was that the wider health authority accepted and supported the benefits associated with a higher proportion of single-bed rooms. Without such support at a high level, there may have been many prolonged dissenting views on peculiarities of children, recurrent cost penalties, and the like. The support addressed several of the project objectives: environments with less chance of infection, amenities for family support, and the value of good rest as part of a healing environment.

10.5.1 Designing a Place Not Like a Hospital

A contextual analysis and literature review were undertaken concurrently with the strategic reference groups. After the benchmarks, standards, and opportunities were explored, master planning began. Because the site is in an urbanized part of the city, expanding vertically was the only viable option for consideration. An exercise researching linkages, topographical limitations, building typologies, and functional collocations was carried out. The main driver of the masterplan became the size and collocation of the operating functions (surgery department) and high-care functions (intensive care unit). Operating or high-care floor footprints typically drive the shape of other clinical floors, thus producing homogenous, dense building forms. However, because of the project vision, opportunities were explored for producing a series of outdoor terraces specific to each floor. The fixed, more rigid program of the lower operating and high-care floors, which covered virtually the entire site, was not restrictive to more malleable programming above, allowing for different sizes of terraces. Each one of the terrace gardens was therefore open to the sky and related to different floor functions as the building stepped inward. Because this opportunity was identified early, an in-house landscape architecture team could be active in the design from the start (an integration further expanded on in the following chapter of this book). The idea combined well with other objectives of keeping a busy and vibrant public portion of the building under the operating floor, and separating the more private, secure-feeling patient care areas toward the upper half of the building.

Several issues revealed themselves with this newly identified approach, which required resolution. The design team grappled with any arising conflicts

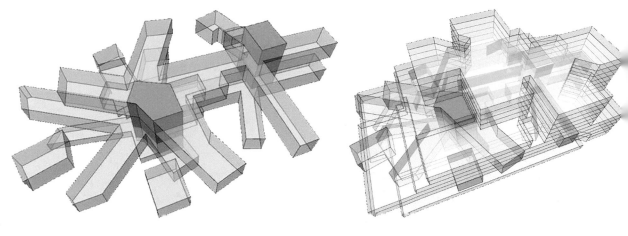

▲ Figure 10.5

Trunk and branches shown inside the facility.
Source: Conrad Gargett Lyons

▲ Figure 10.6

Program arranged around trunk and branches.
Source: Conrad Gargett Lyons

of collocation, orientation, interest, and daylight and explored a number of methods to resolve these conflicts. This was undertaken in parallel with the development of functional relationships. Synthesizing these factors, the design team used an analogy to understand the solution for themselves with language that eventually continued in explaining the concept to others. Eventually the idea developed toward the following design solution: a tree-inspired void could branch across spaces and give form to the many intersecting goals established in the brief.

The building by necessity has a deep plan that fills most of the available urban site. Deep plans have much of their interior spaces devoid of natural light due to the physical distance from the window perimeter. To counteract this, the form of a giant tree could be immersed into the middle of the building, with its trunk reaching vertically and its branches radiating horizontally out to the window walls. Removing this tree form and leaving only the negative imprint of the void would connect spaces spanning all directions. Some of the branches take up the height of two floors and some take up the height of just a single floor. The branches consist of circulation paths, multi-purpose spaces, or special functions. Their ends channel light and views from the perimeter into the core of the building. From this core, the city skyline, the former town hall, or the residential hotel across the road can be referenced.

There are two of these interlinked tree voids inside the final building. The main entrance relates directly to the primary trunk and the vertical circulation is directly adjacent to it. The tree analogy addresses the project vision at several levels. Firstly, its branches bring natural light into the heart of the building, while providing views outward to the surrounding city. The reception point at the base of the trunk has direct lines of sight to each floor lobby so

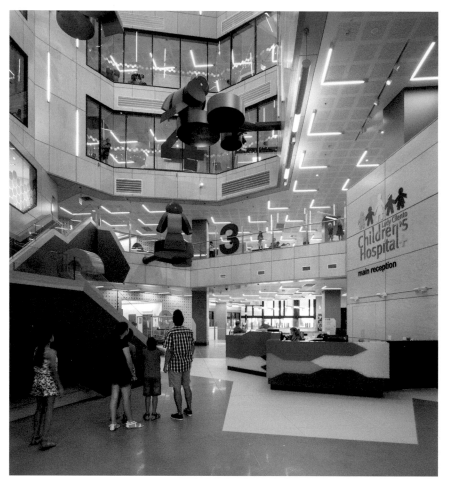

◀ Figure 10.7

Queensland Children's
Hospital—main "trunk"
or atrium.
Source: Christopher Frederick
Jones

that a simple relationship can be used for explaining and relating to destinations. The wayfinding within the building also becomes more intuitive through the mechanism of natural light and reference points. The outside world can see into many of the building's activated areas without breaching privacy. Flexible spaces most open to this visibility can be used for concerts, displays, artworks, markets, parties, school classes, and incidental meetings—all part of an engaging and "normalized" daily life. Pathways through the ground floor function as shortcuts to and from surrounding precincts, thereby encouraging schoolchildren to traverse the hospital space and be seen through the public parts of the atrium. From the more private and upper parts of the atrium, observers can see this life flowing below. The branches, linking different elevations of the building, also force an induction of natural air flow at the bottom public areas of the floors; this natural flow of air maintains high-quality, non-conditioned air at tenable conditions in an otherwise semitropical environment.

Harm Hollander

The tree analogy also helped to inform the expression and character of the trunk and branches. A tree is irregular in shape and its general expression. It can be large but because of its irregularity, it is not overbearing in scale. The trunk inside the building interpreted this nature of a tree; it broke down the scale of its surrounding walls into an irregular pattern of differing facets so that a child would not be overwhelmed by the immense scale of the void.

10.6 Conclusions

The project method for designing the Queensland Children's Hospital allowed a series of opportunities to be imbued into a living brief. This chapter has focused on a few of the core decisions and circumstances within the overall design process. Success in these areas was due to specific conditions of the project, serving as lessons learned for projects of similar scale and scope:

- The briefing team was well informed by leading international trends and expectations.
- The briefing team articulated their aspirations and objectives without attempting to spell out solutions.
- Child patients and the carers held prominence in pre-design planning workshops. This led to the project vision of a place that was "not like a hospital". Client stakeholders had buy-in to this idea and became committed to its execution.
- The brief was viewed as a living document, open to further opportunities.
- There was transparency in the agreement of priorities.
- Throughout the project there was continued communication and collaboration between the executive level and designers.

QCH has resulting qualities that are not like a hospital. As well as serving a clinical function, it provides a stage set for healing: life, interaction, and a relationship with the surrounding environment. Delivering an environment that fosters healing is an ongoing challenge and improvements of processes leading to new benchmarks are encouraged. To advance toward more therapeutic environments, a project method must identify an informed project vision that creatively challenges the default, function-based approaches prevalent in current design practices (Black 2015). This commitment to a more robust pre-design planning stage provides the support needed for successful and innovative architecture for health.

Bibliography

Black, Andy. "Notes on the Design of Hospitals and Their Clinical Organisation". *The Australian Hospital + Healthcare*, Winter (2015): 72–73. https://issuu.com/westwick-farrowmedia/docs/australian_hospital_healthcare_bull_d9dfda0cba6fb1.

Neild, L. Chapters 7–8 in *Changing Hospital Architecture*. London: RIBA Enterprises, 2008.

Pentecost. "A Perfect Storm: The Economic Challenge and The Salutogenic Response." *International Academy for Design and Health*, Key Note Address. The 9th Design & Health World Congress & Exhibition, 2013.

Prasad, Sunand, ed. *Changing Hospital Architecture*. London: RIBA Enterprises, 2008.

Chapter 11

The Efficacy of Healing Gardens
Integrating Landscape Architecture for Health

Katharina Nieberler-Walker, Cheryl Desha, Omniya El Baghdadi, and Angela Reeve

11.1 Introduction

Hospitals are places that are inherently abstracted from the normal course of life—they are places that people go to only in times of exceptional disease, disorder, and crisis. For the majority of the population, the hospital environment is highly unfamiliar in terms of how it looks, feels, smells, and sounds—as well as the emotional and physical sensations elicited by being either a patient or a family member. Patients can experience a range of emotions and physical experiences that often differ from their "normal" circumstances. This may include stress, fear, pain, agitation, boredom, and isolation. As presented in a paper to the European Healthcare Design conference (El Baghdadi et al. 2017), there is an increasing recognition of the importance of patients feeling—at least periodically—"normal", to reduce the physical and emotional strain of being in hospital, which we propose can be facilitated through the design of hospital spaces. This can be achieved through the deliberate inclusion of features that establish a sense of familiarity in the design of hospital spaces.

While research is ongoing to establish quantitative connections between outdoor settings and health outcomes, such as recovery rates and well-being (Cervinka, Röderer, and Hefler 2011; Davis 2011; Cooper Marcus and Sachs 2014; Jiang 2014), we know from cognitive neuroscience and environmental psychology literature that appreciating what is "normal" occurs at varying levels of consciousness. This connection to "normal" is deeply related to the relationships and roles of the different parts of the brain (Williams Goldhagen 2017). Furthermore, what our senses consider normal is at least twofold, relating to both innate preferences that reflect humanity's evolutionary relationship with nature and the compilation of personal memories an individual has experienced from birth.

In this chapter we discuss how healing gardens can be designed to achieve normalcy, improving users' experiences with healthcare settings. Within this context, our use of the term "normalcy" relates to designing an environment that embeds a composition of inherited and learned familiarity related to nature, and allows for the activities of daily life to take place. We offer experiential evidence through the Queensland Children's Hospital (QCH) in Brisbane, Australia (see also Nieberler-Walker 2015, 2017; Reeve, Nieberler-Walker, and Desha 2017), with regards to the role that hospital external environments can play in going beyond conventional landscape design to create "healing gardens" (i.e., therapeutic green spaces designed to promote well-being and emotional and cognitive restoration, to patients, their families, and staff).

A key argument within this chapter is that landscape architecture as a profession has a critical role to play—from concept design through to handover—in championing the integration of healing gardens as a means for health benefits. Addressing the increasing rhetoric of healing gardens as being no more than incidental green spaces in and around buildings, we position them to be intentionally designed for a specific outcome, considering each facility's unique climate, landscape, and context. This positioning encourages healing gardens to transcend simple planter beds, and become programmed space within the hospital, inciting activity or emotion the way any interior space would. The resulting conclusions have immediate implications for designing outdoor spaces in hospitals to promote a sense of "normalcy" for end users, and create conditions conducive to healing.

11.2 Healing Gardens as Vehicles to Promote Normalcy

Landscapes and greenspaces, and more specifically healing gardens, need to be primary elements in the design of hospital projects, particularly in urban contexts. We propose this as a natural next step on a long and established journey into urban greening. Building on Appleton's (1996) work in the 1980s, there is a rich history of the role of nature in health and well-being in general, including Wilson (1984) and Kellert et al. (2008). There is also a rich body of work on the role of nature as a stimulant for therapy or restoration, including Cooper Marcus and Barnes (1999), Ulrich (1984), Kaplan and Kaplan (1989), and Grahn and Stigsdotter (2010).

Significant international attention is now focused on the role of nature in promoting healing, with growing interest specifically in "healing gardens". For our purposes we define healing gardens as therapeutic green spaces designed to promote well-being and foster emotional and cognitive restoration in patients, their families, and staff. Research in various theoretical fields demonstrates that human beings are physically, neurologically, and emotionally responsive to cues in their surrounding environment (Ulrich 1984; Kaplan and Kaplan 1989; Kellert et al. 2008). This has implications for healing, as architectural design has been shown to affect sympathetic (and alternatively the parasympathetic) nervous system (Bengtsson 2015), which in turn has potential to influence the body's ability to heal. Dating back more than 20 years, seminal work in this field has found that higher stress levels reduce the body's healing processes, which points to the underlying reason for accelerated healing rates in hospital patients who have views of natural features (Ulrich 1984; Ulrich et al. 1991). Experiences in these green spaces should—by design—feel more comfortable and conducive to healing for users, and allow them to participate in the familiar activities of play, exploration, discovery, exercise, and more. To achieve this, programming a healing garden in a specific and intentional way is necessary.

11.3 Designing for Normalcy—Insights From the Queensland Children's Hospital (QCH), Australia

The QCH has provided a pivotal opportunity to integrate a number of "healing gardens" that could provide a safe place within the hospital where visitors could seek respite from the hospital environment. Surrounding this opportunity was the vision of designing a hospital that would provide a holistic approach to health and well-being, where the focus of the facility was shifted—at least in part—from one of treating sickness to one of promoting health. The design team therefore sought evidence-based design principles to inform a facility that could nurture body and mind.

The QCH, formerly known as the Lady Cilento Children's Hospital, was opened in 2014, incorporating a community plaza and 13 outdoor spaces, including 11 healing gardens, catering for the needs of patients, their families, and staff, as well as the broader public. The hospital building itself was designed to allow natural light, fresh air, and views to the outdoors. The QCH maximizes the amount of greenery on-site, with only 25% of the site area covered by a conventional roof and the remainder being public open space and roof terraces. Being an inner-city hospital with substantial land constraints, this was achieved through an innovative building design where the steplike building façade allows for roof terraces on many of the building's floors.

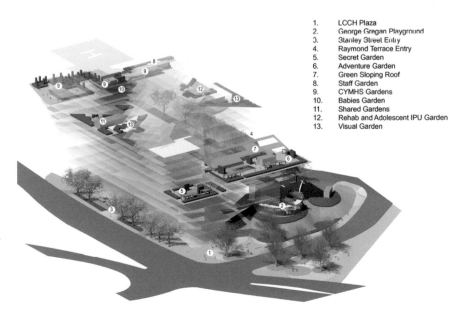

1.	LCCH Plaza
2.	George Gregan Playground
3.	Stanley Street Entry
4.	Raymond Terrace Entry
5.	Secret Garden
6.	Adventure Garden
7.	Green Sloping Roof
8.	Staff Garden
9.	CYMHS Gardens
10.	Babies Garden
11.	Shared Gardens
12.	Rehab and Adolescent IPU Garden
13.	Visual Garden

▶ Figure 11.1

Overview of Queensland Children's Hospital's various healing gardens and outdoor spaces.
Source: Conrad Gargett

Each healing garden at the QCH was designed to promote stress reduction through creating an environment that is resonant with people's innate preference for certain natural settings and features, to facilitate parasympathetic nervous system activity and allow for contemplation, relaxation, and a sense of being grounded and safe. The gardens may also connect with people's individual experiences and feel "familiar" through the use of plants and vegetation from the region. They provide an immersive experience that visually, acoustically, and mentally takes people away from the often highly emotional, disorientating, and unfamiliar experience of being a patient or family member in a children's hospital, to an environment that feels relatively "normal".

It is important to note that the familiarity and connection the gardens seek to evoke in visitors is not necessarily meant to mimic that of the visitors' own gardens or places they visit in their daily lives (although this may be the case, particularly for visitors who are from the South East Queensland region)—but rather to assist the deep, innate affiliation to natural spaces that exists within most, if not all humans (Wilson 1984; Kellert et al. 2008). It is also proposed that this sense of "normal" can be achieved through the kinds of experiences that occur in the gardens. Activities such as having a cup of tea on a park bench, lying on grass, playing basketball, or walking along garden paths can connect people to "normal life" outside of the hospital. In healing gardens, visitors can use the garden by themselves in any way they choose—sit, walk, take a nap, or take part in activities led by a professional therapist, occupational or horticultural.

Design to achieve a sense normalcy is challenging, and on reflection of the design process for the QCH gardens, six emerging design principles were identified that incorporate extant literature, design philosophies, theories, and examined healthcare models (El Baghdadi et al. 2017). Here we explain the principles and use examples from the QCH project.

11.3.1 Design to Support the Target User Group

This principle proposes that healing gardens should be planned around a defined user group and their surrounding environment, culture, and climate. Given that culture and community are so central to day-to-day living, hospitals can be quite removed from these human connections and our personal "context"—for example, home, loved ones, and conversations covering more than medical issues. Recognizing the unique experiences of users is necessary to create spaces that feel familiar to them: What a person with disabilities, someone from a rural region, a teenage patient, or a geriatric volunteer may require for "normalcy" can vary. In addition, the target user may be patients, staff, the general public, or a combination of populations. Healing gardens can soften unfamiliar hospital interiors, providing a physical and social relationship to neighboring institutions, facilities, and even the natural environment.

At the QCH, the community plaza and George Gregan playground spaces bring together people from the hospital, neighboring schools, research facilities, and the Mater Hospital. These spaces can be seen as an extension of the nearby Southbank Parklands and the Grey Street entertainment precinct, and are linked to all forms of public transport. The plaza has become a popular lunch

The community plaza at Queensland Children's Hospital.
Source: Christopher Frederick Jones

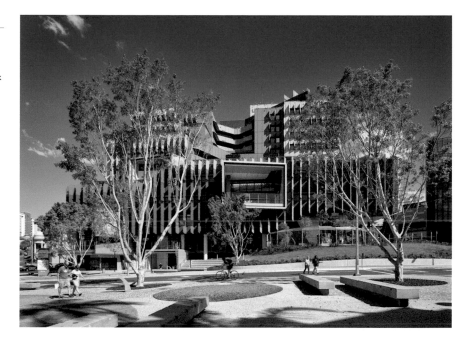

or meeting spot for the broader community, adding a sense of liveliness and connection to the hospital. In this case, these spaces appeal to the public, and more specifically neighboring park visitors, schools, and city workers.

11.3.2 Program for a Variety of Activities

This principle requires that healing gardens be designed to enable visitors to engage in a range of activities that reflect "everyday life". Visitors should be able to exert a certain amount of personal control and choice over how they spend time in the gardens. This includes, but is not limited to, places where people can sit, play, socialize, and eat. The goal is to combine priorities for the functionality or performance of the systems (i.e., activities to cater to various needs) and the safety or engineering aspects (i.e., how safe, well designed, and reliable the system is) with the aesthetics of experience (i.e., how the whole interaction with the service feels or is experienced) (Bate and Robert 2006). Importantly, people should have the ability to decide for themselves (at least to a certain degree) how they will spend time in the space. Allowing for some degree of autonomy can provide a critical sense of personal control that may reduce the sense of helplessness often associated with being unwell.

At the QCH, the composition of healing gardens sought to address a variety of activities, including the need for social interaction, physical exercise, personal time, and meditation. For example, in the Secret Garden, the lawn can be used for a picnic, while the shelters provide a pleasant setting for conversation and mindfulness. This is in contrast to the spaces in the kitchen garden or the gardens tailored to adolescents, where related functional programmatic

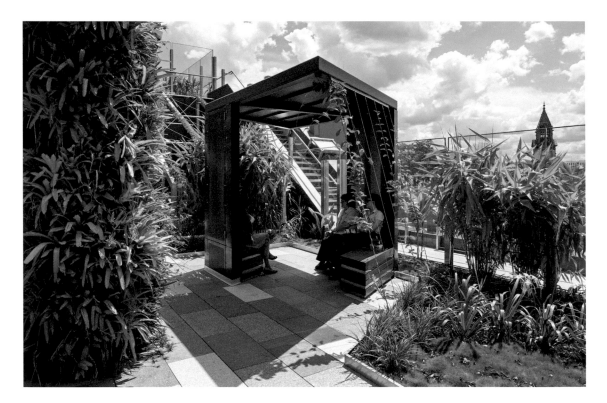

▲ Figure 11.3

Features and furnishings support a variety of activities.
Source: Christopher Frederick Jones

elements are included. Each garden enables a range of activities for its target user and use, including a kitchen garden with fresh herbs, an exercise yard associated with the "outdoor" gymnasium, a barbecue garden for socializing, and an adolescent garden as a youth-oriented interactive space.

11.3.3 Co-locate for Accessibility

A strong link between indoor and outdoor ensures that patients have the opportunity to readily access and engage with the functional features of healing gardens. In home and other familiar environments, indoor living spaces often have views of—and have welcoming connections to—features such as patios, verandahs, lawns, swimming pools, and vegetable gardens. This linking assists with intuitive wayfinding, and reduces disorientation and the sense of unfamiliarity, as experienced and documented by many in the field. A seamless transition between the indoor and the outdoor contributes to the feeling of being connected to the opportunities healing gardens can provide.

At the QCH, the Adventure Garden, which is located adjacent to the physiotherapy and occupational therapy ward, offers outdoor areas for play, entertainment, and rehabilitation. The co-location of hospital functions from inside to

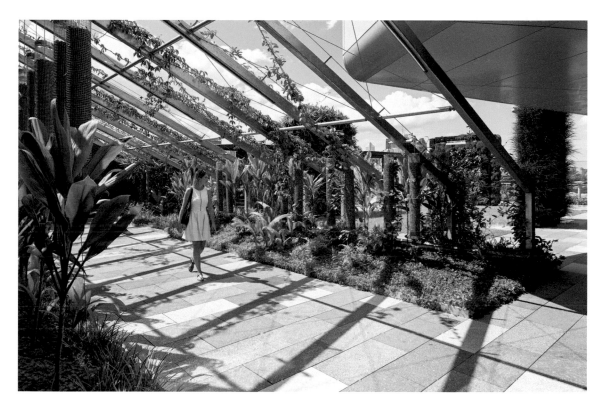

▲ Figure 11.1

Gardens link interior program and are co-located to ensure use.
Source: Christopher Frederick Jones

outside allows for outdoor rehabilitation, including a wheelchair training run and ramp, a climbing wall, a basketball hoop, and an herb garden. Similarly, the Child Youth Mental Health Services (CYMHS) Gardens are located adjacent to the Mental Health unit, and are specifically designed for young children and adolescents to help elevate the mood, calm the mind, and gently stimulate the senses.

11.3.4 Integrate Adequate Green and Open Space

This principle requires healing gardens to go beyond capturing the imagination of users where activities and events are given the space to occur. Knowing what "normal" experiences are expected to occur in the space helps size plantings, direct orientation, and prioritize the hardscapes and greenspaces available to users. In day-to-day life, we experience a mix of indoor and outdoor environments, in contrast to hospital stays, where we are often restricted to internal spaces. Studies have suggested that gardens provide a restorative setting where users can recuperate and find reprieve from stressful environments (Cooper Marcus and Barnes 1999; Whitehouse et al. 2001; Sherman et al. 2005). Adequate green and open space is critical to contrast adjacent clinical spaces that often include bright lights, white walls and hard floors, sterile rooms, and large equipment.

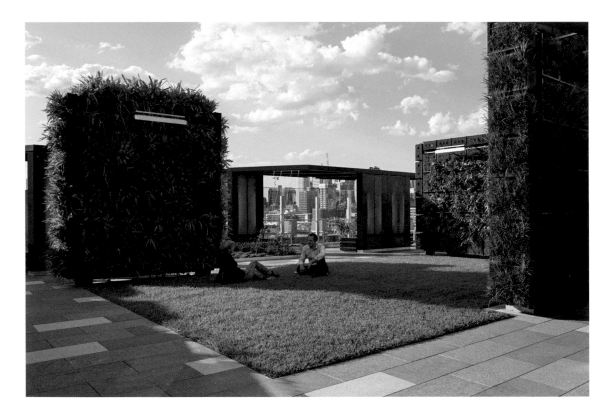

▲ Figure 11.5

Adequate green and open space allows for lounging and relaxation.
Source: Christopher Frederick Jones

At the QCH, open space is maximized by stepping back the façade and thereby using roof terraces to provide the opportunity for experiences like running, cooking, lounging, or gardening. The 11 green and open spaces were strategically allocated to a variety of end-user needs, spanning publicly accessible, private, and therapeutic settings.

11.3.5 Design for Prospect and Refuge

The importance of our evolutionary history in defining our innate preferences for particular settings and views was addressed more than 30 years ago by Jay Appleton. Appleton defined prospect and refuge theory, which has subsequently underpinned an approach to design that recognizes the importance of natural landscape settings in stimulating neurological, physiological, and emotional responses in the majority of people—which in turn is recognized as providing restorative, therapeutic, and rehabilitative benefits (Appleton 1996). Others such as Söderback, Söderström, and Schälander (2004) and Cooper Marcus (2007, 2016) have considered how particular designs may resonate with an individual's memories and preferences (relating to his or her individual sense of normality), with a particular focus on the importance of outdoor settings to deliver this.

Katharina Nieberler-Walker et al.

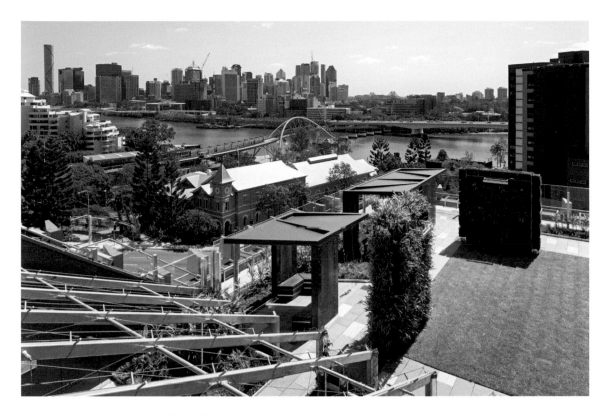

▲ Figure 11.6

Prospect over the surrounding city of Brisbane from the Queensland Children's Hospital.
Source: Christopher Frederick Jones

At the QCH, various healing gardens were designed for specific users and therapeutic benefits in mind, with all of the healing environments more broadly incorporating design elements for conscious and subconscious comfort and an element of surprise. Vegetated monoliths and epiphyte columns mimic trees on roofs, and the gardens are located to provide uninterrupted views over the city and distant landscape. Garden spaces are open, and integrate with the building to facilitate visitor access. Built infrastructure is inconspicuous, and the gardens are designed to connect with the surrounding landscape while also obscuring the building itself to convey a sense of immersion and spaciousness.

11.3.6 Stimulate All Senses

In familiar environments, we often find ourselves engaging the five senses, including smelling flowers and freshly cut grass, tasting food from the herb garden, touching leaves as we walk past, hearing the trickle of water and the sound of wind in the trees, and noticing and looking for where the bird calls are coming from. In hospitals, however, tastes are dulled, touch sensations are often painful or uncomfortable, sounds are mechanical, smells are sterile, and sights are pale. Using a combination of diverse

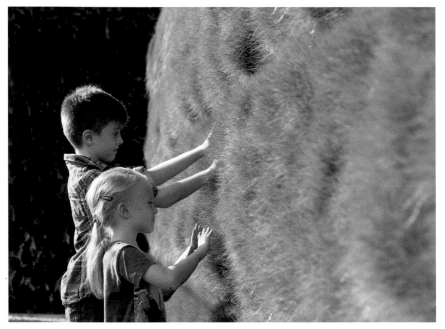

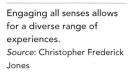
◀ Figure 11.7

Engaging all senses allows
for a diverse range of
experiences.
Source: Christopher Frederick
Jones

and attractive visual, auditory, and olfactory stimuli, gardens can provide critical distraction from prevailing concerns about the reasons for being in the hospital.

At the QCH, outdoor spaces were designed to provide places for contemplation, relaxation, and calm, with vertical greenery used strategically to provide sheltered seating that feels removed from the hospital environment. The Secret Garden is potentially the most well-used garden in this regard, possibly due to its character, orientation, and views. The proximity of the Secret Garden to the parents' retreat allows its use as a calming sanctuary in often difficult and stressful times.

11.4 Detailing the Role of Landscape Architecture in Healthcare Design

There is a commonly observed gap between the vision for hospital design, and indeed healing garden design, and what is actually achieved in practice, highlighting a crucial need to also consider the process by which such visions become reality. Currently hospitals are often designed more through the ideas, needs, and priorities of healthcare staff, architects, and designers according to preexisting standards. The project vision may have a clear overall outcome in mind; however, it is often high level and open to interpretation, and will mean different things to different people depending on contexts such as their background, knowledge, professional priority, and personal values. Design teams meet this myriad of expectations and contexts often with a limited budget, constrained timeframe, and add-on rather than integrated landscape components.

In their day-to-day professional work landscape architects enter this arena with a variety of design techniques to meet the client briefs, offering solutions to various externalities, such as pollution, building performance, and noise

Katharina Nieberler-Walker et al.

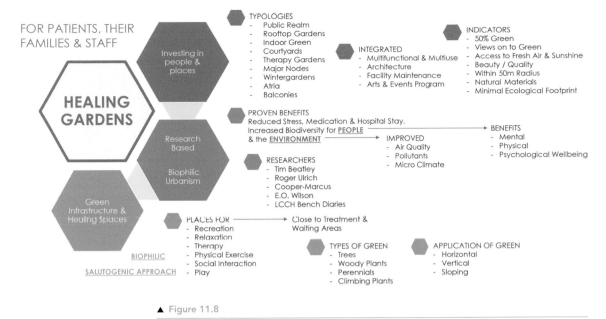

FOR PATIENTS, THEIR
FAMILIES & STAFF

HEALING
GARDENS

Investing in
people &
places

Research
Based

Biophilic
Urbanism

Green
Infrastructure &
Healing Spaces

BIOPHILIC

SALUTOGENIC APPROACH

TYPOLOGIES
- Public Realm
- Rooftop Gardens
- Indoor Green
- Courtyards
- Therapy Gardens
- Major Nodes
- Wintergardens
- Atria
- Balconies

INTEGRATED
- Multifunctional & Multiuse
- Architecture
- Facility Maintenance
- Arts & Events Program

INDICATORS
- 50% Green
- Views on to Green
- Access to Fresh Air & Sunshine
- Beauty / Quality
- Within 50m Radius
- Natural Materials
- Minimal Ecological Footprint

PROVEN BENEFITS
Reduced Stress, Medication & Hospital Stay.
Increased Biodiversity for PEOPLE
& the ENVIRONMENT

IMPROVED
- Air Quality
- Pollutants
- Micro Climate

BENEFITS
- Mental
- Physical
- Psychological Wellbeing

RESEARCHERS
- Tim Beatley
- Roger Ulrich
- Cooper-Marcus
- E.O. Wilson
- LCCH Bench Diaries

PLACES FOR
- Recreation
- Relaxation
- Therapy
- Physical Exercise
- Social Interaction
- Play

Close to Treatment &
Waiting Areas

TYPES OF GREEN
- Trees
- Woody Plants
- Perennials
- Climbing Plants

APPLICATION OF GREEN
- Horizontal
- Vertical
- Sloping

▲ Figure 11.8

Emergent design approach for healing gardens.
Source: Omniya El Baghdadi, Cheryl Desha, Katharina Nieberler-Walker, and Jenny Ziviani

insulation. However, normalcy as a healing garden outcome is still ad hoc, champion-based, and highly variable. To overcome this, we recognize the need for a rigorous design approach to healing gardens, which clearly identifies design objectives (normalcy or otherwise) and implements clear design strategies to achieve them. Responding to the need for transdisciplinary teams to understand and apply this knowledge, we have developed design considerations to create effective healing gardens, as shown in Figure 11.8. As shown, this provides the landscape architecture profession with a fortified foundation to ensure presence within design processes, from concept through to construction.

Furthermore, to guide design team thinking, we have also developed a landscape design lens (Figure 11.9). This design lens puts the wellness outcomes of the healing garden at the center, and focuses all design drivers on "nature for well-being". It remains outcomes focused, rather than being prescriptive, recognizing that design is a creative process not unlike the creation of a painting or the making of a sculpture.

With this context and pathway in mind, it is possible for multidisciplinary teams to realize the design brief vision or idea, through firstly considering the design approach, and then analyzing the design objectives and synthesizing this into a holistic design outcome. This process for healing garden design is illustrated in Figure 11.10. While this diagram shows a linear progression, design is in fact an organic and often cyclical process that requires regular evaluation with regard to its key objectives and potentials for innovation.

Through knowing how to go about designing healing gardens, design teams can ensure that they produce effective green spaces within the myriad of project parameters.

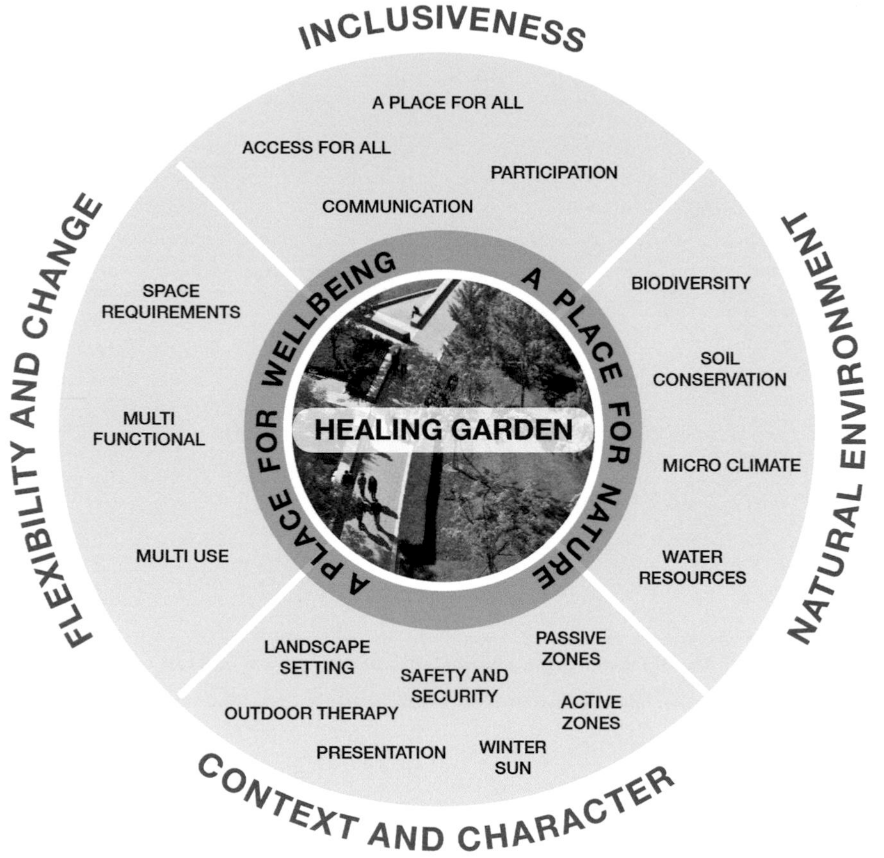

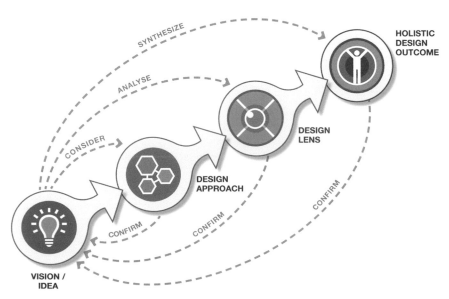

INCLUSIVENESS

A PLACE FOR ALL

ACCESS FOR ALL

PARTICIPATION

COMMUNICATION

A PLACE FOR WELLBEING

A PLACE FOR NATURE

HEALING GARDEN

BIODIVERSITY

SOIL CONSERVATION

MICRO CLIMATE

WATER RESOURCES

NATURAL ENVIRONMENT

FLEXIBILITY AND CHANGE

SPACE REQUIREMENTS

MULTI FUNCTIONAL

MULTI USE

LANDSCAPE SETTING

OUTDOOR THERAPY

SAFETY AND SECURITY

PRESENTATION

WINTER SUN

PASSIVE ZONES

ACTIVE ZONES

CONTEXT AND CHARACTER

◀ Figure 11.9

Emergent design lens.
Source: Katharina Nieberler-Walker

SYNTHESIZE

ANALYSE

CONSIDER

CONFIRM

CONFIRM

CONFIRM

HOLISTIC DESIGN OUTCOME

DESIGN LENS

DESIGN APPROACH

VISION / IDEA

◀ Figure 11.10

Emergent design process.
Source: Katharina Nieberler-Walker

Katharina Nieberler-Walker et al.

11.5 Conclusions

In this chapter we have advocated for an integrated landscape architecture strategy from the beginning of a hospital project, with the end goal of creating opportunities for patients, their families, and staff to experience a sense of normalcy within often intimidating and foreign institutional settings. Enabled with this strategy, we have noted the significant potential for healing gardens to foster improved wellness outcomes, normalcy or otherwise. We have presented six emergent design principles for healing gardens in healthcare design, which can provide rigor and transparency in the journey of ideating, documenting, and implementing healing gardens.

Landscape architects play a critical role in applying these design principles strategically, holistically, and in collaboration with other professions. This provides a significant opportunity to fill the knowledge gaps and to raise awareness through the documentation of holistic precedents and their benefits, the creation of optimal design specifications, and formulation of policy and good practice guidelines to move industry forward.

Finally, we reflect on the importance of the design process to promote practical strategies for facilitating high-quality healing garden design. Within the process, the six design principles for normalcy in healthcare facilities provide practical guidance for connecting users to familiar experiences to promote health and well-being. Together, the design process and principles have the potential to fundamentally shift understandings of healing gardens in healthcare settings, establishing their efficacy and improving health.

Acknowledgments

The author team would like to thank colleagues from the following companies and organizations who have contributed their valuable time in our research journey: Queensland Government (Queensland Health), the Queensland Children's Hospital, Centre for Children's Health Research, Aurecon, Conrad Gargett, Lyons, Lendlease, Landscape Solutions, the Queensland University of Technology, Griffith University, and the University of Queensland. The authors would also like to specifically thank Professor Jenny Ziviani (Children's Heath Queensland) for her contributions with regard to the projects cited.

Bibliography

Antonovsky, Aaron. *Health, Stress, and Coping*. San Francisco, CA: Jossey-Bass, 1979.

Appleton, Jay. *The Experience of Landscape*. Chichester: Wiley, 1996.

Bate, Paul, and Glenn Robert. "Experience-Based Design: From Redesigning the System Around the Patient to Co-Designing Services with The Patient." *BMJ Quality & Safety* 15, no. 5 (2006): 307–310.

Becker, Craig M., Mary Alice Glascoff, and W. Michael Felts. "Salutogenesis 30 Years Later: Where Do We go from Here?" *International Electronic Journal of Health Education* 13 (2010): 25–32.

Bengtsson, Anna. *From Experiences of the Outdoors to the Design of Healthcare Environments*, no. 66 (2015).

Beyer, Hugh, and Karen Holtzblatt. *Contextual Design: Defining Customer-Centered Systems*. San Francisco, CA: Morgan Kaufmann Publishers, 1997.

Cervinka, Renate, Kathrin Röderer, and Elisabeth Hefler. "Are Nature Lovers Happy? On Various Indicators of Well-Being and Connectedness with Nature." *Journal of Health Psychology* 17, no. 3 (2012): 379–388.

Cooper Marcus, C. "The Future of Healing Gardens, Health Environments." *Research & Design Journal* 9, no 2 (2016): 172–174.

Cooper Marcus, C., and N. Sachs. *Therapeutic Landscapes: An Evidence-Based Approach to Designing Healing Gardens and Restorative Outdoor Spaces*. New Jersey: John Wiley & Sons, Inc., 2014.

Davis, Brad E. "Rooftop Hospital Gardens for Physical Therapy: A Post-Occupancy Evaluation." *HERD: Health Environments Research & Design Journal* 4, no. 3 (2011): 14–43.

El Baghdadi, Omniya, and Cheryl Desha. "Conceptualising a Biophilic Services Model for Urban Areas." *Urban Forestry & Urban Greening* 27 (2017): 399–408.

El Baghdadi, Omniya, Jenny Ziviani, Katharina Nieberler-Walker, Angela Reeve, and Cheryl Desha. "Normalcy in Healthcare Design: An Extension of the Natural and Built Environment." *European Healthcare and Design* (2017): 11–14.

Frumkin, Howard, ed. *Environmental Health: From Global to Local*. 3rd ed. Hoboken, NJ: John Wiley & Sons, 2016.

Goldhagen, Sarah Williams. *Welcome to Your World: How the Built Environment Shapes Our Lives*. New York: HarperCollins, 2017.

Grahn, Patrik, and Ulrika K. Stigsdotter. "The Relation Between Perceived Sensory Dimensions of Urban Green Space and Stress Restoration." *Landscape and Urban Planning* 94, no. 3–4 (2010): 264–275.

Jiang, Shan. "Therapeutic Landscapes and Healing Gardens: A Review of Chinese Literature in Relation to the Studies in Western Countries." *Frontiers of Architectural Research* 3, no. 2 (2014): 141–153.

Kaplan, Rachel, and Stephen Kaplan. *The Experience of Nature: A Psychological Perspective*. Cambridge: CUP Archive, 1989.

Kellert, Stephen R., Judith Heerwagen, and Martin Mador. *Biophilic Design: The Theory, Science and Practice of Bringing Buildings to Life*. Hoboken, NJ: John Wiley & Sons, 2008.

Marcus, Clare Cooper. "Healing Gardens in Hospitals." *Interdisciplinary Design and Research e-Journal* 1, no. 1 (2007): 1–27.

Marcus, Clare Cooper, and Marni Barnes, eds. *Healing Gardens: Therapeutic Benefits and Design Recommendations*. Vol. 4. Hoboken, NJ: John Wiley & Sons, 1999.

Nieberler-Walker, K. "Designed for Healing—The Gardens of the Lady Cilento Children's Hospital." In *11th World Congress for Design & Health*. Hong Kong, 2015.

Nieberler-Walker, K., C. Desha, A. Reeve, K. Thompson, and O. El Baghdadi. "Working in Partnership to Mainstream Green Spaces in Healthcare Settings: Case Study of Conrad Gargett." World Health Congress, Vienna. Brisbane, Australia, 2017.

Reeve, Angela, Cheryl Desha, and Omniya El Baghdadi. "Nature-Based Design for Health and Well-Being in Cities." In *Routledge Handbook of Sustainable Design*, 399–414. New York: Routledge, 2017.

Reeve, Angela, Katharina Nieberler-Walker, and Cheryl Desha. "Healing Gardens in Children's Hospitals: Reflections on Benefits, Preferences and Design from Visitors' Books." *Urban Forestry & Urban Greening* 26 (2017): 48–56.

Sherman, Sandra A., James W. Varni, Roger S. Ulrich, and Vanessa L. Malcarne. "Post-Occupancy Evaluation of Healing Gardens in a Pediatric Cancer Center." *Landscape and Urban Planning* 73, no. 2–3 (2005): 167–183.

Söderback, Ingrid, Marianne Söderström, and Elisabeth Schälander. "Horticultural Therapy: The 'Healing Garden' and Gardening in Rehabilitation Measures at

Danderyd Hospital Rehabilitation Clinic, Sweden." *Pediatric Rehabilitation* 7, no. 4 (2004): 245–260.

Ulrich, R. S. "Effects of Gardens on Health Outcomes: Theory and Research." In *Healing Gardens—Therapeutic Benefits and Design Recommendations*, edited by C. Cooper Marcus and M. Barnes, 27–86. Hoboken, NJ: John Wiley & Sons, 1999.

Ulrich, Roger S. "View Through a Window May Influence Recovery from Surgery." *Science* 224, no. 4647 (1984): 420–421.

Ulrich, Roger S., Robert F. Simons, Barbara D. Losito, Evelyn Fiorito, Mark A. Miles, and Michael Zelson. "Stress Recovery During Exposure to Natural and Urban Environments." *Journal of Environmental Psychology* 11, no. 3 (1991): 201–230.

Whitehouse, Sandra, James W. Varni, Michael Seid, Clare Cooper Marcus, Mary Jane Ensberg, Jenifer R. Jacobs, and Robyn S. Mehlenbeck. "Evaluating a Children's Hospital Garden Environment: Utilization and Consumer Satisfaction." *Journal of Environmental Psychology* 21, no. 3 (2001): 301–314.

Wilson, Edward O. *Biophilia*. Cambridge, MA: Harvard University Press, 1984.

Chapter 12

Lean Design
The Everett Clinic at Smokey Point

Barbara Anderson, Melanie Yaris, and Julia Leitman

12.1 Introduction

With the Affordable Care Act's major provisions taking effect in 2014, the new Accountable Care Organization (ACO) model designed to achieve a "triple aim"—better care for patients, better health for populations, lower cost per capita—shifted varying degrees of financial responsibility for patient outcomes from the payer level to the provider level. Healthcare organizations would be reimbursed based on outcomes, not volume. This was a significantly different way of thinking and operating, and The Everett Clinic (TEC) wanted to get ahead of the curve.

As the healthcare paradigm began to shift, new models of care delivery were emerging, profoundly affecting the built environment. Clinical care was becoming increasingly team-based and highly collaborative, with greater emphasis on preventative care. Outpatient volumes were increasing, but care was still being administered in clinics designed around outdated care delivery models. Lean methods offered a clear solution, helping providers to understand their current state of operations and inform ideal care processes that would, in turn, enable them to design clinics around streamlined workflows. These developments set the stage for the design of TEC's Smokey Point Medical Center. Completed in 2012, the Smokey Point Medical Center is an example of how healthcare delivery models have evolved over the last decade—and how healthcare facility design has evolved with it.

12.2 Applying Lean Thinking to Healthcare Design

It is well known that the U.S. healthcare system is highly inefficient, and there have been several attempts to address these issues at a national scale. Based on the model developed by Toyota, Lean thinking was first introduced into the

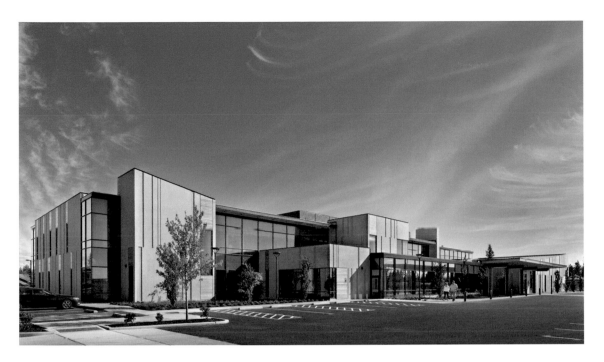

▲ Figure 12.1

South-facing exterior entry.
Source: Benjamin Benschneider

manufacturing sector and greatly influenced corporations such as Ford, Boeing, and Nike. Lean thinking focuses on reducing waste and maximizing operational efficiency and productivity through process improvement. Recognizing that humans are not widgets and delivering healthcare is not an assembly line, the tenets of Lean can still be applied to the planning of healthcare facilities. More importantly, Lean provides a conceptual framework for tackling the problem of waste in healthcare.

The concept of developing the most efficient use of staff time and resources is integral to the design of the physical environment. When Lean processes are in place within the healthcare setting, patients benefit from quality physician time, improved safety, and fewer delays in receiving care. In the case of TEC's Smokey Point Medical Center, these results are evidenced by a reduction in patient cycle times (the time between arrival and discharge) from 52 to 38 minutes, a 26% improvement. Staff also benefit from fewer non-value-added steps and by having what they need, where they need it, when they need it, which allows them to focus fully on patient care.

12.3 Achieving Lean Design Through Integrated Design Events

In order to achieve Lean outcomes, a series of workshops called integrated design events (IDEs), which address operational planning concurrent with conceptual and functional design, are held. IDEs are staffed with consistent, cross-functional clinical and nonclinical representatives charged with exploring and identifying how care will be delivered and how processes will be modified to support these new ideas. The events are tailored for the specific project and structured to guide participants through quantitative and qualitative decisions, focusing not only on data and metrics but also on the importance of elements such as natural light, color, and furniture. Engaging cross-functional teams ensures everyone who has a role in making and sustaining these changes is at the table. Working with cross-functional teams also provides the greatest value to problem solving because every step is important to the good of the whole, and investment from each participant is key to identifying and sustaining change.

Operational planning is the foundation for functional design and the key to creating a well-designed, patient-centered environment. By investing in this process, participants work together within IDEs to develop how the space and workflows are intended to function. They, in turn, are often best equipped to educate and lead their colleagues during the implementation phase of the project.

Throughout the IDE process, the design team helps clinicians and staff visualize, assess, and test their existing and future work processes using a variety of tools and strategies. Together, participants track the "seven flows of medicine" widely recognized by Lean experts as an important exercise and lens through which to identify waste. These seven flows involve patients, families, staff, supplies, equipment, medications, and information. This ensures that the result is both a team and a facility that brings everything together in the right place, at the right time to safely and efficiently deliver care (with added flexibility for the future). Keys to a successful IDE include the following:

- Trust in the process: Lean results are driven by guiding principles, clear visioning, continuity of stakeholder involvement, leadership guidance, and constant validation of design results. Lean results are achieved using IDEs as a vehicle.
- Ensure consistent participation of an integrated team: The team should include organizational leadership, clinical stakeholders, design team, contractor, and key partners and owner representatives.
- Establish a project management processes: Define roles/responsibilities, schedule, decision making, communications, and protocols for the project.
- Identify shared assumptions: Determine the constraints on the functional planning work—budget, structural grid, building size, mechanical, electrical and plumbing systems, and program. There should be a clear understanding of project goals and parameters.
- Structure the IDE activities: Teams should be provided with an understanding of the goals, issues, and constraints; support free thinking of ideas; and provide opportunities to test and simulate. Evaluate ideas and concepts to reach recommended solutions.
- Create report-outs: Summarize work completed during each IDE and all relevant findings. These reports keep the entire group informed, including those who did not attend the IDE, and cultivate accountability with leadership. Questions and discussions are encouraged, documented, and incorporated when appropriate.

Barbara Anderson et al.

12.3.1 Lean Thinking in Action for Continuous Improvement

Part of an IDE is determining where Lean design can be implemented, which depends on the organization's appetite for change. Some organizations wish to rebrand and rethink their model of care, while others wish to address key inefficiencies yet keep many existing processes in place. Following these methods typically challenges traditional architectural phases. Successful IDEs occur at the beginning of the design process, shifting time and resource allocation to bring all stakeholders into the discussion early. It is important for all stakeholders to understand that a higher level of commitment, as well as respect, honest communication, and transparency, forms the foundation of an effective team.

Ensuring Lean thinking is present in the IDE, planning, and design process requires five sequential steps that move clients from thinking about how they currently operate—current state—to how services can be improved in the future state:

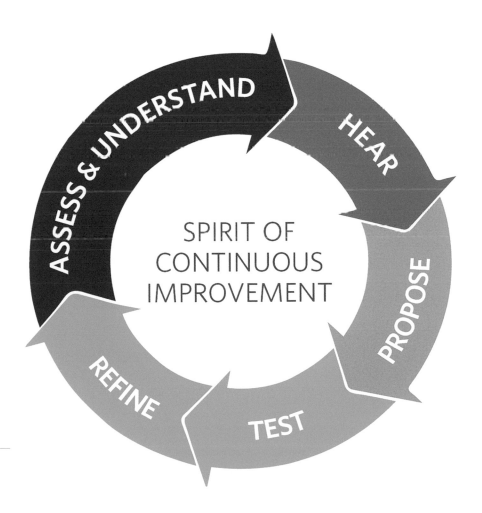

▶ Figure 12.2

Five steps to ensure Lean thinking.
Source: ZGF

1. Assess and understand the current state: Assess and document the current state of operations and space through the lens of what to "keep", "change", or "add". Identify key areas that work well, those that require improvement, and where there are gaps. Through a guided tour of the actual place of operation (called a Gemba walk), in this case the existing clinic, the team sees where and how the work occurs (not how it should be). During this visit, the team identifies and documents areas for improvement—where there are variation, waste, errors, and frustration—and, most importantly, prioritizes which issues can be addressed through architecture. Those that are operationally focused are listed for the client to address internally.

2. Hear the voice of stakeholders: Identify the wants and needs of patients, families, clinical staff, and TEC leadership to provide a baseline for evaluating ideas for improvement. Often the various stakeholders are surprised to hear they share common needs and wants, and this process helps build consensus around key concepts and requirements.

3. Propose improvements to space and operations simultaneously: Ensure that all participants have a clear understanding of the overall process and how they can make an impact. It is helpful to provide participants with concrete examples so they can make the connection between Lean strategies and spatial ideas and how the two inform and impact one another. When people can make a direct correlation between concepts and improved outcomes for patients and staff, there is often a high level of team engagement and opportunity for innovation.

4. Test improvement proposals: Create a "living lab" (in TEC's case, this took place within a large, empty warehouse), where innovation and testing occur throughout design development. Mock-ups provide opportunities to test scenarios and socialize ideas with stakeholders who are not directly involved in the design process. The scale varies for each client and project, from full units to individual modules and rooms.

5. Refine improvements to create standard work: Making work more predictable and reducing variability are both Lean tenets that result in minimizing waste throughout the system and increasing value for patients, staff, and the clinic as a business enterprise. "Pilots" can be used to test and refine ideas in real time and make improvements along the way.

12.4 Overview of The Everett Clinic

Founded in 1924, The Everett Clinic (TEC) is a nationally recognized physician group providing care to more than 330,000 patients throughout Washington State each year. With approximately 2,400 employees, including nearly 600 specialty and primary care providers, it also is one of the largest employers in Snohomish County.

In the early 2000s, TEC grew its market share in north Snohomish County, an hour's drive north from Seattle, and was well positioned to serve an influx of new residents moving into the area. Its current facilities were aging and overtaxed, while competition entered the market. With the Smokey Point Medical Center, TEC had, for the first time in its nearly 90-year history, the opportunity to develop a new prototype multi-specialty clinic from the ground up. The project team included ZGF Architects, J.R. Abbott Construction, Inc., Alliance Project Advisors, Joan Wellman & Associates, Inc., Affiliated Engineers, Inc., Coughlin Porter Lundeen, and Michael Courtney Design, Inc.

The vision was clear. When TEC embarked on the journey to build this new facility, it was a chance to dramatically reimagine the workplace and streamline and enhance the patient experience by reducing wait times and providing comprehensive care for over 20 specialty clinics in a single, easy-to-access location. In addition to primary care, the clinic offers specialty care in behavioral health, cardiology, oncology, obstetrics and gynecology, urgent care, diagnostic imaging, and more. At the time of the planning, the goal was set to cut the time that a patient spends waiting by more than 25%, meaning patients would be in an exam room and talking to a medical assistant about two minutes after arriving at the clinic.

The new facility would enable TEC to create a hub for the region that delivers 90% of patient care services outside of the main campus. With a projected three- to five-year volume of 160,000 patient visits per year, this new space also would help attract new talent, reduce costs, and increase revenue potential.

12.5 Lean Planning and Design Process

TEC had been on a Lean journey several years prior to the planning and design of Smokey Point, enabling improvements in existing clinics and a shift in culture. Leadership understood that their continued dedication to the Lean process was crucial to this project's success. ZGF used a Lean design approach to the programming and design of the clinic, working with a team of care providers, physicians, nurses, medical assistants, laboratory and radiology technicians, receptionists, supply chain staff, and patients. The team worked collaboratively with the architect, contractor, project manager, and clinic leadership to create a facility fully focused on TEC's number one core value: "Do what is right for the patient".

The process began with a kick-off core team workshop to establish a governance structure, a shared vision, and guiding principles and objectives centered around the client's core values. Results from this workshop were assembled in a project charter, an iterative document that became a road map for the project. The charter outlined the required project resources, budget schedule, and the organization's goals and expectations in one place. The charter was continuously updated and shared among team members, ensuring that all stakeholders worked together in unison.

Through eight IDEs held over the course of eight months, the team worked together to collectively make decisions in pursuit of a common goal: create the most efficient means of delivering safe, quality care while keeping the "voice of the patient" at the heart of every decision. The team started the process by going to TEC's existing clinic and mapping the steps involved for each key clinical process (the current state). This window into current operations revealed areas of waste and highlighted opportunities for increased efficiency, most notably the fact that each clinical specialty was equipped

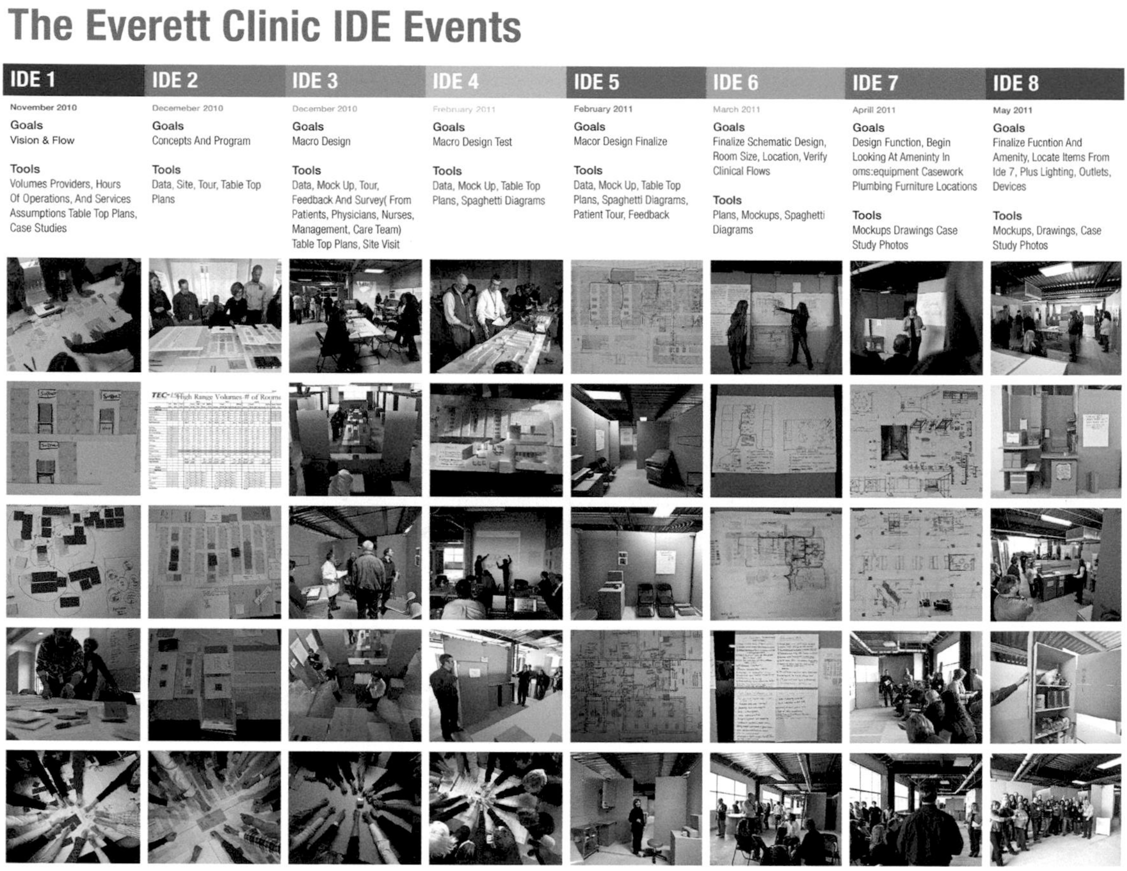

The Everett Clinic IDE Events

IDE 1	IDE 2	IDE 3	IDE 4	IDE 5	IDE 6	IDE 7	IDE 8
November 2010	Decemeber 2010	December 2010	February 2011	February 2011	March 2011	Aprill 2011	May 2011
Goals Vision & Flow	**Goals** Concepts And Program	**Goals** Macro Design	**Goals** Macor Design Test	**Goals** Macor Design Finalize	**Goals** Finalize Schematic Design, Room Size, Location, Verify Clinical Flows	**Goals** Design Function, Begin Looking At Amenity In oms:equipment Casework Plumbing Furniture Locations	**Goals** Finalize Fucntion And Amenity, Locate Items From Ide 7, Plus Lighting, Outlets, Devices
Tools Volumes Providers, Hours Of Operations, And Services Assumptions Table Top Plans, Case Studies	**Tools** Data, Site, Tour, Table Top Plans	**Tools** Data, Mock Up, Tour, Feedback And Survey(From Patients, Physicians, Nurses, Management, Care Team) Table Top Plans, Site Visit	**Tools** Data, Mock Up, Table Top Plans, Spaghetti Diagrams	**Tools** Data, Mock Up, Table Top Plans, Spaghetti Diagrams, Patient Tour, Feedback	**Tools** Plans, Mockups, Spaghetti Diagrams	**Tools** Mockups Drawings Case Study Photos	**Tools** Mockups, Drawings, Case Study Photos

▲ Figure 12.3

The Evert Clinic's eight integrated design events.
Source: ZGF

with its own dedicated space and staff. The siloed arrangement translated to duplication of resources, erratic utilization of space, staff delays, and long patient wait times.

Turning the traditional design process inside out by first identifying strategies for operational improvement allowed the team to optimize the building program and develop appropriate architectural solutions in parallel to support the program. Working in a "living lab" environment where team members could challenge current thinking and quickly cycle through ideas, they tested and simulated each potential solution, mapping flows and travel distances with spaghetti diagrams, creating tabletop exercises to examine various ways of arranging program elements, and building full-scale mock-ups. The team also invited community members and patients to test the mock-ups and report their experiences through on-site surveys so that the team could immediately incorporate their feedback into the design. In total, over 120 patients and staff reviewed and tested mock-ups throughout the process.

Barbara Anderson et al.

12.6 Vision, Guiding Principles, and Goals

The guiding principles for Smokey Point, established in the project charter, included the following:

- Define value in patient terms
- Identify processes that enhance and add value
- Eliminate all non-value-added steps
- Make the remaining value-added steps flow smoothly
- Pursue perfection by continuous improvement

These principles were then distilled into two overarching design goals focused on creating the optimal care environment for the clinic:

1. Create an operationally efficient clinic design that supports the delivery of the most effective patient-centered care that can be replicated easily in future facilities
2. Utilize a holistic approach to design to enhance value and the user experience

These overarching goals were then used to structure a series of subgoals and design strategies and solutions, discussed in the next section.

12.7 Create an Operationally Efficient Clinic Design That Supports the Delivery of the Most Effective Patient-Centered Care That Can Be Replicated Easily in Future Facilities

Using a patient-first lens, the team identified elements that patients value most in a clinic and explored architectural solutions that would enhance their experience. With a focus on minimizing waste and any non-value-added steps, the clinic was designed to optimize patient flows, allowing care providers to move through the stages of care efficiently. The team also recognized the clinic had to be designed for flexibility so space could be easily reconfigured to meet changing patient needs.

12.7.1 Ease of Wayfinding Through Centralized Check-In

Understanding that the patient experience begins with arrival and check-in, the team developed strategies to maximize efficiency in these operations. When studying the clinic's current state, we found that check-in procedures were performed by staff who were also dedicated to several other functions and that patients frequently did not arrive with completed paperwork, records, insurance information, and other critical items. This caused delays and longer wait times. To address this issue, the team shifted check-in responsibilities to the off-site resource center staff, streamlining the amount of space and time required to properly prepare patients for their appointment. This strategy also provided patients with clear wayfinding and a welcoming arrival.

Medical assistants stationed in clinic team spaces were electronically notified when patients had checked in and were ready to be brought to an exam room. These solutions reduced patient visit lead times from 53 to 40 minutes,

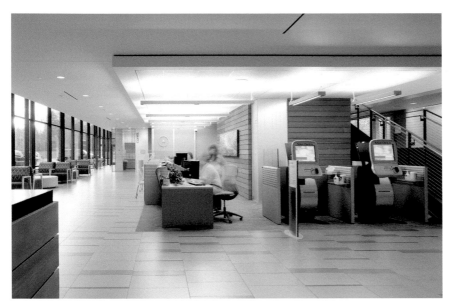

◀ Figure 12.4

The team anticipated advancements in kiosk technology by incorporating a "plug-and-play" modular furniture system in the check-in area, allowing workstations to be easily transformed into electronic kiosks as the adoption rate grew.
Source: Doug J. Scott

which minimized the need for large waiting areas. Instead, the team provided small "pause areas" designed for momentary breaks, leading to a 23% reduction in non-patient care space and contributing to overall savings of $2.1 million.

12.7.2 Create Flexibility Through a Standardized Clinical Module

After analyzing exam room utilization rates, service demand, clinic schedules, and flows and synergies between specialties, the team identified an ideal exam room size and layout that would function as a universal standard, eliminating the need for dedicated exam rooms for each specialty. The exam rooms were right-sized, growing from 80–100 square feet to 120 square feet, allowing them to accommodate intake functions, such as weights and measures, and the needs of all specialists. Additionally, the layout was designed to maximize transparency and open space, and minimize the number of fixed monuments, encouraging eye contact between care providers and patients.

The team went two steps further. First, they recognized that shared exam rooms among the different specialties reduced the exam room need overall, from 80 to 60 rooms. By mapping the 60 exam rooms over the site, the team discovered the optimal clinical care module, which was then replicated throughout the building. Second, in concert with a calming patient experience and clear wayfinding, exam rooms were double-sided and team spaces were located on the inside of the module.

Flexibility was a key driver in the design of the exam rooms, which were planned as same-handed rooms with equipment housed in identical locations, allowing care providers to be instantly oriented and familiar with operations in any given space. The rooms were tested for each specialist, ensuring optimal performance, and were supplemented by multi-purpose rooms that could be used for additional services, consultations, non-assigned workstations, or

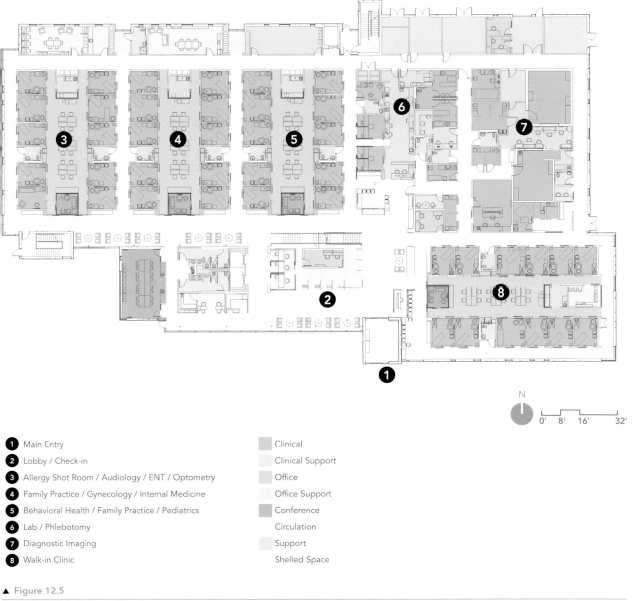

1 Main Entry

2 Lobby / Check-in

3 Allergy Shot Room / Audiology / ENT / Optometry

4 Family Practice / Gynecology / Internal Medicine

5 Behavioral Health / Family Practice / Pediatrics

6 Lab / Phlebotomy

7 Diagnostic Imaging

8 Walk-in Clinic

Clinical

Clinical Support

Office

Office Support

Conference

Circulation

Support

Shelled Space

N

0'   8'   16'   32'

▲ Figure 12.5

TEC first-floor plan.

telemedicine. This standardization and sharing among specialists led to an increase in exam room utilization from 55% to 75%.

The resulting clinical care module became the "DNA" of the clinic—the foundational piece around which team workspaces, circulation, and support spaces were placed. Each clinical module was composed of team space, eight exam rooms, two procedure rooms, two restrooms, and one multi-purpose room. The team determined the number of modules that were needed to serve the initial volumes of patients and provided shelled space for two additional modules, which were fitted out for increased capacity as needed. By creating a shared, universal module that eliminated the need for designated space for each specialty, the team was able to reduce the total number of exam rooms by 25%. The efficient footprint, coupled with the reduction in non-patient care space, enhanced collaboration among care providers, reduced patient visit cycle times by 25%, and improved patient and staff satisfaction, recruitment, and retention rates.

12.7.3 Avoid Distractions and Inefficiencies Through Onstage and Offstage Circulation Paths

Circulation and wayfinding are key elements of the patient experience. In analyzing the current state, the team observed a lack of separation between onstage functions (those that involve interaction with patients) and offstage functions

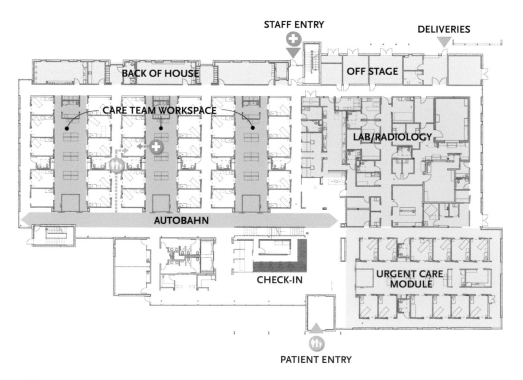

▲ Figure 12.6

Distinct circulation paths for staff and patients maximize efficiency and create a calm, soothing experience for both groups. Double-sided exam rooms with team space located inside the module help maintain onstage/offstage separation.

Barbara Anderson et al.

(the work that goes on behind the scenes). This lack of separation created distraction and inefficiencies for both patients and staff.

Once the clinical module was established, the team created a major circulation path that leads all patients directly from the entry to each clinical specialty with the aid of wayfinding graphics, color cues, and natural light. Referred to as the Autobahn, this separation of flow minimized travel distances and created a calm, soothing environment. The team created a back-of-house staff entrance, which connects directly to work and support spaces, to maintain offstage circulation. Materials and waste also enter and exit the building from this offstage zone.

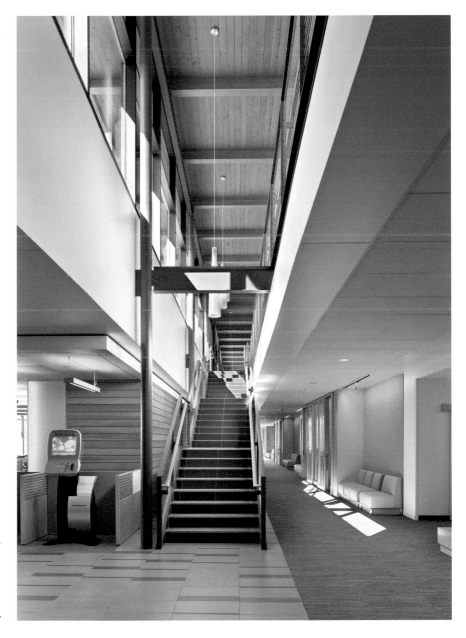

▶ Figure 12.7

The Autobahn provides clear wayfinding on both levels, leading patients directly to exam rooms for each specialty.
Source: Benjamin Benschneider

12.7.4 Enhance Communication Through Collaborative Teaming Areas

Committed to optimizing operations and enhancing patient-centered care, TEC physicians and leadership championed an organizational shift from a collection of siloed specialties to an integrated, collaborative network characterized by systemic thinking and team-based care. Seeing opportunities to improve upon traditional workspace arrangements, which housed each physician in his or her own private office and grouped medical assistants in a different part of the clinic, the team designed open, collaborative workspaces where physicians and medical assistants now work side-by-side. This co-location improved communication, productivity, and patient safety.

In lieu of private offices, the team provided a "green room" for physicians—a dedicated place of respite—to account for the reduction in privacy inherent in the shift to a collaborative workspace. However, once the physicians adapted to the new model of team-based care, utilization of the green room was so low that the space was repurposed for clinical function.

The implementation of team-based care, in combination with more efficient facilities, allowed care providers to perform "standard work", meaning the sequence of tasks is standardized and repeated in the same manner by each team member. This is a Lean tool for minimizing waste, improving patient safety, making work as predictable as possible, and forming the baseline for continuous improvement. At TEC, key elements of standard work include completing patient charting in real time at the conclusion of each patient visit and providing each patient with an after-visit summary. This practice supports physicians in keeping their work "in flow" and reducing delays by completing required paperwork as they go, rather than in large batches at the end of the day. The team also implemented a daily management system in which morning huddles promote situational awareness and communication, preventing delays to the clinic schedule later in the day.

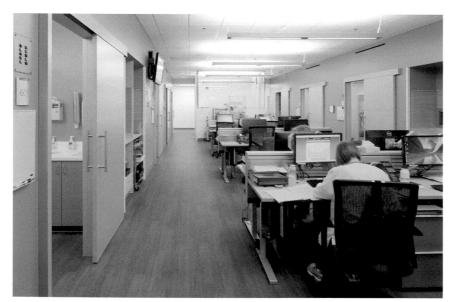

◄ Figure 12.8

The facility has no dedicated physician offices. Instead, care teams are co-located to encourage collaboration across care specialties.
Source: Doug J. Scott

Barbara Anderson et al.

12.7.5 Address All Patient Healthcare Needs in One Visit Through a One-Stop Shop Concept

Feedback from patients throughout the design process revealed the desire to have the clinic serve as a one-stop shop where they could address all their healthcare needs in one visit. One major obstacle to this was blood draws, which patients typically had to travel to before or after their clinic visit. Committed to bringing phlebotomists into the exam rooms, the team worked closely with laboratory representatives on the team to identify processes and equipment that would allow them to travel from room to room as needed. The team implemented a standard process to summon phlebotomists to the exam rooms and designed an offstage phlebotomy workstation where equipment and supplies are housed for easy access. Specimens are immediately transported to the lab through the back-of-house corridor. Nicknamed "water striders" because of their mobility, these phlebotomists drastically reduced the patient cycle time, increased patient satisfaction, and improved clinical operational efficiency by ensuring that patients were prepared for future appointments.

In the end, defining operational changes prior to space requirements, and then testing those changes in parallel with design solutions, was a successful approach. Instead of starting with a list of program spaces and arranging those to fulfill adjacency and square footage requirements, the operational process and the space for that process were designed simultaneously. A program on its own has little meaning or value relative to process and flow; rather, space is shaped and defined by operations just as operations are shaped and defined by space. The Lean process integrates traditionally linear programming and schematic design phases into a consolidated, iterative effort where proposed operational and space plans are tested, analyzed, refined, and then tested again. The engagement of patients, staff, and leadership results in alignment around future operations, a program, and design that is within the scope and budget. This is an outcome of the work, not a starting point.

12.8 A Holistic Approach to Design Enhances Value and the User Experience

12.8.1 Create Attractive Aesthetics That Are Low Cost Through an "Affordable Elegance" Concept

The design of the clinic is largely driven by the budget and goals for the project. A modest tilt-up concrete shell provides a low maintenance, durable finish that was produced on-site using local sand and gravel and accented by Northwest-harvested cedar. Vertical reveals irregularly spaced across the concrete façade create visual impact, scale, and texture to mitigate the mass of what is essentially a "big box".

Northwest-harvested wood accents provide a sense of inviting warmth and contrast to the concrete. To bring the warmth inside, ZGF took advantage of shorter ceiling spans to create an exposed heavy timber roof above the entry.

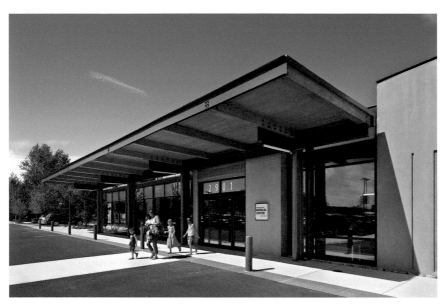

The entry on the south side is flanked by a steel and wood canopy surrounded by storefront windows, welcoming patients to the facility.
Source: Benjamin Benschneider

The glass curtain wall and storefront windows allow natural daylight to penetrate deep into the building. As a result, the entry is washed with daylight toward the public circulation space, which is situated just beyond the check-in area. Amenities are available off the main entry lobby, including comfortable seating along the window, a self-serve Starbucks coffee machine, and a warm fireplace with seating and artwork.

Modularity and flexibility are recurring themes throughout the building. Healthcare is changing so rapidly that facilities need to "flex" to allow the healthcare provider or building owner to reconfigure spaces to meet the needs of physicians and patients—in a cost-efficient manner. For this project, it was important to balance the first cost with the long-term value of flexibility. Demountable partitions and systems furniture are used in key areas with the highest likelihood for change, such as workspaces, patient check-in, and registration.

The Lean process also resulted in features that were both innovative and flexible, such as pivoting tables in each exam room developed to support consultation and education or to provide a functional area for blood draws and blood pressures. When not in use, the tables are positioned against the wall, removing a barrier between care providers and patients. The tables also conceal printers for after-visit summaries, while panels designed to mount computers, blood pressure cuffs, and educational materials hide the wiring and cables within, resulting in a clean, clutter-free aesthetic.

Another Lean principle is to make things visible. The rooms are intentionally devoid of fixed cabinets or casework. They rely instead upon a daily supply cart provided and stocked for the specific clinics of the day, making it easy to replace for another specialty. This has translated into a more efficient and denser

Barbara Anderson et al.

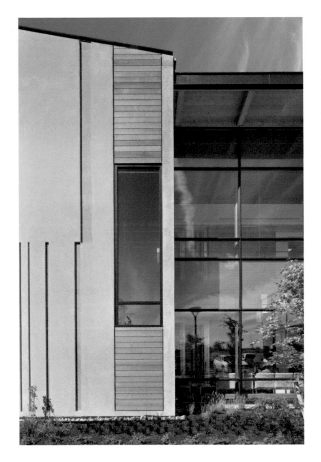

▲ Figure 12.10

Inspired by Italian mathematician Fibonacci, the sequence of vertical reveals provides a subtle but intentional connection to nature that carries through the building from the outside in.
Source: Benjamin Benschneider

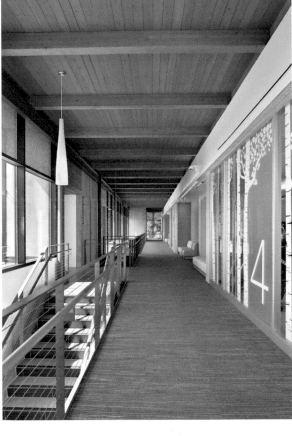

▲ Figure 12.11

Windows at the end of corridors help with orientation and wayfinding, providing views to adjacent green spaces.
Source: Benjamin Benschneider

use of the rooms because specialty services can be easily scheduled in almost any room.

12.8.2 Create a Calming Interior Through Therapeutic and Sustainable Material Choices

The interior palette is intentionally straightforward. Materials were sourced locally, manufactured, and assembled for maximum value, durability, and minimal environmental impact. As users move through the space, intuitive wayfinding and environmental graphics reflect a healing environment that soothes and connects with nature. Onstage areas (check-in, procedure scheduling, and triage departments) are clearly labeled with a variety of decals and raised lettering on glazed panels and doors.

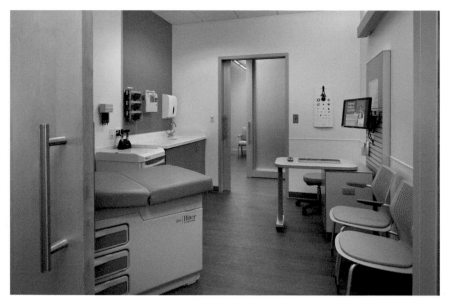

◀ Figure 12.12

Enlarged exam rooms allow care to be easily brought to each patient and accommodate a wide range of specialties.
Source: Benjamin Benschneider

12.9 Conclusions

To date, the Smokey Point Medical Center has received numerous design awards, including the American Institute of Architects (AIA) National Healthcare Design Award and the Healthcare Interior Design Competition's Citation of Merit in Healthcare Design. The continued success of the organization as a highly efficient, patient-centered, flexible, and sustainable facility is rooted in the operations of TEC clinicians and staff, who were partners in the restructuring of their care model. Also critical were the structure and support provided by TEC leadership, who championed the process and were actively engaged in the IDEs.

After establishing a successful Lean prototype at Smokey Point, ZGF partnered again with TEC to design a two-story, 44,000-square-foot clinic—which repurposed an existing grocery store—in Shoreline, Washington. Based on the Smokey Point module, the Shoreline clinic was designed in just six weeks using a Lean, cross-functional approach. It opened its doors in 2016, with many of the same spatial relationships as the Smokey Point Medical Center.

Today the Smokey Point Medical Center still serves as a prototypical state-of-the-art ambulatory, urgent care, and multi-specialty clinic, designed to incorporate Lean principles from the ground up. The planning and design process, and consequent changes to operational efficiency, highlights how integrating Lean thinking into facility development provided an opportunity for TEC to define a new model of care. Outcomes demonstrate that the resulting model continues to improve the health of patient populations, reduce the cost of healthcare on a per capita basis, and increase the number of patient visits each day. The new paradigm also aligns with the ACO's triple aim, and its de-siloed nature continues to foster close interaction between patients, providers, and staff.

Chapter 13

Employee Wellness
The Dan Abraham Healthy Living Center at Mayo Clinic

Peter G. Smith and Stephen N. Berg

13.1 Introduction

The National Institute for Occupational Safety and Health has studied workplace stress in the healthcare industry for almost two decades. It is common knowledge that healthcare workers often work long hours, have heavy workloads, and face high expectations. These factors can lead to occupational distress, burnout, and even physical illness. In a 2014 survey by CareerBuilder, healthcare providers reported higher levels of stress than any other industry, with 69% of workers reporting moderate stress and another 17% claiming high stress levels.

Healthcare organizations need to address this problem head on to ensure that employees are engaged and have a positive sense of well-being. Organizations that realize the importance of employee well-being and have incorporated wellness programs are seeing benefits beyond lowered healthcare costs and employee satisfaction. In one study, employees leveraged wellness programs to make lifestyle changes, and ended up saving their companies on average $353/year per employee due to 10.3 hours of recouped productivity (Mitchell, Ozminkowski, and Seth Serxner 2013). Wellness programs can reduce absenteeism, increase productivity, reduce stress, and promote a culture of support and engagement, ultimately fostering the camaraderie that is required for employee retention.

For Mayo Clinic to successfully promote wellness to the public, it is essential that its employees reflect the healthy lifestyles they are advocating. Healthcare is a people-centric industry, where employees play a critical role in the services exchanged. As the U.S. population ages, the demand for healthcare services makes it difficult for providers to deliver consistently high levels of care. Healthcare administrators are continually dealing with the recruitment and retention of experienced professionals, delivering quality care, and patient satisfaction. In a Gallup study (Paller and Evan 2004), it was found that hospitals employing the least engaged nurses spend $1.1 million more per year in malpractice claims than those with the most engaged nurses.

Mayo Clinic's commitment to wellness is evident through one of the nation's largest wellness centers that serves not only employees and their families but also the public. The Dan Abraham Healthy Living Center (DAHLC) was originally built in 2007 to provide fitness and wellness programs to employees and their families. In 2014 the building was expanded to offer wellness services to the public as well. The DAHLC is an inspiring and accessible center that combines the best knowledge, equipment, and research in fitness, nutrition, and clinical care. Environments like the DAHLC that promote wellness continuously and proactively can help maximize an individual's physical, mental-emotional, and social functioning.

13.2 Mayo Clinic's Journey to Wellness

Mayo Clinic is a nonprofit organization dedicated to clinical practice, education, and research. Its flagship campus, and home to the Dan Abraham Healthy Living Center (DAHLC), is in Rochester, Minnesota. Additional Mayo Clinic campuses are in Arizona and Florida, and the Mayo Clinic Health System has dozens of locations in several other states (Mayo Clinic, n.d.). Mayo Clinic has approximately 40,000 employees in its Rochester location, and another 46,000 dependents, totaling $350 million in healthcare costs per year (Olsen and Warren 2011). Providing a state-of-the-art wellness center not only helps reduce healthcare costs but also improves employees' ability to maintain healthy and balanced lives. Since its creation, the DAHLC has received recognition as a national leader among corporate wellness programs.

With the financial help and vision of businessman and philanthropist Dan Abraham, Mayo Clinic began a journey to better the lives of its employees. For many years, Mayo Clinic managed employee health and wellness through a suite of offerings, including health risk assessments, online telephonic coaching, a 24-hour nurse care line, individualized web-based health risk management, education programs, treatment tools, benefit incentive programs, a healthy living newsletter, disease management programs, and comprehensive general and specialty healthcare. In addition, the Rochester campus had two small on-site fitness centers. These two satellite fitness centers were introduced in 1995 and 1998 as an amenity to employees. Following the success of these centers, Mayo Clinic started the planning process for the DAHLC. It opened in 2007, dramatically changing the worksite wellness offerings to employees.

The timeline of wellness offerings at Mayo Clinic is outlined in Figure 13.1, beginning in 1994, when Dan Abraham first committed to fund a wellness center for employees. Later phases were completed in 2007 and 2014.

The DAHLC first opened in 2007 as a three-story, 110,000-square-foot building providing access to state-of-the-art physical fitness areas, nutrition guidance, and an abundance of wellness programs. Membership is open to not only employees but also their spouses and adult dependents ages 18–24. Spouses make up 15% of the membership and adult dependents account for 2%. Thirty percent of employees on the Rochester campus are DAHLC members. Current

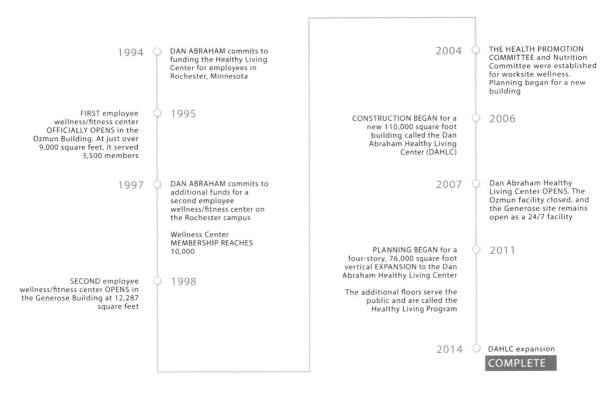

1994 — DAN ABRAHAM commits to funding the Healthy Living Center for employees in Rochester, Minnesota

FIRST employee wellness/fitness center OFFICIALLY OPENS in the Ozmun Building. At just over 9,000 square feet, it served 3,500 members — 1995

1997 — DAN ABRAHAM commits to additional funds for a second employee wellness/fitness center on the Rochester campus

Wellness Center MEMBERSHIP REACHES 10,000

SECOND employee wellness/fitness center OPENS in the Generose Building at 12,287 square feet — 1998

2004 — THE HEALTH PROMOTION COMMITTEE and Nutrition Committee were established for worksite wellness. Planning began for a new building

CONSTRUCTION BEGAN for a new 110,000 square foot building called the Dan Abraham Healthy Living Center (DAHLC) — 2006

2007 — Dan Abraham Healthy Living Center OPENS. The Ozmun facility closed, and the Generose site remains open as a 24/7 facility

PLANNING BEGAN for a four-story, 76,000 square foot vertical EXPANSION to the Dan Abraham Healthy Living Center — 2011

The additional floors serve the public and are called the Healthy Living Program

2014 — DAHLC expansion **COMPLETE**

▲ Figure 13.1

Project timeline.
Source: BWBR

membership is approximately 15,545 people, with employees making up 73% of that total and the remainder being family members. Some of the most popular services at the DAHLC are drop-in group fitness classes (over 150 classes are offered per week) and small group training services. In total, there are nearly 4,000 users every day.

Mayo Clinic extended its wellness mission in 2014 when the DAHLC received a four-story, 76,000-square-foot vertical expansion for wellness programs to serve the public. Referred to as the Healthy Living Program, this service of Mayo Clinic provides a unique and revolutionary experience to people who wish to achieve and sustain wellness. For many people, finding a practical healthy lifestyle program they can maintain over time can be difficult. Mayo Clinic launched the Healthy Living Program as a comprehensive wellness program based on research, not based on current trends. The goal is for people to adopt healthy behavioral changes in diet, exercise, and stress management/resiliency, therefore improving their overall quality of life. The Mayo Clinic Healthy Living Program is organized by teams of experts, including physicians, therapists, health and wellness coaches, dieticians, fitness instructors, child care providers, researchers, and many other positions that support the mission of the DAHLC. They use clinical experience and research to help people break down barriers, dispel myths, and give participants a comprehensive wellness experience tailored to their individual goals. What makes the program unique is that it offers ongoing support long after the person returns home.

13.3 DAHLC Goals and Objectives

Mayo Clinic's goal is to improve the health status and well-being of employees on the Rochester campus by implementing effective wellness practice, education, and research strategies. Mayo Clinic's vision for worksite well-being is to be the healthiest workforce in America, understanding that healthy employees translate to a better patient experience and increased productivity. Wellness programs were designed with outcome-based measurements to promote continuous improvement that would lead to engagement and behavior change over time. The leadership at Mayo Clinic recognizes the importance of healthy living in prevention and treatment of many chronic diseases. They believe employees are the greatest asset to the organization, therefore, the leadership is committed to improving employee health.

To achieve this overarching goal, Mayo Clinic examined five strategic initiatives for the creation and operation of the wellness programs being offered to employees and the public. These were: (1) assess the population for health risks, considering preferences and unmet needs; (2) develop organizational policies that support a healthy living culture; (3) maximize workforce engagement and behavior change strategies; (4) design and deliver appropriate targeted healthy living interventions; and (5) measure effectiveness of initiatives.

13.4 Project Team and Process

BWBR and design partner Dewberry, selected to design the new Center, utilized an interactive client-centered project approach to begin the programming and design process. Along with the design team, Mayo Clinic gathered world-class experts from various medical fields to discuss program elements included in this groundbreaking wellness center. The project approach began with visioning sessions to engage Mayo Clinic employees and experts, empowering them to make critical decisions and build consensus. This was accomplished through active listening, asking questions, testing assumptions, and proposing new parameters to validate project needs and budget. The project was then refined through the space program, conceptual plan diagrams, and exterior design concepts. The project approach yielded a collaborative spirit, effective communication, and a common vision.

13.4.1 Programmatic Elements

During the visioning sessions, Mayo Clinic introduced its three pillars of wellness, which were used to develop programs, services, spatial adjacencies, and the overall character of the spaces. As defined earlier in this anthology, wellness is a relative state where one maximizes their physical, mental, and social functioning in the context of supportive environments. Using the definition of wellness as a starting point, Mayo Clinic introduced nutrition, physical fitness, and resiliency as its three pillars of wellness. All the programmatic elements focus around these pillars in the planning and design of the DAHLC.

Mayo Clinic's three pillars of wellness.
Source: BWBR

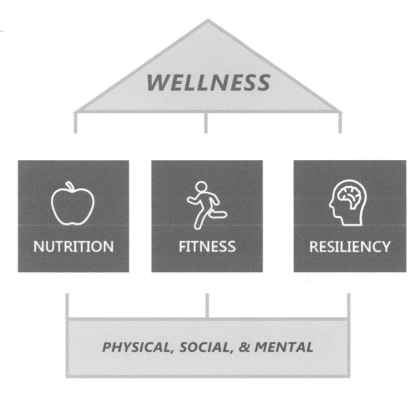

Nutrition is the first pillar because a healthy diet can benefit an individual's physical, mental, and social well-being in considerable ways. Eating well has positive effects on your body, including disease prevention, restful sleep, and weight control. Healthy eating has also been linked to mental state by keeping moods balanced and energy levels up, making it more likely for an individual to seek and enjoy social activities. Within the DAHLC facility, several spaces are dedicated for people to receive personalized nutrition recommendations and guidance to make positive changes in their diet, as well as offer places for people to gather, socialize, and relax.

The second pillar is physical fitness. Mayo Clinic encourages everyone to become more comfortable adding exercise and movement into their daily routines. Fitness areas are provided for individuals to improve on core strength, balance, and flexibility. Introducing exercise not only helps with improving the body's physicality but also offers the promotion of social interaction, teamwork, and bonding. Program elements that support physical fitness include a natatorium, cardiovascular equipment areas, strength training zones, and group fitness rooms of various sizes.

The third pillar is resiliency. Resiliency is defined as the capacity to recover quickly from difficulties (Oxford English Dictionary 1989). To be resilient, it is necessary for a person's emotions and mood to be in a healthy, balanced state. To keep the mind and body primed to deal with all types of situations, a person must develop a sense of resiliency by paying attention to one's needs and feelings, engaging in activities that are fun or relaxing, and exercising regularly (American Psychological Association n.d.). Thus, meditation and relaxation areas are provided to allow mind and body practices to focus on creating awareness, easing stress, and improving overall quality of life. Program elements that support resiliency include wellness evaluation and assessment rooms, meditation rooms, seating alcoves, outdoor spaces, and a spa complete with a massage room, steam room, and whirlpool.

13.5 Design Goals and Solutions

The DAHLC acts as a gateway building for Mayo Clinic, and provides an experience that educates, inspires, and motivates all who visit the facility. Every effort was made to ensure the program is genuine and tailored to accommodate

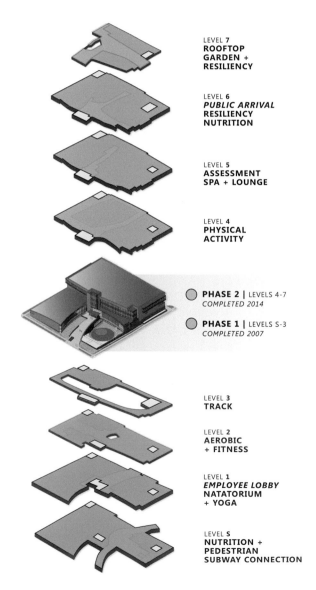

LEVEL **7**
ROOFTOP GARDEN + RESILIENCY

LEVEL **6**
PUBLIC ARRIVAL
RESILIENCY NUTRITION

LEVEL **5**
ASSESSMENT SPA + LOUNGE

LEVEL **4**
PHYSICAL ACTIVITY

○ **PHASE 2 |** LEVELS 4-7
COMPLETED 2014

○ **PHASE 1 |** LEVELS S-3
COMPLETED 2007

LEVEL **3**
TRACK

LEVEL **2**
AEROBIC + FITNESS

LEVEL **1**
EMPLOYEE LOBBY
NATATORIUM + YOGA

LEVEL **S**
NUTRITION + PEDESTRIAN SUBWAY CONNECTION

◀ Figure 13.3

Building axonometric showing programs across levels.
Source: BWBR

lifestyles of the users. Design inspiration revolved around creating a welcoming and calming environment, one that builds confidence and hope in its users without being intimidating or ostentatious. Throughout each level, there are spaces offering healthy nutrition, physical fitness, and resiliency. To illustrate how the planning and design of the Center aimed to achieve the three programmatic pillars, eight design goals and corresponding design solutions are introduced.

13.5.1 Design Goal 1: Create a Facility that is Accessible and Encourages High Utilization

The building is carefully sited along a main pedestrian corridor between parking ramps and the adjacent medical facilities where employees work. With seven stories

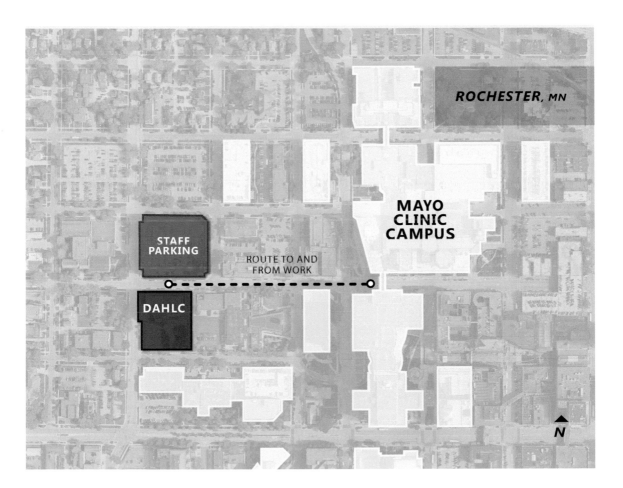

▲ Figure 13.4

Mayo Clinic campus.
Source: BWBR

above-grade and one below, the building is connected to the larger Mayo Clinic subway system via underground pedestrian tunnels. DAHLC's convenient campus location is key to employee utilization of the building.

13.5.2 Design Goal 2: Establish a Building Infrastructure to Allow Vertical Expansion to the Existing Building While Maintaining Cohesiveness and Beauty

The original building designed in 2007 was planned to accommodate a future vertical expansion. Structural elements were sized to allow for additional floors, and elevator shafts were planned for expansion as well. It was important to select an exterior cladding material that could be easily adapted for a cohesive future expansion, making the terracotta rainscreen system a strategic choice. The vertical expansion of the Dan Abraham Healthy Living Center was completed in 2014, and nearly doubled the size of the original building by adding 76,000 square feet divided between four stories and a 20,000-square-foot rooftop terrace.

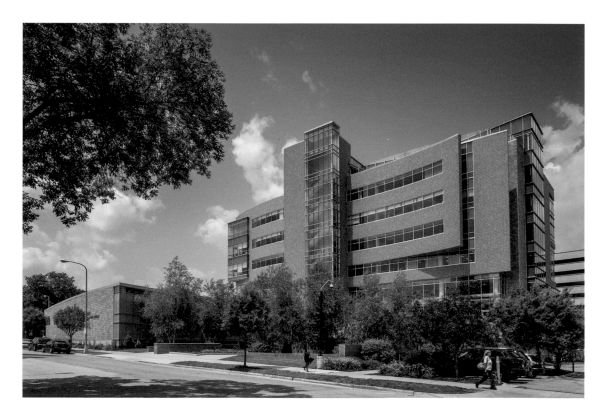

▲ Figure 13.5

Completed vertical expansion—Phase 2.
Source: Brandon Stengel, www.farmkidstudios.com

Peter G. Smith and Stephen N. Berg

13.5.3 Design Goal 3: Create a Landmark Building That Showcases the Promotion of Wellness by Allowing People to View Healthy Activities Inside and Encourage Inspiration

Clad in terracotta panels with expanses of fritted and clear glass curtainwall, the building represents the quality that people associate with Mayo Clinic. The exterior façade conveys a dynamic expression of stretching, tension, and movement. The floor to ceiling glass wall of the running track is cantilevered out beyond the terracotta, thereby putting energy and movement on display. Through the implementation of warm materials and bold building forms, the design of DAHLC is noticeable unique and conveys the importance of health on the Rochester campus. To signify the importance of wellness in the Center, there is an expansive glass curtain wall to allow people outside of the building to view the healthy activities inside, encouraging inspiration and curiosity.

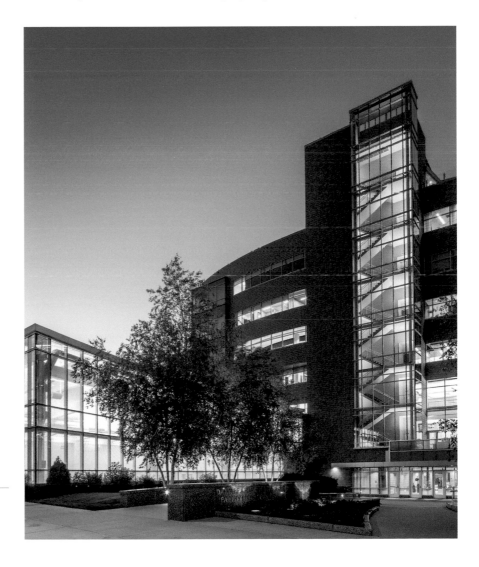

▶ Figure 13.6

Primary building entrance and natatorium.
Source: Brandon Stengel, www.farmkidstudios.com

13.5.4 Design Goal 4: Accommodate Flexibility and Adaptability as Needs, Opportunities, and Ideas Arise

A research-based organization like Mayo Clinic requires a building with flexibility to maintain state-of-the-art wellness programs. Structural bay dimensions were maximized to offer potential for the reconfiguration of spaces. Individual areas were designed to allow Mayo Clinic to adapt offerings as programs progress into the future. For example, the fitness studio spaces incorporate mechanical systems that allow for a range of thermal conditions required for hot yoga, meditative fitness classes, or active exercise requiring a cooler environment.

13.5.5 Design Goal 5: Create a Welcoming, Light-Filled Environment With Connections to Nature

Natural daylight and a connection to nature are paramount to the project, and nearly all occupied spaces have access to natural daylight. The site was excavated on the south side to unearth a portion of the building, therefore allowing natural daylight into the building's subway level. The excavated area was

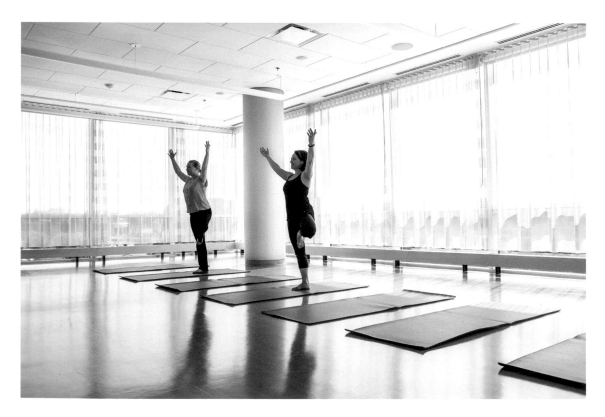

▲ Figure 13.7

Yoga and meditative fitness studio.
Source: Brandon Stengel, www.farmkidstudios.com

Peter G. Smith and Stephen N. Berg

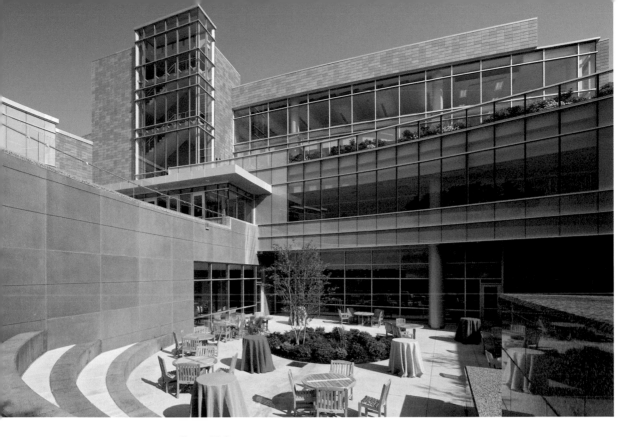

▲ Figure 13.8

Courtyard and outdoor café—Phase 1.
Source: Don F. Wong

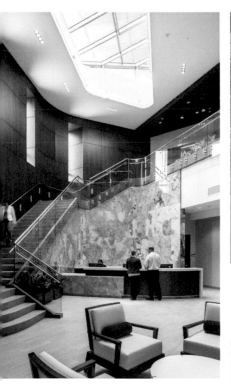

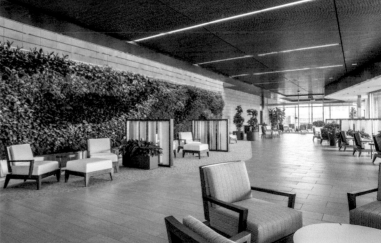

▲ Figure 13.10

Resiliency area with living wall.
Source: Brandon Stengel, www.
farmkidstudios.com

◀ Figure 13.9

Main lobby of the Healthy Living Program.
Source: Brandon Stengel, www.farmkidstudios.com

designed as a terraced courtyard so people can enjoy the outdoors and have access to the benefits of fresh air and sunlight.

The cardiovascular/fitness area is open to the jogging track above, creating a large two-story volume with generously sized windows flooding the space with daylight. Daylight from the skylight on the upper most floor floods into the lobby of the Healthy Living Program on Level 6, where guests begin their inspiring journey to long-lasting wellness. Bringing nature indoors, as seen with a 60-foot-long "living wall" and skylight, reflects the importance of access to natural features.

13.5.6 Design Goal 6: Encourage Physical Activity

DAHLC features a natatorium, which contains a four-lane, 25-yard lap pool, a warm-water therapy pool, and steam rooms. The facility contains many fitness amenities including aerobic exercise studios, yoga and meditative studios, a three-lane jogging track around the building perimeter, and several other fitness areas. A teaching studio with treadmill workstations promote learning/training while simultaneously achieving non-strenuous physical activity. In addition to programmed fitness spaces, other design elements were used to promote physical activity. Open staircases rich with daylight were strategically placed to encourage choices in vertical movement, and outdoor courtyards/terraces used for fitness activities can be seen by those passing by.

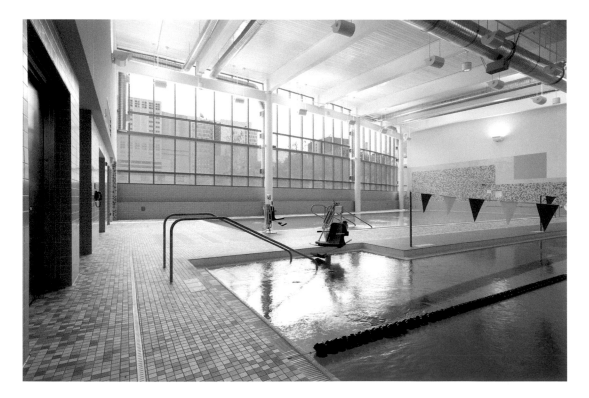

▲ Figure 13.11

Natatorium.
Source: Don F. Wong

Peter G. Smith and Stephen N. Berg

▶ Figure 13.12

Teaching studio with
treadmill desks.
Source: Brandon Stengel,
www.farmkidstudios.com

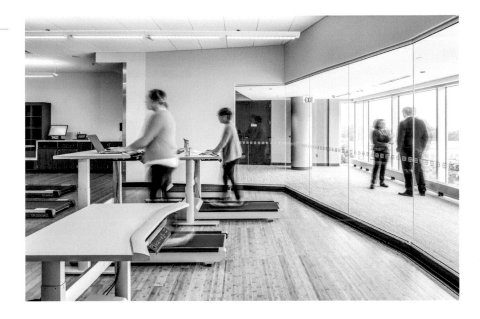

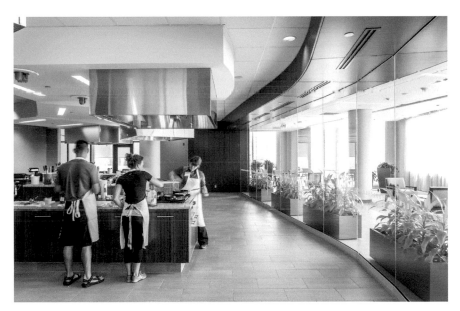

13.5.7 Design Goal 7: Promote Healthy Eating Habits and a Holistic Understanding of Nutrition

A centrally located café serving healthy meal options is directly adjacent to an outdoor courtyard for access to natural daylight and fresh air. The outdoor courtyard is used for socialization, relaxation, and a seasonally operated farmer's market. Individuals taking part of the Healthy Living Program can make their own meals in a state-of-the-art participation kitchen. There is a dining room adjacent to the kitchen, so groups can not only learn to cook healthy meals, but also enjoy the

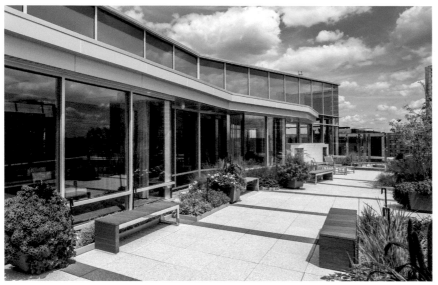

◄ Figure 13.14

Exterior resiliency area on
the rooftop terrace.
Source: Brandon Stengel,
www.farmkidstudios.com

meals that they have prepared together. For those who are on the go, nourishment stations are located throughout the facility to provide water and healthy snacks.

13.5.8 Design Goal 8: Achieve a Sense of Resilience and Regeneration by Relaxing the Mind and Soul

There are many program elements that support resiliency, including an employee wellness evaluation and research clinic, assessment rooms, meditation rooms, relaxation studios, and a spa complete with massage room, steam room, and whirlpool. The meditation rooms were designed with low ambient lighting, natural stone, and sapele wood panels to create a calming interior. Resiliency spaces are located on Levels 6 and 7 so they are not only away from potentially disruptive areas but support easy access to the outdoors via the rooftop terrace.

13.6 Evidence of Successful Design

Mayo Clinic prides itself on building strong relationships between employees and patients. By creating a profound experience, Mayo Clinic respects the emotional and personal connections that become present between patients and employees. These connections are a solid foundation for the ongoing success of people in their personal and professional lives.

Key objectives of the project were to maximize employee engagement and achieve sustainable results. With the target audience being the non-traditional exerciser, an incentive program was introduced to reduce the membership cost for more frequent use. Mayo Clinic has studied how frequency of use has affected health outcomes and healthcare costs of employees. Frequent users (those who visit the facility three times per week or more) enjoyed 36% lower healthcare costs and 13% lower body mass index (BMI) than infrequent users. Therefore, wellness center attendance was associated with significantly lower healthcare costs and BMI improvement.

Mayo Clinic considers the project to meet and continue to exceed its objectives. Return-on-investment (ROI) data supports statistically significant changes in healthcare costs and reduced BMI for frequent users. Mayo Clinic reports also indicate successful outcomes, high utilization of available services, and high satisfaction rates of employees.

13.7 Conclusions

The DAHLC provides a high level of wellness through a balance of care, fitness, nutrition, and natural and spiritual awareness, all in the heart of a city's urban core. It is a model for how organizations can encourage their employees and the public to enjoy a positive lifestyle that incorporates the best practices of exercise and nutrition. The DAHLC is conducting research and education on healthy living so the Center can serve as a corporate wellness program exemplar to help people and organizations throughout the United States and around the world.

Healthcare organizations are becoming more focused on overall wellness, not just medical event-based treatments. By providing both medical care and wellness programs in one location, care teams can collaborate to provide services that address the whole person. Research has made clear that being physically fit is not enough, and that nutritional, mental, and social health are equally important. Healthcare facilities are an asset to the community, not just a place to be treated for illness but also a place where people can receive whole-person care.

Acknowledgments

Special thanks to Mayo Clinic; the Dan Abraham Healthy Living Center design partner Dewberry; the project team, including Alvin E. Benike, Damon Farber Associates, IMEG Corp./LKPB Engineers, and Meyer Borgman Johnson; and the many individuals of BWBR, all of whom were instrumental in creating a building that allows Mayo Clinic to flourish as a leader in healthcare and wellness.

Bibliography

American Psychological Association. "The road to resilience." n.d. www.apa.org/helpcenter/road-resilience.aspx.

Mayo Clinic. "Dan Abraham Healthy Living Center." n.d. https://dahlc.mayoclinic.org/hubcap/dan-abraham/.

Mayo Clinic. "Mayo Clinic Locations." n.d. www.mayoclinic.org/about-mayo-clinic.

Mitchell, Rebecca J., Ronald J. Ozminkowski, and Seth Serxner. "Improving Employee Productivity Through Improved Health." *Journal of Occupational and Environmental Medicine*, 55, no. 10 (2013): 1142–1148.

Olsen, Kerry D., and Beth A. Warren. "Integrating Health and Health Care." *ACSM Health and Fitness Journal* 15, no. 4 (2011): 29–34.

Oxford English Dictionary, 2nd ed., 20 vols. Oxford: Oxford University Press, 1989. Available at http://www.oed.com/.

Oxford English Dictionary. Oxford: Oxford University Press, 2014.

Paller, Deborah A., and Perkins, Evan. 2004. "What's the Key to Providing Quality Healthcare?" *Gallup Business Journal* (2004). https://news.gallup.com/businessjournal/14296/whats-key-providing-quality-healthcare.aspx.

Chapter 14

From Vice to Wellness
Defining a New Typology in Healthcare Retail Design

Megan Stone

14.1 Introduction

The legal medicinal cannabis industry is a worldwide phenomenon. This chapter will trace the industry's evolution, from its origin in the nineteenth century to modern-day society, where it is gaining widespread acceptance by medical professionals, patients, lawmakers, and consumers. A result of this evolution is the creation of a new building typology, one that combines health, wellness, and education into a unique retail storefront. This holistic approach to design has revolutionized the customer experience and, more importantly, it has increased health and healing outcomes for patients in the United States who rely on medical cannabis to alleviate their health symptoms and treat disease.

14.2 Cannabis History and Evolution

14.2.1 What Is Cannabis?

Cannabis is an ancient, plant-based medicine that has been used worldwide for thousands of years. It was described in the *United States Pharmacopeia* for the first time in 1850 and was widely popular in the U.S. during the nineteenth and early twentieth centuries (Bridgeman and Abazia 2017). The federal government began regulating cannabis in 1937 with the Marijuana Tax Act and dropped it from the *United States Pharmacopeia* in 1942. The Marijuana Tax Act essentially outlawed the possession or sale of marijuana and more stringent federal regulations followed, criminalizing the use of cannabis and restricting its procurement for research purposes (Martin 2016).

In the 1970s, a grassroots movement began promoting the decriminalization of medical marijuana at state and local levels because there were credible reports that cannabis provided relief for a variety of ailments and health symptoms (Martin 2016). These efforts paid off more than 20 years later in 1996, when the state of California passed the Compassionate Use Act, permitting legal access and use of botanical cannabis for medicinal purposes under physician supervision. In agreement with its healing effects, other states followed California's lead, and by November of 2018, 30 states and the District of Columbia enacted laws that allow for limited use of medical cannabis under certain circumstances and for a variety of treatments. Nine of these 30 states and the District of Columbia have also legalized cannabis for recreational use (National Cannabis Industry Association 2018).

In October 2017, a Pew Research Center survey reported that about six in ten Americans (61%) believe the use of marijuana should be legalized, nearly double what that number was in 2000 (31%). Generational and partisan differences in views of marijuana legalization remain, with younger generations of millennials (70%), Gen Xers (66%), and baby boomers (56%) saying the use of marijuana should be legal (Geiger 2018). The trajectory of this acceptance with each generation, compounded with the medicinal benefits of cannabis being more widely recognized, will fuel continued growth in the cannabis industry in the years ahead. This growth creates the context for the design challenge we face today: How can design work with business growth so that patient and consumer health is not affected negatively?

14.2.2 The Rise of Alternative Therapies

According to WebMD and the National Institutes of Health, about 40% of adults in the United States say they use some sort of alternative medicine as a complement to, or replacement of, traditional (mainstream) therapies (Healthcare Global 2015). Examples include probiotics, melatonin, acupuncture, chiropractic care, reiki, fish oil supplements, roseroot, coconut oil, and cannabis. All are believed to possess a variety of healing properties, only some of which have been well studied, which is why practitioners and researchers continue to debate their efficacy (National Center for Complementary and Integrative Health 2008).

Regardless, the mainstreaming of these alternative and complementary therapies can be explained by the shift in the individual's role in his or her own health. Patients and the general public believe deeply in the health benefits of certain therapies, whether they are looking for a natural solution to an ailment or are trying to avoid the oftentimes more financially burdensome traditional healthcare system. Beyond general wellness and illness prevention, spiritual/religious/cultural motivations and the often lower cost compared to prescribed medications appeal to patients as health consumers. As consumers existing within a health marketplace, it is in their best interest to be financially smart, educated about their treatment plan, and willing to explore natural means to alleviate symptoms, reduce pain, and treat disease.

14.2.3 Cannabis Today

Of all the alternative therapies, cannabis arguably is the biggest disruptor to hit cultures and the economies the world over. According to the 2017 edition of the United Nations' World Drug Report, approximately 183 million people (3.8% of the world's population) use marijuana, making it the most commonly used drug globally. Roughly 22% of this global total represents the nearly 40 million cannabis consumers in North America (United Nations' World Drug Report 2017). While these statistics represent both recreational and medicinal users, the impact of cannabis in today's culture is profound.

In some parts of the western United States where medical use and recreational use are legal, cannabis sales are rising dramatically. The roots of this emerging alternative health field lie in underground subcultures rather than mainstream life. Once considered simply an addictive vice, cannabis now is used to treat a wide range of medical conditions, such as cancer, epilepsy, glaucoma, PTSD, multiple sclerosis, and chronic pain.

The *New England Journal of Medicine* polled physicians and clinicians worldwide on cannabis and found that 76% were in favor of the use of marijuana for medicinal purposes, even though marijuana use is illegal in most countries. This study, along with more recent comprehensive reports, concluded that more research needs to be done to move cannabis discussions forward toward an even stronger basis of evidence in regards to health effects (National Academies of Sciences, Engineering and Medicine 2017).

Increased study within the field matches the increase in retail sales of medical and recreational cannabis in the United States, which are projected to hit $8–$10 billion in 2018 (a 50% increase from 2017) and continue rising (Marijuana Business Daily 2018). Throughout the rest of North America, this translates to profits in the tens of billions of dollars, now that legalization has taken effect in Canada. Cannabis today is big business. What once was promoted by a surreptitious world of outlaw independent sellers has developed into a semi-legal network of collectives, now emerging as viable medical and recreational retail establishments. Cannabis as an industry, of course, is subject to ever-changing regulations, medicinal product offerings, patient preferences, and predictions about the future. Medical marijuana dispensary owners constantly seek ways to adapt to the evolving landscape, while being smart about how they serve their customers' health, as well as the needs of the communities in which they exist.

14.2.4 Retail Dispensaries

Today's cannabis dispensaries are a hybrid specialty concept store and holistic therapeutic practice. Market regulations vary widely depending on location, and they have great impact on both the patient experience and retail operations. That being said, there is a set of best practices in design that must be considered when planning and creating cannabis consulting environments for retail. Why best practices? Because design changes perception and experience. Applying holistic design thinking to the medicinal cannabis industry is altering thoughts, feelings, and behaviors worldwide. The four key areas of focus are as follows:

1. Brand design: Developing an identity for the dispensary as well as its expression across various patient touchpoints or areas that support and inform patients

2. Interior design: Creating and documenting the space to accommodate patient, employee, and product flows
3. Retail design: Integrating architecture, industrial design, ergonomics, environmental graphic design, merchandising management, and consumer behavioral psychology
4. Security-led design: Specifying privacy and safety frameworks, along with crime and loss prevention features that have minimal negative impact on the healing experience

This chapter will present guidelines for the four pillars of design that both respond to and craft culture. The guidelines are supported by case study examples of real projects that integrate the health and patient experience with the overall design. How future design professionals approach this new frontier that is at the intersection of retail and healthcare will create a precedent for how alternative medicine can integrate into everyday society as an acceptable and holistic option for individuals.

14.3 Brand Design: Transforming Cannabis Retail

As Dr. Richard Farson asserts in his book *The Power of Design*, design can be harnessed to influence human behavior and effect change (Farson 2008). Since the early twentieth century, the use of cannabis as a plant-based medicine was demonized, criminalized, and defamed despite cannabis's historical use as a natural healer. Today, with effective branding that combines retail, hospitality, education, and healthcare design, cannabis retailers are professionalizing their industry and bringing it out of the shadows of its past while also differentiating their businesses from competitors. The result is a modern medicinal cannabis industry that is altering thoughts, feelings, and behaviors, connecting patients and health seekers to reputable growers and distributors in new legal markets throughout the world.

Modern consumers seek to connect and identify with experiences and people on a deeper level to make more meaningful and memorable connections. Branding today is much more than logos and simple color palettes. Rather, it delves into the core purpose and story behind and within the business. How can the business be an integral part of the patient's health experience? Does the retailer stand for quality? Does it empathize or specialize in a particular product or ailment? Is it locally owned and reputable? Does it have selections that are organic or vegan? Every touchpoint where the patient interacts with the dispensary, whether virtual or physical, must have the application of its visual identity consistently presented. Furthermore, visual identity systems created specifically for the medicinal cannabis industry should be appropriate, memorable, and consistently applied to everything related to it in the dispensary. Identities that portray cannabis in elegant and modern new ways help lift the industry away from the visual clichés of its clandestine past.

Because medicinal cannabis dispensaries face heavy restrictions on how they can market their practices, traditional advertising and promotional activities are often not allowed. This increases the importance of having a well-designed and uniquely branded dispensary environment. Dispensaries need to incorporate aspects of the brand story along with identity elements that are powerful and compelling. Within the space, branding plays an essential role in attracting and engaging patients and facilitating their health and healing journey.

Examples of brand touchpoints in the dispensary environment:

- Exterior storefront: Whether it is discrete or bold, exterior signage must clearly identify the dispensary, be positive and hospitable, while conforming to all legal codes. Restrictions on public views into the dispensary must also be thoughtfully considered.
- Lobbies and waiting areas: The visual identity should be applied in a welcoming, approachable way that sets the tone for the interaction between patient and staff. Seating areas can feature digital signage, promotional materials, and displays that inform and entertain patients as they are waiting to be served. Providing information in these places helps patients understand their various treatment options. The materials specified and design details in these areas establish a distinct first impression.
- Product showrooms: Displays of the cannabis stock, as well as packaging and take-home materials, offer an opportunity for enhancing and extending the patient experience. These showcases make natural plant therapy choices visible in a way that traditional pharmaceuticals, with their chemical ingredient compounds, cannot.

14.3.1 Texas Original Cannabis Company/Texas Original Compassionate Cultivation (TOCC)

Texas Original's Manchaca, Texas, storefront exemplifies a fully branded environment that goes beyond just the placement of branding logos and packaging. All elements of the space connect to the epilepsy-focused design, building on a brand story and its patient-centric values.

The brand identity development drew upon strong Texan iconography to create a logo that conveys a true sense of Texas pride, quality medicine, and professionalism, crucial to establishing itself as reputable in a state with rigid cannabis laws. The investment in the retail space further communicates the brand's dedication to serving the special needs of their epileptic customers and families. A clearly identifiable entrance provides a warm greeting for patients and establishes a distinct sense of arrival.

Material selections were particularly critical for TOCC as patients and families immediately assess their surroundings to ensure safety in case of an epileptic seizure. Hard surfaces, sharp edges, and tripping hazards were minimized in the lobby and throughout the space. Residential-inspired furnishings and décor instill a cozy, comfortable feel. Beyond providing an aesthetically pleasing environment, a sense of comfort and safety is achieved. Every detail communicates the brand's commitment to these specific patients and establishes a level of trust that makes this a memorable and meaningful experience.

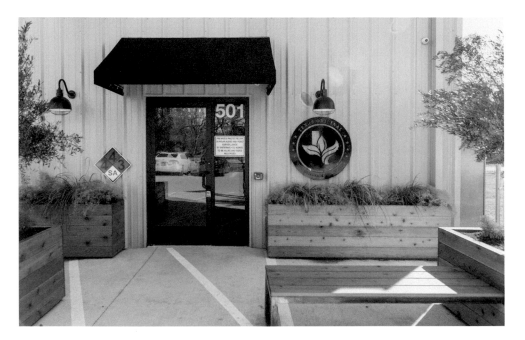

▲ Figure 14.1

Main entrance of TOCC. An activated retail entry adds ambience to the nondescript metal agricultural structure.

Source: Sum and Substance

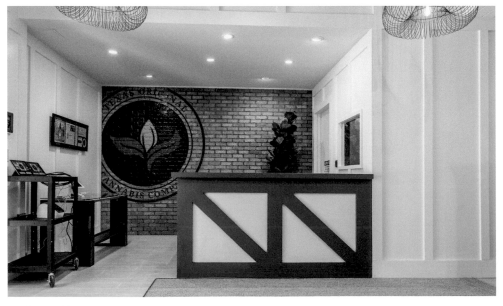

▲ Figure 14.2

The 350-square-foot lobby and dispensary area were designed to instill the comforts of a residential living room (2018).

Source: Sum and Substance

Megan Stone

14.4 Interior Design: Safe Healing Environments

A new frontier in the retail arena, medicinal and adult recreational use cannabis is one of the fastest-growing industries in the United States. Due to its recent legalization, sales are projected to top $20.2 billion by 2021, assuming a compound annual growth rate of 25% (Arcview Market Research 2016). The only consumer industry categories to reach $5 billion in annual spending and post anything near to a 25% compound growth rate were the cable television industry (19%) in the 1990s and the broadband Internet industry (29%) in the 2000s.

Design firms have much to offer this new health sector. Because dispensaries are a retail experience with medical value, they are a new typology at the intersection of retail and healthcare design. Setting a higher standard for this new typology involves carefully considered space planning that addresses both the retail and healthcare experiences of patients, along with their associated privacy, security, and legal necessities. Programmatic requirements, such as public restrooms, private consultation rooms, and vaults, need to be located with this sense of privacy in mind. Air filtration and odor mitigation are other environmental concerns that need to be addressed in the design process. By strategizing to enhance the patient experience, improve business function, and reinvent stereotypes about the use and users of the products, designers play a key role in shifting opinions and developing the future of legalized cannabis.

Key areas to be addressed through space planning and interior design are as follows:

- Decompression zones: Physical and emotional transitional spaces between outside and inside the dispensary that psychologically signal to patients that their well-being and privacy are paramount.
- Reception desk: A safe space for both patients and staff that facilitates all intake activities. Discretion and ease are important factors here as patients surrender identity verification materials and are welcomed into the dispensary.
- Seating areas: Waiting for service is an inevitable part of most consulting practices. Since studies have shown that time spent waiting can have negative impacts, providing music, videos, and literature that educate and entertain can mitigate this issue. Views to the outdoors, access to natural light, and infusion of natural elements into these areas, such as green walls or water features, create a more positive waiting experience and support the health and well-being of both patients and employees. Seating must be comfortable, yet hard-wearing, and accommodate patients with a variety of mobility or ADA issues.
- Private consultation rooms: Private rooms that accommodate a variety of patient types, some of which may have mobility or ADA issues, and their guests (family members or others), should be calm, efficient areas to receive information, education, and consultation that are specific to the individual patient's needs.

- Retail showrooms: Showrooms should be designed to guide customers efficiently and with discretion, through the consultation, product selection, and check-out process. Address ergonomics and accessibility, as universal design is also important for dispensaries. Effective space planning will minimize the number of steps for employees to enhance customer service. Interactions between customers and staff should have minimal interruptions so patients feel well cared for and at ease. Showrooms should also be designed to cater to the more experienced patients who are looking for a consistent and expedited experience. Consider incorporating express order placement and/or check-out areas.
- Back-of-house: Loading bays, storage areas, inventory stockrooms, and employee areas must be designed to support smooth and efficient operations behind the scenes. Prevention of product diversion through open space planning, use of glass-front cabinetry, integration of employee locker rooms and break areas, and electronic access and surveillance systems is imperative, as with any retail business.

Dispensaries can regularly see hundreds of patients and guests daily. This necessitates environments that are durable, yet look clean and polished. Add to this an ever-changing roster of treatment products on the market and dispensaries need to be designed with flexibility in mind as well. As with any interior design for medical environments, the psychology of the patient experience must be considered. Whether it is a first-time patient who is fearful and most likely on sensory overload, or seniors, who are the fastest-growing cannabis consumer demographic, or women, who are an increasingly important customer segment, or the seriously ill and their emotional family members, design can help meet the needs of all guests served.

In all areas, color should be uplifting and convey neither sterile clinic nor dingy "head shop". Lighting should help create an environment that is inviting and memorable. Furnishings need to be commercially durable and easy on the eyes. Taking design cues from retail banks and coffee shops, as well as contemporary medical offices, works well for dispensary interiors.

14.4.1 Level Up Dispensary

With an alluring environment of European-inspired sophistication coupled with a one-on-one consultative experience akin to a fine jeweler, the Level Up dispensary in Tempe, Arizona, showcases best-in-class products and patient education. Programming the space to cater to privacy and efficiency in both the patient experience and business operations was critical to maximize customer service and throughput.

Custom display cases and illuminated shelving showcase products and inform patients about available selections. Designed with a circular customer flow to eliminate bottlenecks in this high-volume store, patients are able to move through the dispensary experience at their own pace while not impacting the flow of the other patients and employees.

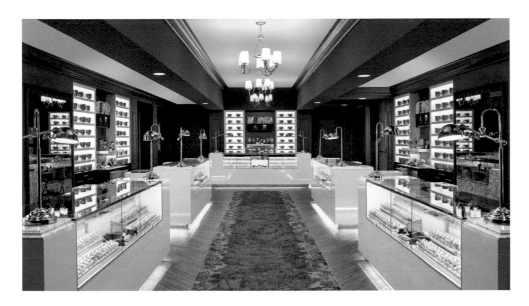

▲ Figure 14.3

Custom display cases and illuminated shelving showcase products and engage customers (2017).

Source: Richard Cadan Photography

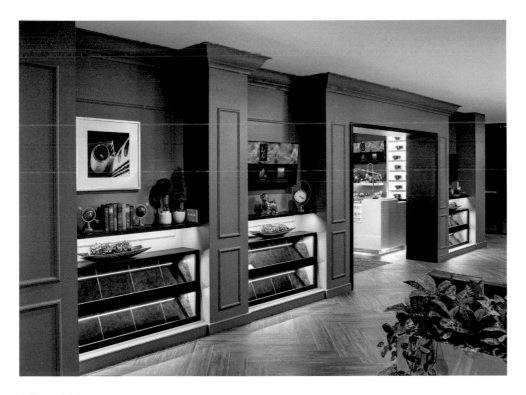

▲ Figure 14.4

Rich, deep tonal colors welcome and calm (2017).

Source: Richard Cadan Photography

14.5 Retail Design: Mixing Health and Comfort

Medical retail cannabis has gone from a consumer base of medical card-carrying individuals with specific needs and tastes to a consumer base of virtually anyone over the age of 21. Leveraging established retail design principles and consumer behavior insights helps dispensaries maintain the professionalism of cannabis retail despite a mixed consumer base of both medical and recreational users.

Through effective design, dispensaries should introduce new patients to all of the healthcare options available to them, help educate them about what is being offered, facilitate selection of treatment, and connect with them emotionally to create informed healthcare recipients who are interested in fully understanding the care they receive.

Merchandising techniques inform the location of cannabis and cannabinoid products on the shelves, determine their adjacencies, and make them easier to understand and select. Cases and fixtures that showcase the treatment options in a secure, well-lit, and comfortable viewing manner (well edited, organized, and ideally located between waist and eye levels) lead to a friendly environment that prompts and promotes patient discussions with health providers.

Here are things to consider for improving the healing experience through effective design in dispensary showrooms:

- Product display fixtures: Because of the size and delicate nature of cannabis, product displays require fixtures that have varying degrees of security and accessibility. Modular components (including shelves, stands, and hanging options) that offer flexibility are able to display a variety of flavors and sizes of products. Secure-access features are often required so the employee can handle a product first before the patient can inspect it. Shelving and displays should be designed with scale in mind, so they never look too empty or overly cluttered. The specified materials and finishes should align with the brand and achieve a cohesive environment.
- Visual merchandising: Products should be displayed to help facilitate education, discovery, and purchasing. Position products at eye level for easy viewing and accessibility for sampling when appropriate. Minimize clutter to maintain the product as the hero while using signage and visual props to create emphasis where needed and to help tell a story. Popular medical options should be displayed within easy reach by the employees, without making the consultants turn their backs on patients. Dispensaries provide the ability to interact directly with products. Display cases that are uniquely designed and arranged can effectively promote all of the product options for consumers. This level of engagement is distinctly different from pharmacies, where health products cannot be sampled, demonstrated, or supplemented with accessories.
- Environmental graphics: Powerful graphics can immerse customers in the brand story. Using lifestyle images or well-photographed product images in dispensary showrooms helps facilitate a deeper connection to the space and adds a level of sophistication to the retail environment.

- Point of sale: Efficiently designed casework helps facilitate speedy trans-actions. This space supports the final moment in the customer journey, so reinforce the brand while providing opportunities to leave a lasting impression.

Surroundings that promote browsing, have unobstructed views of product transactions, and a pleasant ambience that is coupled with skilled and knowl-edgeable sales staff create a well-executed retail experience. Shopper insight consultant Anne Marie Luthro feels strongly that "dispensaries should be com-mitted to educating patients because legal medical cannabis is new and there is a steep learning curve". To her point, there are a variety of cannabis strains and product delivery methods. Plus, there are a range of benefits and drawbacks to each cannabis option. Good retail design aids in providing space and communi-cation strategies that help patients absorb information and make well-educated health decisions (Luthro 2017).

14.5.1 Tru|Med Dispensary

Tru|Med Dispensary in Phoenix, Arizona, was the first-of-its-kind retail space ded-icated to displaying and selling premium concentrates. The goal was to create an approachable yet high-end experience that focuses on high-quality products.

A dedicated display for this modern category of options allows staff the proper space and setting for more intimate consultations, deeper explanations, and

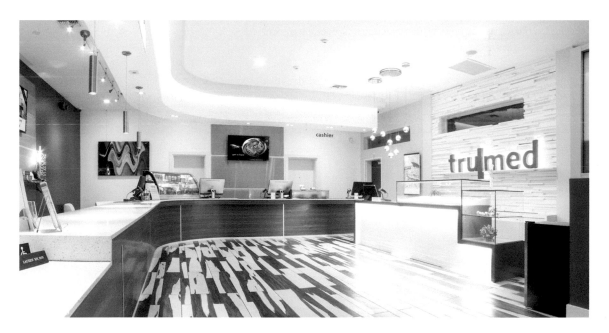

▲ Figure 14.5

A jaw-dropping showcase and feature wall make patients, stop, ask, browse, and learn (2015).
Source: Tien Frogget Photography

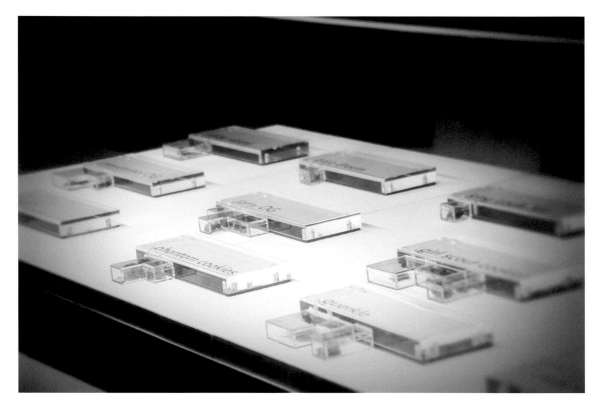

▲ Figure 14.6

The concentrate bar features LED-lit glass displays at counter level (2015).
Source: Tien Frogget Photography

thorough demonstrations. Due to the smaller physical size, this product can be merchandised in a case format similar to jewelry rather than on a shelf behind the counter like other products. In this setting, environmental graphics on digital signage screens flank a feature wall behind the display. Macro photography of concentrate products is used to elevate the product and further brand the display as "concentrates".

14.6 Security-Led Design: Dealing With Safety and Well-Being

Loss prevention, commercial protection, and personal safety are important in any retail business, but even more so at medicinal cannabis dispensaries. In these shops, most transactions are cash-based and require vigilance, unlike other healthcare industry providers. Dispensary design must facilitate discrete private interactions and transactions so that patients and staff can feel at ease, much like a traditional pharmacy. In many markets, the state and/or local regulatory bodies are explicit when it comes to what is required for surveillance, monitoring, and security; but the level of requirements varies greatly state by state. A blend of hardware and software security, along with security-focused design practices, safeguards cannabis dispensaries and their patients.

Megan Stone

Tony Gallo, managing partner of Sapphire Risk Advisory Group LLC, which specializes in loss prevention and security for high-risk retail, likens current cannabis dispensaries to pawn, alcohol, tobacco, and firearms stores, where there is a need to consider both external and internal security (Gallo 2017). In order to mitigate concerns and define these healing practices as part of a safe and approachable new typology, measures must to be taken to provide welcoming environments where security safeguards are seamlessly blended into the fabric of the retail experience. Design helps create this positive perception.

The following security dimensions must be integrated seamlessly into the retail design:

- Access control: Traffic flow and access into and out of the facility itself are an important consideration. Bullet-resistant glass designed to blend with interiors and feel approachable must be used at critical moments of interaction with the public. Limited access zones, and restricted access to back-of-house and other private areas, must also be programmed into the design.
- Surveillance: Lighting must be appropriate to detect and mitigate fraud while also creating a healing mood. Unobtrusive, yet effective, security camera placement throughout the space, but especially at check-in and point-of-sale areas, provides important video surveillance. High-resolution imagery helps identify suspects and ensure employees are adhering to protocols, from on-site or off-site.
- Security systems: Break-ins, shoplifting, theft, and suspicious activity during and after hours may be problematic. Including posted warnings, sensor lighting, vaults, locks, and alarms in the dispensary design program is integral to scaring away would be criminals but not patients. Security guards should be uniformed consistent with the dispensary visual identity.

Dispensaries need to be beautiful spaces that convey a medical tone and adhere to HIPAA regulations for patient privacy. Strictly enforcing security measures is more than good business—it is an essential governmental regulation in many locations.

14.6.1 The Healing Center

The highest level of security is delivered in a mere 335 square feet at The Healing Center in San Diego. In order to conform with some of the most stringent security requirements of any legal cannabis market in existence at the time, all exterior walls, as well as all interior rooms in which employees or product are present, had to be bullet resistant. In this case, every wall, including the interior glass partition system, is bullet resistant. High design can still be achieved under such constraints. The small space feels open and larger due to the lack of solid interior walls. By running the bullet-resistant glass from counter to ceiling, the reception window feels inviting rather than off-putting and clandestine. This application changes the perception of a space with bullet-proof glass while providing employees with a clear view of anyone coming in the front door.

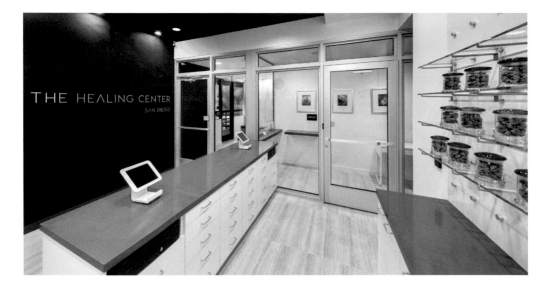

▲ Figure 14.7

Silver-framed bullet-resistant glass partitions—required by local ordinances—separate functional areas but keep the space feeling open and visually accessible (2016).

Source: Richard Cadan Photography

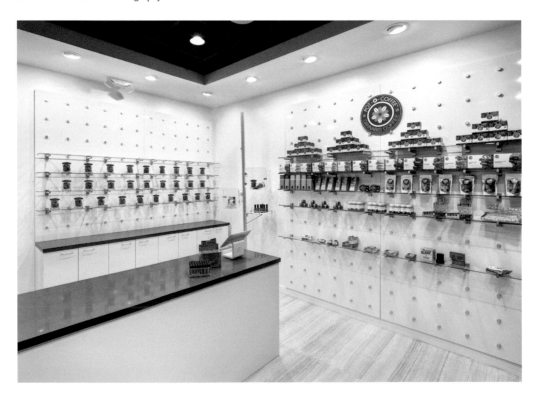

▲ Figure 14.8

Flexible merchandising fixtures utilize vertical space for product displays and provide a more comfortable shopping experience (2016).

Source: Richard Cadan Photography

Megan Stone

14.7 Conclusions

Design changes perception and experience. Applying design thinking to the medical cannabis industry is altering thoughts, feelings, and behaviors worldwide. Since the early twentieth century, the use of this plant-based medicine has been demonized, criminalized, and defamed despite its historical use as a natural healer. The reintroduction of medical cannabis into society continues to battle a unique hypocrisy—people accept the plant as medicine, but they do not accept the industry around the plant as safe and professional. This dichotomy can be addressed by a holistic approach to designing cannabis dispensaries.

The merging of brand, interior, retail, and security-led design makes legal medicinal cannabis retail experiences unlike any others within the health industry. There will come a point in time, many industry leaders believe, where medical cannabis retail will be as accepted and ubiquitous as other health-focused product retailers, such as supplement or juice shops. Forging a positive connection to the cannabis community by creating extraordinary storefront medical practices that are cutting-edge, clean, and professional will transform the patient experience. Further, by considering design's impact on culture, designers can keep health at the center of all design choices for new markets. This is an unparalleled opportunity to change people's perceptions of cannabis by applying design thinking to all aspects of the store environment and patient experience.

The cannabis industry supports hundreds of thousands of jobs, tens of millions of dollars in tax revenue, and billions in economic activity globally, and is poised to continue its growth (National Cannabis Industry 2017). Design is proving to be a powerful tool in altering negative perceptions of this once clandestine industry. Elevating the value of a patient-driven healthcare experience using these practices can enhance the entire community.

Bibliography

"Annual Marijuana Business Factbook." *Marijuana Business Daily*, 2018 Edition. mjbizdaily. com/factbook/.

Arcview Market Research. *The State of Legal Marijuana Markets*. Report. 5th ed. Arcview Group, BDS Analytics, 2016.

Bridgeman, Mary Barna, and Daniel T. Abazia. "Medicinal Cannabis: History, Pharmacology, and Implications for the Acute Care Setting" *P & T: A Peer-Reviewed Journal for Formulary Management* 42, no. 3 (2017): 180–188.

Farson, Richard. *The Power of Design: A Force for Transforming Everything*. Georgia: Greenway, 2008.

Fix, J. (Director of Patient Services, Copperstate Farms). Personal Interview, March 2018.

Gallo, T. (Managing Partner of Sapphire Risk Advisory Group LLC). Personal Interview August, 2017.

Geiger, Abigail, and Hannah Hartig. "62% of Americans Favor Legalizing Marijuana." *Pew Research Center*, October 08, 2018.

Luthro, A. M. (Retail Strategist and Shopper Insight Expert). Personal Interview, August 2017.

Martin, Scott C. "Marijuana in the United States: How Attitudes Have Changed." *Time. com*, April 20, 2016.

National Academies of Sciences, Engineering, and Medicine. *The Health Effects of Cannabis and Cannabinoids: The Current State of Evidence and Recommendations for Research.* Washington, DC: The National Academies Press, January 2017. https://doi.org/10.17226/24625.

The National Cannabis Industry, 2017. Associationthecannabisindustry.org

National Center for Complementary and Integrative Health. "The Use of Complementary and Alternative Medicine in the United States." 2008. https://nccih.nih.gov/research/statistics/2007/camsurvey_fs1.htm.

"State Policy Map." National Cannabis Industry Association, 2018. https://thecannabisindustry.org/ncia-news-resources/state-by-state-policies/.

"TOP 10: Emerging Trends in Alternative Medicine." *Healthcare Global*, June 01, 2015. www.healthcareglobal.com/top-10/top-10-emerging-trends-alternative-medicine.

United Nations Office on Drugs and Crime. "World Drug Report 2017". www.unodc.org/wdr2017/.

WebMD Medical Reference, reviewed by David Kiefer, MD. "What Exactly is Alternative Medicine?" November 2016. www.webmd.com/balance/guide/what-is-alternative-medicine#1.

Part 3 | **Global Health**

This domain is based on the belief that the design of architectural settings should be sustainable, preserve ecosystems connecting geographic areas, and enhance the global environment. An architecture for health at this scale recognizes that the consequences of a project extend far beyond the project itself. People and other living organisms are all directly and indirectly affected by the built environment.

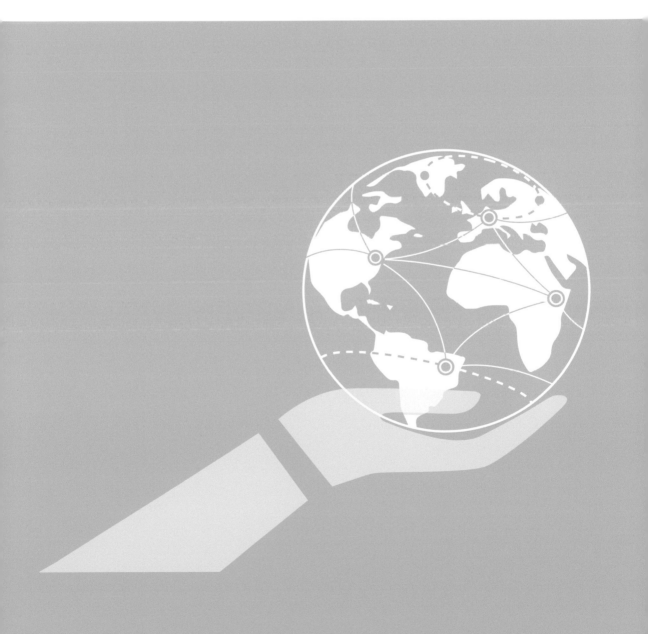

Chapter 15

Outdoor Oncology
A Nature-Inclusive Approach to Healthcare Delivery

Bart van der Salm

15.1 Introduction

The summer of 2015 saw the inauguration of Project Chemotherapy Outdoors, also known as the "Chemotuin" (Chemo-Garden), on the grounds of the Tergooi Hospital in Hilversum (NL). This pavilion offers patients of the oncology department the possibility to receive chemotherapy treatments in the open air. Challenging the idea that healing environments must remain controlled, sterile, and free of outside influence, this progressive project has generated a great deal of interest, both nationally and internationally: firstly, because of its pioneering character from a medical perspective, and secondly, through the symbiosis between architecture and landscape that is manifested within the project. This chapter explores this symbiosis and describes the mutual necessity and reciprocal dependence between architecture and landscape as essential ingredients in realizing healing environments.

15.2 Nature and Healing

While Western medicine primarily focuses on the cure of a disease as the ultimate goal (pathogenesis), complementary (holistic) medicine focuses instead on factors that promote health and well-being (salutogenesis). The immediate environment contributes in this case to disease prevention and quality of life, whereby stress factors and health are in balance with one another (Agnes van den Berg 2005). The effects of restorative feelings can be described by the biophilia hypothesis (Kellert 1993), among other things. As human beings we have an innate affiliation with nature because, as a species, we evolved in a natural environment. In the case of biophilia, natural elements and the natural environment are assigned a healing character (a concept that is expanded upon in later chapters of this book).

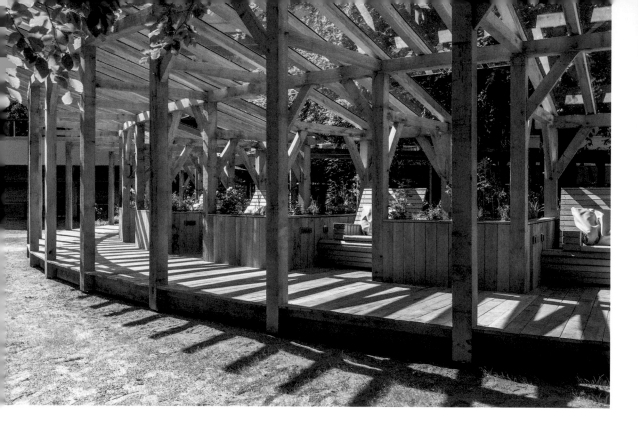

▲ Figure 15.1

The Chemotuin, a pavilion for open-air chemotherapy on the grounds of the Tergooi Hospital in Hilversum (NL).
Source: Design by VANDERSALM-aim; photography by Milad Pallesh

Considered the first healthcare centers in Europe (Agnes van den Berg 2005), the asclepieia (healing temples) of ancient Greece were often erected in wooded valleys near cold and hot sources of water. The narrow, elongated rooms of the dormitories were open on the south side, so that patients could stay in a well-ventilated area warmed by sunlight. Likewise, in the monasteries of the Middle Ages, the position of the central courtyard and botanical garden played an important role, and rooms for convalescence were explicitly designed around these outdoor spaces. Patients were placed in spaces with a direct view outside, in order to take advantage of nature's healing properties. The garden also produced medicinal herbs used in treatment. One of Europe's first "pavilion-style" hospitals was constructed in the eighteenth century in France. From this, a new connection with the natural environment surrounding the hospital emerged. It was assumed that such an environment, with its sunlight and fresh air, would have a therapeutic effect and positively influence patients' health.

The healing effect of fresh air was nonetheless a revived discovery in healthcare during the nineteenth century. Besides a new organizational structure for hospitals, this also brought about the first sanatoria. These were largely built in the first half of the twentieth century for curing patients with tuberculosis and include well-known sanatoria, such as the Zonnestraal in Hilversum (Jan Duiker 1928), the Sanatorium Joseph Lemaire (Fernand and Maxime Brunfaut 1937), and the Paimio Sanatorium (Alvar Aalto 1933). Outside of healthcare, a similar appreciation for fresh air also became apparent in educational institutions in the first half of the

Bart van der Salm

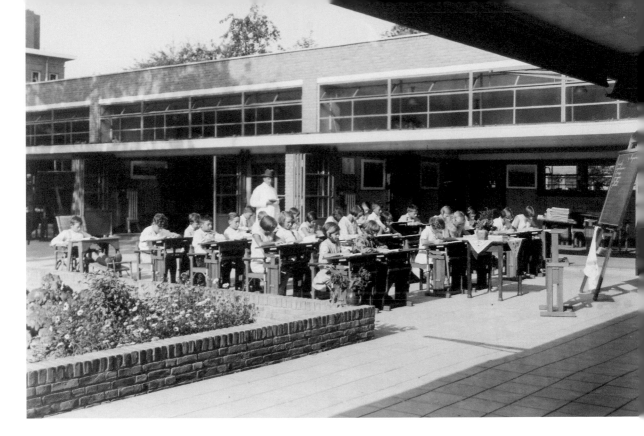

▲ Figure 15.2

At the Dordtse Buitenschool in Dordrecht (NL) the sidewalls of the classrooms could slide open, so that lessons could be taught outdoors in nice weather.
Source: Regionaal Archief Dordrecht, 552–301195

twentieth century, such as at the Elizabeth McCormick Open Air School (Chicago, 1911), École de plein air de Suresnes (Suresnes, 1932), and the Open Air School for the Healthy Child (Amsterdam, 1930). Classrooms were constructed in such a way that the exterior walls of the learning spaces could be opened or pushed aside.

In the late 1970s patients and nursing staff became increasingly dissatisfied with the sterile and unfriendly design of hospitals of the time (Van den Berg, 2005). This led to the creation of Planetree, a nonprofit organization in the United States founded by Angelica Thieriot. In 1978 she wrote,

> As a patient I rebelled against being denied my humanity, and that rebellion led to the beginnings of Planetree. We should all demand to be treated as competent adults, and take an active part in our healing. And we should insist on hospitals meeting our human need for respect, control, warm and supportive care, a harmonious environment and good, healthy food. A truly healing environment.
>
> (Planetree 2017)

Planetree provides guidelines for the design and organization of healthcare institutions and is based on a care environment that combines a domestic character with the presence of natural elements, such as gardens and water elements.

These examples demonstrate how the presence of nature and natural elements has been used to varying degrees for centuries to realize healing environments. Historically, themes like daylight, fresh air, and rest have played an important role in establishing such environments. With today's knowledge, a new element can be added: living with life—that is to say, all types of life. Yet from what design methodology or school of thought would one be able to approach the question of designing a new healthcare environment?

15.3 Nature-Inclusive Design

One methodology closely linked to the creation of an integrated design concept between architecture and landscape (meaning all types of life) is designing from a nature-inclusive perspective. In this design methodology the architectonic spatial task is inherently linked to facilitating opportunities for animals and plants to live and grow.

An advocate of nature-inclusive design is Maike van Stiphout, director of DS Landscape Architects (DSLA) and head of landscape architecture at the Academy of Architecture in Amsterdam. In order to provide insight regarding principles for nature-inclusive designs, DSLA has developed, among other things, a "program of requirements" for animals. This entails an overview in which a wide variety of animal species are linked to the architectural conditions that they require for nesting and habitation. Such conditions relate to the height, orientation, and size of a place. As a practical overview it shows how a large potential to attract various animal species can emerge through relatively simple architectural resources.

Nature provides a variety of needs for us which are vital in importance. Consider, for instance, things like food, fuel, medicine, and clean air. In order to maintain this system, it is crucial to stimulate biodiversity as much as possible (Maike van Stiphout 2014). This is, in essence, a straightforward premise; what we, as humans, seek in our environment, plants and animals need as well—a safe and comfortable habitat with enough food to survive. The question, then, is how to embed these conditions in the design requirements in such a way that we increase the biodiversity of a place through our built environment.

▼ Figure 15.3

The programmatic requirements needed by various animals can be seen in the amenities integrated in the structure's outer perimeter through relatively simple means, in order to provide local species with places to shelter and nest. *Source*: DSLA, Maike van Stiphout

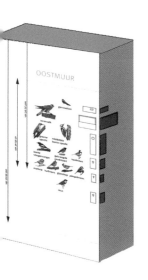
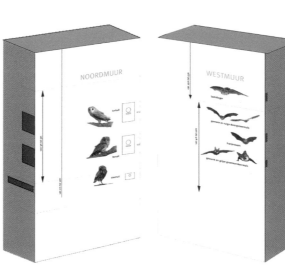
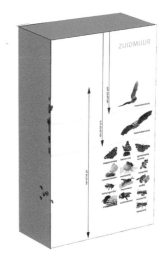

Bart van der Salm

Moreover, the dietary requirements of these animal species are just as relevant as the necessity for habitation. After all, if there is no food, then there is no life. To grasp this concept, it is important to understand the natural food chains that exist between species found on and around a given site. These findings can ultimately be traced back to the smallest "ingredient". Thus, it is possible to determine which plant species attract the smallest animals, which in turn become food for the larger species (e.g., aphid → ladybird beetle → finch, etc.). Because these plants form the basis of new food chains, the specific dependencies between these species is essential. If this cohesion is suitably manifested, then the right conditions will arise and an increase in biodiversity will be achieved. Nature-inclusive designs do not happen by chance; agreeable and location-specific environments for plants and animals are created by means of targeted design tools.

15.4 Grounding: A Marriage Between Architecture and Landscape

Understanding historical exemplars, biophilia, and nature-inclusivity, a healing environment can arise only through an intimate relationship between architecture and landscape; in other words, from physical manifestations of all types of life. We can speak of a healing environment only when that environment positively contributes to improved well-being—to a better quality of life. This is a broad concept, and based on this description it can apply to different situations. When we apply this thinking to a controlled medical environment, or to the individual perspective of a patient, the terminology can become more specific. Of course, the consequences of being sick or remaining in a medical environment involve practical, legal, and operational frameworks as well, especially in relation to the free-radical of nature.

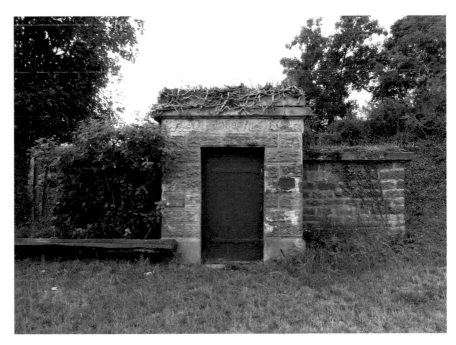

▶ Figure 15.4

A marriage between architecture and nature; this is an example of a structure where both entities are equivalently relevant. Here architecture is nature and nature is architecture; each is inseparable from the other. *Source*: Photography by VANDERSALM-aim

Nevertheless, it is this field of tension in which a marriage between architecture and landscape proves to be of both mutual necessity and reciprocal dependence. This perspective indicates a situation in which a spatial design is anchored in its own network of service and operation. On one hand, both entities need each other; on the other, they also provide one another with content.

If we consider architecture as a static entity and landscape as a dynamic entity, a friction, or energy, emerges at their interface. The manner in which this energy manifests in a design stands in direct relation to the pieces of the whole. This can lead to a number of different outcomes. Firstly, it can be the sum total of different starting points (1 + 1 = 2). Secondly, the result can be more than the sum of the parts (1 + 1 = 3). Thirdly, the outcome of a spatial design can fuse into a single gesture (1 + 1 = 1).

The first outcome is a symbol of the practical solution—a situation where the potential between architecture and landscape remains unused. This results in the merging and stacking of outcomes within the context of the question. The outcome is logical and sound, and follows the program of requirements, yet lacks innovative character in achieving a better outcome than that posed by the design task itself. In the second outcome an intelligent interpretation of the assignment is sought, along with an elaboration upon the question to achieve a better result. Landscape and architecture come together here in an organized visual language that is both pleasant and comfortable. The final point of view leads to a significantly different outcome; here, a connection linking the assignment to the landscape's intrinsic qualities and the architectural appearance is sought. Neither can be considered independently of the other, as both serve one another and are designed based upon a single methodology.

Something special happens in the physical-spatial experience of this last scenario, defined here as the phenomenon of "grounding". This feeling of grounding occurs when, as a user, one not only gains a visual perception of space but also experiences a sensory experience that is all-encompassing—an environment where smell, sound, taste, and touch, together with sight, provide a new spatial dimension. Within architectural theory such sensory spatial experiences are grouped under the concept of phenomenology. An outspoken proponent of this form of architecture is Juhani Pallasmaa, a Finnish architect and former professor of architecture.

In his book *The Eyes of the Skin*, Pallasmaa (2012) describes the ability of our body to observe space versus the unilateral faculty of visual perception. Pallasmaa argues that the body is able to remember space through sensory experiences. Consciously or unconsciously, the body reads "atmospheres" and incorporates these into itself. Through these experiences, memories are stored in a personal spatial "library". This library forms the basis of how we experience our present environment. This will be different for each individual as well; in which spatial environments, for example, do we feel comfortable, lonely, or strengthened?

This sensory experience of space is intensified through the merger of architecture and landscape. A completely new palette of elements arises in relation to single spatial (architectonic) experiences. Take, for instance, the scent of wet leaves, the light warmth of the sun on your chair, the rustling of branches, the tang of the autumn air, a vista over the fields: all in all, it is an experience that appeals to every sensory perception. Such a collective experience adds a memory to our physical and mental consciousness, and synchronizes these elements into (the internal creation of) gestalt—in other words, experiencing a physical connection with a place or experience. The most intense sensory experiences could be described as "primitive spatial experiences". These experiences are so strong that they can mentally bring one back to the place where the sensory experiences were gained. A moment when this connection between sensory elements takes place can be described as "grounding", or being "grounded" in the moment. Thus, the smell of wet leaves, for example, can return one's mind once again to that special place in the forest.

In short, previously gained physical-spatial experiences in our lives have a strong imprint on the experience value of our current living environment. Through a combination of architecture and landscape, these experiences can be intensified in a positive way. Such principles are used as a guideline in the design of the Chemotuin. There, a natural environment is created that appeals to these memories, in order to reduce stress and discomfort during chemotherapy.

15.5 Project Chemotherapy Outdoors: The "Chemotuin"

The Chemotuin is a pavilion that has been developed according to a nature-inclusive design methodology. The Tergooi Hospital in Hilversum is located in a parklike setting abutting the Goois Nature Reserve. The potential to incorporate this outdoor space in the hospital's activities, however, had not yet been actualized. At Tergooi Hilversum, thousands of chemotherapy treatments are administered to patients with cancer each year, and the duration of these therapies is typically longer than just one day. The hospital wanted to give patients the opportunity to receive chemotherapy in the open air, thereby making optimal use of the existing healing environment (hospital facility as well as surrounding parklands).

In order to offer these patients a comfortable place in the oncology department's outdoor space, VANDERSALM-aim conceived a design for a pavilion. The organization of the pavilion is based on the spatial principle of an old-fashioned beach chair, which can be seen as a way to establish a place in a scenic open space. The envelope of a beach chair lends its user a feeling of shelter and privacy, while the surrounding environment can still be experienced. The pavilion consists of three collective and four individual seating places that are integrated into an earthen embankment. Grasses, shrubs, and flowers provide an enclosure for these seats, allowing the patient to remain completely relaxed during chemotherapy. The pavilion is set up in such a way that these seating places serve as small rooms in the landscape, whereby the patient is literally enveloped by nature.

Nesting boxes and wintertime shelters for birds and butterflies are an integral part of the wooden structure. In choosing specific types of flora, a source of nourishment is provided for all kinds of animals. This supplies nectar, seeds, and berries, and offers an ideal living environment for butterflies, birds, bees, and other pollinators. In order to optimize this alignment, the landscaping plan was established in close consultation with a horticultural expert. The pavilion thereby enhances the biodiversity of the site, augments the variety of life, and wraps nature like a "jacket" around the patient.

Apart from this implementation, the architectural, practical, and safety considerations that influence the pavilion's daily use should also be guaranteed. The boardwalk that runs from one of the treatment rooms toward the veranda provides a logistical connection with the hospital and offers a protected and dry

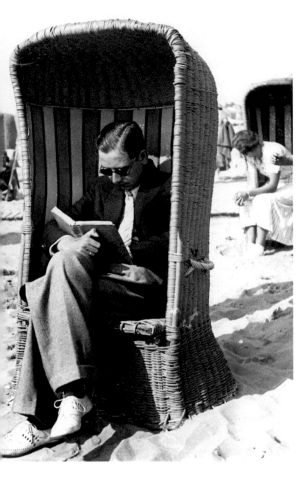

▲ Figure 15.5

The spatial significance of an old-fashioned beach chair as a new typology for creating places to spend time in an open area or scenic landscape.

Source: Nationaal Archief/Collection Spaarnestad/het Leven/ Kees Hofker

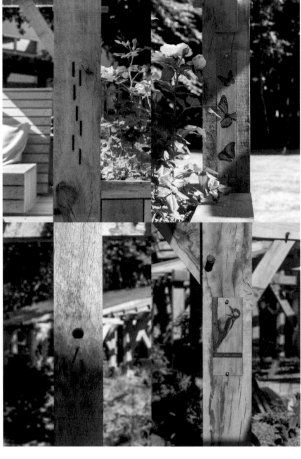

▲ Figure 15.6

Various nesting places for birds and butterflies are integrated in the main wooden support structure. The images on the back of the posts show how each type is intended to be used.

Source: Design by VANDERSALM-aim; photography by Milad Pallesh

link that passes between two monumental beech trees. The construction of the pavilion comprises a prefabricated oak structure, which is placed on a screw pile foundation to spare the root ball of the beeches. The roof is made of tempered glass plates with an "active coating", which eliminates the buildup of dirt and tarnishing through sunlight and rain. The glass roof of the wooden structure provides enough necessary shelter that sitting outside is still possible even when the weather turns for the worse. Caregivers can be summoned using an alarm system situated at each of the seats.

The furniture's upholstery is resistant to cytostatics, and a liquid-proof zone has been installed beneath the boardwalk so that, in case of spills, the cytostatics will never come into contact with the underlying soil surface. To further reduce this risk, the intravenous infusion used for the treatments is administered to patients in the adjoining indoor room, making it unnecessary to perform

Bart van der Salm

Area plan of Tergooi
Hospital with the
Chemotuin addition.
Source: Drawings by
VANDERSALM-aim

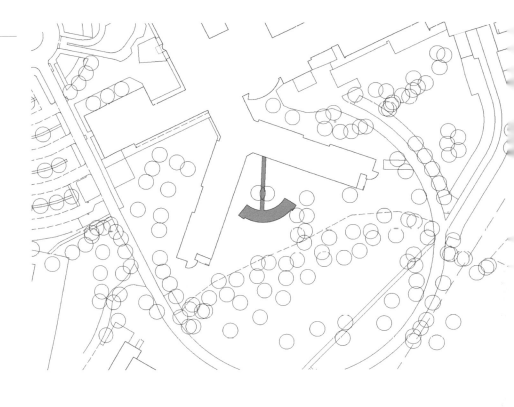

Plan view of Chemotuin
addition.
Source: Drawings by
VANDERSALM-aim

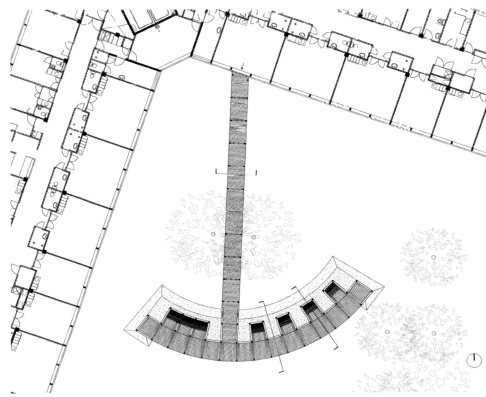

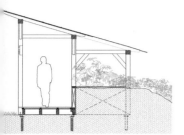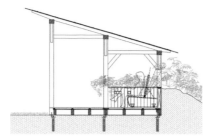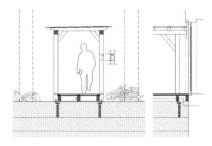

medical procedures once outside. Following this, patients can then proceed on their own with an infusion pole to one of the seats.

Certain medical scenarios and settings are obviously not conducive to being transplanted outdoors (e.g., intensive care units, operating rooms). However, healing processes that are both long-term and transportable, such as IV drips, blood transfusions, and childbirth recovery monitoring, all have the potential to follow this project as a model for a suitable and alternative approach to delivering healthcare. Working together with healthcare professionals, architects can identify spaces in a hospital as having the potential to be placed outdoors and/or be nature inclusive. In the case of the Chemotuin, the project served as a relatively small-scale intervention in an already existing chemotherapy program, feasible due to the hospital's proximity to a wildlife refuge and the Chemotuin's proximity to the necessary support systems of a large-scale healthcare center. In addition to this favorable location, the support of the involved medical oncology teams ensured a firm embedding of the project within the hospital structure. As an additional honor, the Chemotuin was nominated for the 2016 Hedy d'Ancona Prize for excellent healthcare architecture. The project was ultimately awarded second place at a ceremony in the restored Zonnestraal sanatorium in Hilversum.

Within this project, the principles of nature-inclusive design create an inseparable triangle between patient, architecture, and the surrounding life—nature. This means that the new structure not only is a place where people can temporarily stay but also provides a dwelling place for local flora and fauna, giving these a lasting habitat. The option to receive this kind of chemotherapy in the open air is innovative from a medical standpoint. To investigate what kind of effect this outdoor situation has on patients, the pavilion is linked to scientific research.

▲ Figure 15.9

Sections depicting various seating and treatment arrangements in which the user is always surrounded by nature.
Source: Drawings by VANDERSALM-aim

15.6 Research

The pavilion became operational in the summer of 2015, and the case study that has since been conducted by the Vrije Universiteit Amsterdam and the University of Groningen was completed in June 2017. Central to this investigation was the question of whether such a place in nature can contribute to the attainment of more positive emotions and a reduction of stress, thus improving patients' well-being. Even the idea of building the pavilion itself garnered a favorable reception. Of the total group of 60 patients who participated in the survey, an overwhelming 94.7% were positive to very positive about the initiative to build the pavilion. Since its completion, 56.4% of patients have used the pavilion, and another 30.9% say they would like to use it if they could. Furthermore, the

Bart van der Salm

option to be physically outdoors during treatment was also met with an encouraging response. Of the subjects surveyed, 49.1% prefer to be outside in the hospital's garden during their chemotherapy, while 25.5% have a preference to remain inside. Only 12.7% of study participants did not make use of the pavilion, and did not want to either. The remaining patients indicated no preference or were undecided. Aside from the survey results this case study provides, a number of interesting findings also emerged from the research:

- Patients in the pavilion had an overall more positive experience of their environment.
- Patients reported slightly more positive/restorative feelings (effects of nature).
- Patients felt better connected with nature.
- A majority of patients preferred to remain in the garden during their chemotherapy. The main reasons for this were: enjoyment of beautiful weather, privacy, stress reduction, getting in touch with oneself, nature, and fresh air.

The significance of having a natural vista became apparent through the research. This was not only valued by the patients in the garden but also positively evaluated by patients who remained indoors but had a view of the garden. This shows that when patients are unable to go outside, a view of nature can still make a positive contribution to well-being. However, it is important to underline that simply the visual perception of nature is not equivalent to the physical experience of nature. When other sensory experiences besides sight are excluded, such a situation cannot lead to the grounded "living" environment that can be so valuable to patients' well-being. Similar conclusions are also highlighted in another recent study, which found that a natural environment is associated with more positive emotions, stress reduction, and an improvement of the cognitive domain (Van den Berg and Van den Berg, 2012).

In conclusion, the following indications and recommendations from the pilot study are noteworthy:

- One should be attentive to the physical environment in which care is administered.
- Exposure to nature has a positive effect on health and well-being.
- Making use of nature in interior spaces is beneficial, but consider whether certain care can also be given in outdoor spaces (i.e., developed for this purpose).
- Patients themselves express support for receiving care in a natural outdoor space.

15.7 Conclusions: The Outdoor Room as New Typology

For centuries there has been a strong belief in the healing power of the natural environment. Since the 1980s (Ulrich 1984; Kaplan 1987) such findings have been scientifically affirmed; nature (in various forms/likenesses) and health are inextricably linked. Despite this knowledge, the average healthcare facility today focuses on efficiency, practical use, and internal logistical flows. The connection with the surrounding environment and outdoor spaces is often of secondary importance.

The completion of the Chemotuin, therefore, petitions for a new typology that will inspire and augment the existing healthcare environment: the outdoor room, a place in the landscape where the maximum potential for patients, plants, and animals is sought. In principle this kind of thinking about architecture and land-scape is without scale—it can occur on a single square meter, but can also be applied to an entire healthcare complex. An outdoor room is an additional low-tech integration and can be constructed with minimal impact on the existing structures within a care environment. Yet this setup requires a certain amount of indepen-dence from the patient, as well as the willingness to temporarily remain in an envi-ronment different from that of the medical staff (who can be summoned remotely). The outdoor room is therefore particularly suitable for lighter forms of care in this manifestation, wherein patients are partly self-reliant and do not require constant medical supervision (e.g., rehabilitation, long-term care, residential care). These

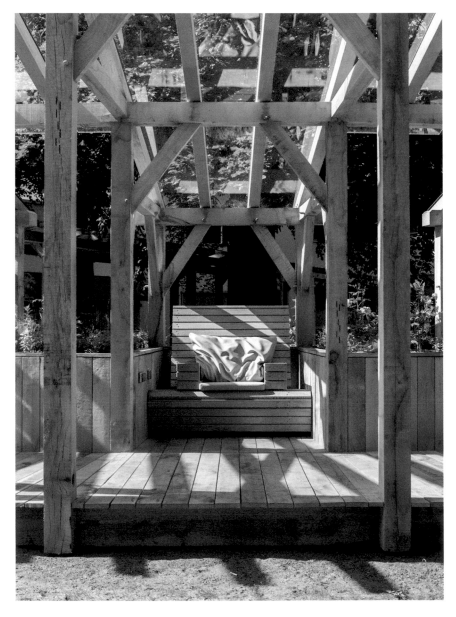

◀ Figure 15.10

The outdoor room as a new typology for receiving medical care in a healing environment.
Source: Design by VANDERSALM-aim; photography by Milad Pallesh

Bart van der Salm

outdoor rooms can be an external extension, situated adjacent to the healthcare institution, or even realized on the roof of a complex—a place where the increase in biodiversity is a logical consequence of a nature-inclusive design methodology. The resulting grounded spatial experience stimulates all the senses so that every-day affairs can fade into the background. What is created is a room with plants and animals, the sun and the wind—a place for living with life.

Acknowledgments

Translation services provided by Dutton-Hauhart of Amsterdam, the Netherlands.

Bibliography

"Green Inspirations—An interview with Maike van Stiphout, DSLA." *Column Gevelbouw Magazine*, no 2, 2014, Weert, The Netherlands.

Kaplan, Stephen. "Aesthetics, Affect, and Cognition: Environmental Preference from an Evolutionary Perspective." *Environment and Behavior* 19, no. 1 (1987): 3–32.

Kellert, Stephen R., and Edward O. Wilson, eds. *The Biophilia Hypothesis*. Washington, DC: Island Press, 1993.

Pallasmaa, Juhani. The Eyes of the Skin: Architecture and the Senses. Hoboken, NJ: John Wiley & Sons, 2012.

Planetree, Inc. *Patient and Family Partnership Councils and Beyond: Solutions for Making Good on the Promise of Partnering with Patients*. Derby, CT: Planetree Inc., 2017.

Tanja-Dijkstra, Karin, van den Berg, Agnes, Maas, Jolanda, Bloemhof-Haasjes, Janet, and van den Berg, Pieter. "Chemotherapy in the Garden—Pilot Study." *Vrije Universiteit Amsterdam and the University of Groningen* 5 (2017, July): 175–181.

Ulrich, Roger S. "View Through a Window May Influence Recovery from Surgery." *Science* 224, no. 4647 (1984): 420–421.

Van den Berg, Agnes E. *Health Impacts of Healing Environments: A Review of Evidence for Benefits of Nature, Daylight, Fresh Air, and Quiet in Healthcare Settings*. Groningen: UMCG, 2005.

Van den Berg, Agnes E., and Magdalena MHE van den Berg. "Health Benefits of Plants and Green Space: Establishing the Evidence Base." In *XI International People Plant Symposium on Diversity: Towards a New Vision of Nature, 1093*, 19–30, International Society for Horticultural Science, 2012.

Chapter 16

Living Buildings
The Bullitt Center

Steve Doub, Jim Hanford, Margaret Sprug, Chris Hellstern, and Katherine Misel

16.1 Introduction

The design of the built environment can greatly influence our collective well-being. Ideally, the strategies that we use to achieve highly sustainable, regenerative, and holistic design solutions support human health at multiple levels and scales. For example, proper daylighting design with adequate illumination and control of glare can improve the psychological well-being of building occupants, while also reducing energy consumption and air and water pollution associated with energy production. Producing food on-site using treated graywater for irrigation can bring nutrition and happiness to building users, while reducing regional water demand for agriculture.

This chapter explores how the advanced, regenerative design standard of the Living Building Challenge (LBC) can improve human health. Unique to the LBC, certification is given after a one-year performance period and relies on data demonstrating proven performance. At the time it was completed, the Bullitt Center, located in Seattle, Washington, was the seventh, and largest, certified Living Building in the world. In this case study, we explore how applying the LBC to an ordinary, urban commercial office building can lead to both desired and unexpected results.

16.2 The Bullitt Foundation and the Bullitt Center

16.2.1 The Bullitt Foundation

In 2009, The Miller Hull Partnership was selected by the Bullitt Foundation and its development partner as the architect for its new headquarters, the Bullitt Center. Having outgrown its previous office, the Foundation purchased an urban block to develop a new headquarters that would embody its core principles as an environmental non-profit working to advance the ecological health of the Cascadia region.

Denis Hayes, president of the Bullitt Foundation, organizer of the first Earth Day, and former director of the Solar Energy Research Institute, stated, ". . . our desire is to open a wedge into the future so that we, and others, can see what is possible in a contemporary office building" (Carter 2011). Because of his history with renewable energy, Hayes's original focus was on building a Net-Zero Energy facility that followed a replicable model for urban commercial development. While evaluating potential sites, the Foundation discovered the International Living Future Institute (ILFI) and the Living Building Challenge (LBC) and saw it as the ideal and comprehensive environmental framework to realize a new building. Hayes and the Foundation felt that if a building on an urban site in Seattle could meet ILFI's Challenge—a city with low solar exposure, but adequate rainfall—it would demonstrate "If Living Buildings can be built and operated in Seattle, the cloudiest major city in the contiguous 48 states, they can and should be built anywhere" (Living Proof Blog 2015).

16.2.2 The Bullitt Center

The Bullitt Center is a 52,000-square-foot commercial office building containing six stories of leased space over a partial basement. The building's base is constructed from reinforced concrete, with the top four floors from heavy timber post-and-beam construction, using structural steel for lateral support. The building expresses a dynamism, with automated windows and exterior blinds, metal cladding, large glazed openings, and a glazed main stairway that projects from the north façade. A defining feature is the large overhanging solar PV array. Currently, the Bullitt Foundation

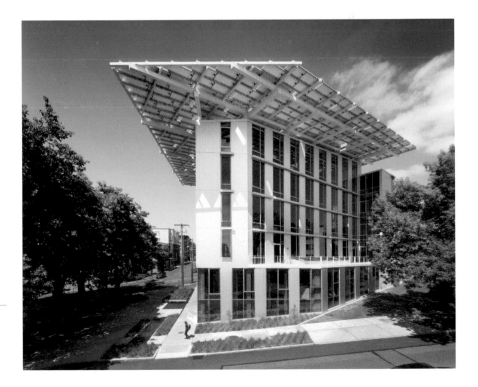

▶ Figure 16.1

View from the south across East Pike Street, the Bullitt Center, Seattle, Washington.
Source: Nic Lehoux

occupies half of the top floor. The remainder of the building is leased to a diverse set of like-minded organizations, both for-profit enterprises and nonprofit institutes.

For Miller Hull, working collaboratively with the Foundation and a diverse array of consultants to achieve this vision brought forth a new era in design. The performance-based approach of the LBC required greater conviction and greater thought toward long-term performance. The regenerative design approach required the firm to use its history of creative problem solving, while bringing in new tools around building performance and occupant engagement.

16.3 The Process

16.3.1 The Living Building Challenge

Sustainable building certifications typically assess to which degree a project meets specified prescriptive requirements and performance standards relative to a defined baseline. In 2006, Jason McLennan and the International Living Future Institute (ILFI) had a simple but profound vision: Instead of simply making buildings "less bad" for their occupants and the environment, would it be possible to make buildings that could have zero occupant and environmental impact, or even be restorative? The result was the Living Building Challenge (LBC), arguably the world's most rigorous sustainability benchmark. Using the metaphor of a flower, the framework is organized into a series of performance areas, or petals: Place,

▼ Figure 16.2

Living Building Challenge petal and imperative summary matrix.
Source: International Living Future Institute, Living Building Challenge Standard v2.0

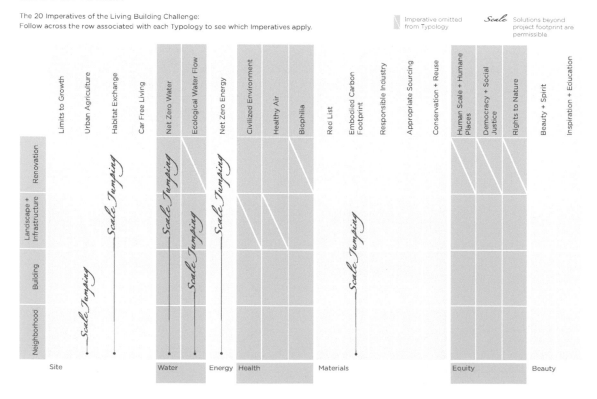

SUMMARY MATRIX

The 20 Imperatives of the Living Building Challenge:
Follow across the row associated with each Typology to see which Imperatives apply.

Steve Doub et al.

Water, Energy, Materials, Health and Happiness, Equity, and Beauty. The petals are subdivided into more specific sub-requirements, or imperatives (ILFI 2010).

Unlike other benchmark rubrics, the LBC has no prescriptive checklists or projected performance. Instead, it requires one year of performance data prior to certification and third-party verification that all imperatives have been reached.

16.3.2 The Bullitt Center Design Process

When design of the Bullitt Center began in 2009, there was no precedent for a commercial building of a similar scale and complexity that had been built to meet the LBC. To ensure success, the Foundation and its development partner assembled a team of architects, engineers, contractors, and consultants that not only were leaders in the most sustainable methods and technology available but also knew success depended on an open and continual exchange of information and strategies. While the method of delivery was a typical construction manager at risk model, it was the vision of Denis Hayes that inspired the team to commit to an unprecedented level of collaboration required for this project.

To chart a path for the design process, a comprehensive two-day eco-charrette was conducted before any design work began. This included the traditional owner/architect/developer/contractor team, but also included representatives from the City of Seattle who would be permitting the project, representatives from the community and the neighborhood where the project would be built, and over 30 research and design professionals from all over the country. This created a deep bench of experts who could give critical feedback as the project progressed. Using the input from the charrette, the team was able to synthesize the best ideas and methods for achieving the LBC goals. Roughly 80% of the project's design was established during those two days. The breakthrough that guided the project was defining the carrying capacity. In other words, determining how much of the building can be supported indefinitely with the available natural resources found in the site's ecosystem. By calculating solar income, annual rainfall, and carbon, the team determined the site could support approximately 50,000 square feet of office use. Figuring out the remaining 20% of the design concept took another two years, using energy and comfort simulation, daylighting studies, ventilation modeling, and of course, cost analysis, to vet every conceivable alternative solution that might offer better performance or cost.

16.3.3 Outcomes

The Bullitt Center opened in 2013, was certified in 2014, and remains the largest commercial Living Building at the time of this publication. Since it opened, the project has been recognized with 17 awards for sustainable design, published nationally and internationally, and continues to be referenced as the "world's greenest office building" (Living Proof Blog 2015), which helps draw approximately 5,000 visitors a year.

Despite the LBC premium being estimated to cost about 25% more than a standard office building, the Bullitt Center was 75% leased when it opened. The premiums are primarily found in the high-performance, triple-pane curtain walls, gray and blackwater treatment systems, rainwater to potable water systems, and over 14,000 square feet of PV array. When the Bullitt Foundation was seeking financing for the project, most lenders saw the project as too risky. Appraisals based on comparable projects did not exist. The building was appraising for about $14 million and it would take close to $20 million to build. In 2017, the now occupied project was appraised at $32 million.

16.4 The Bullitt Center and LBC: Specific Design Responses and Project Performance

16.4.1 Place: Restoring a Healthy Coexistence With Nature

With an increase in populations moving to urban areas, cities must accommodate growth by becoming denser, which increases congestion and pressure on existing services, or by increasing in area, which compounds sprawl and reduces natural habitat and arable land. Each of these conditions creates challenges for human health and well-being. One of the goals for sustainable design is to create balanced urban developments using existing sites with developed pedestrian networks that are served by public transportation and incorporate diverse uses and opportunities.

To address this double bind, the LBC imperatives for the Place petal require projects to redevelop brownfields or previously developed sites so as not to decrease density. The project must also promote urban agriculture and sequester natural habitat elsewhere, which is equal to the size of the developed site. This land must be purchased through an accredited land trust that will hold and protect the land in perpetuity, thereby offsetting the very development of the project itself. The petal also promotes the use of human-powered transportation to reduce the reliance on fossil fuels, while supporting healthy activities. The requirements include strategies designed to support walkable communities and bicycle infrastructure and facilities.

The site selected by the Bullitt Foundation was a gently sloping lot on Capitol Hill, a vibrant mixed-use Seattle neighborhood. The site was an underdeveloped location that originally consisted of a surface parking lot and a one-story building adjacent to McGilvra Park. Close to both downtown and public transportation, the site has walkable access to more than 20 bus routes, a streetcar, and Link Light Rail station, making it possible for most tenants to commute car free.

Unlike most new developments in Seattle, the Bullitt Center has no on-site parking except for a single shared loading space in the recycling and bike room. While parking is not required by Seattle's zoning code for this site, it was an unorthodox move and a deterrent for some tenants. Ultimately, the building was fully leased within the first two years, attracting tenants whose values aligned with those of the Foundation and the project. Over time, building occupants have shaped their commuting behavior favoring modes other than cars. A survey of tenants by the University of Washington's Integrated Design Lab indicated a 12% decrease in time traveling by car, a 65% increase in public transportation use and a 58% increase in travel time by bike (Burpee et al. 2015).

Based on the Seattle location—amid a robust network of neighborhood farmers markets supporting local urban and ex-urban farming—the project did not have to provide additional space for on-site agriculture.

Steve Doub et al.

Aerial view of the Bullitt
Center looking southeast
away from downtown.
Source: Andrew Buchanan/SLP

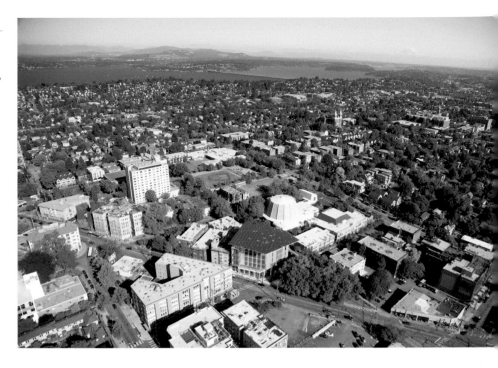

View from the west
through McGilvra Park with
pedestrian entrance to
ground-floor tenancies and
sliding doors at upper floor.
Source: Nic Lehoux

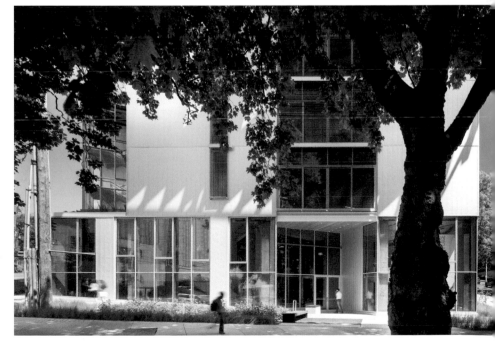

16.4.2 Water: Creating Water Independent Sites, Buildings, and Communities

The World Health Organization points out that 10% of the global "disease burden" could be prevented by increasing access to safe drinking water, improved sanitation, and improved water management. In addition, safe water could reduce annual mortality by over 3 million globally (WHO 2008). In 2004, 850 billion gallons of untreated wastewater and stormwater were released as combined sewer overflow and between 3 billion and 20 billion gallons of untreated wastewater were released from sanitary sewer overflows in the U.S. (USEPA 2004). Clearly, water supply and waste treatment in built environments have a clear and direct connection to the health of individuals and communities.

The LBC imperatives for the Water petal require projects to use only as much water as can be collected on-site from annual precipitation, or an otherwise closed-loop water system (Net-Zero Water). All water flow must be treated on-site, allowing only outflow equal to predevelopment levels (Ecological Water Flow). The goal is to develop new water resources and modes of treatment that don't stress existing infrastructure.

The Bullitt Center uses only a fraction of the water typical for an average commercial office building. The average commercial building in the U.S. uses 20 gallons of water per square foot per year. In contrast, the Bullitt Center uses just one gallon per square foot per year, a 95% reduction in water use. Using a rooftop catchment, the building collects all rainwater and delivers it to a 56,000-gallon cistern in the basement. This "water income" sets the water budget for the project. The significant reduction in water use is due in large part to composting toilets, which require only a few tablespoons of water per use and eliminate sewage outflow from the building entirely. By doing this, the Bullitt Center restores the natural cycle of soil fertility, rather than depending on a system that continually depletes soil fertility and relies on chemical fertilizers to restore these depleted nutrients.

The Bullitt Center's black water (waste from toilet fixtures) is treated by ten composters in the basement that treat the waste by the same processes typical of any garden compost pile. Under current occupancy levels, the composters are emptied once a year. The liquid portion of this waste is recovered in several leachate tanks that are pumped out of the building on a monthly basis. Meanwhile, gray water (water from sinks) is treated by the green roof, which acts as a "constructed wetland", filtering the flow to a level acceptable for infiltration into the aquifer/groundwater. Infiltration infrastructure built into the landscaping between the building and McGilvra Park allows this flow to infiltrate into the water table. As a result of these strategies, the Bullitt Center has the same water footprint as the Douglas fir forest that would have originally occupied the site.

From 2013 until 2018, regulatory requirements at the county, state, and federal levels prevented commercial office buildings from consuming captured rainwater. After years of advocacy, testing, and design documentation, the Bullitt Center obtained approval for potable use of collected rainwater, thereby closing the water cycle. It is important to recognize that if all new commercial buildings used water in the way the Bullitt Center uses it, existing supplies of water would go much further in meeting future demand, even with significant growth in population.

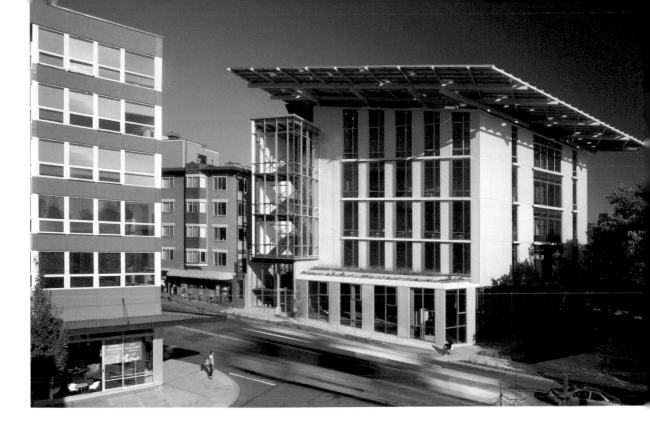

▲ Figure 16.5

View from the northwest across East Madison Street with the constructed wetland, the main entry, and the irresistible stair.
Source. Nic Lehoux

16.4.3 Energy: Relying Only on Current Solar Income

If unchecked, global climate change has the potential for disastrous effects on public health within our lifetime (UNIPCC 2018). The primary sources of emissions that lead to climate change are current energy systems, where buildings play a significant role. In 2015 alone, U.S. electricity production generated 1.2 billion metric tons of carbon emissions, 1 billion of that from coal. Overall, building operational energy consumption accounts for 28% of global CO_2 emissions (Architecture 2030, 2019). Particulate pollution and resource extraction are more localized health impacts of building energy use, but these impacts have become less of an issue as climate change has become the dominant effect.

The LBC goal is to move toward carbon-neutral energy systems for buildings, while recognizing that connection to the energy grid is needed in most cases. The Net-Zero Energy (NZE) imperative for the Energy petal requires projects to use only as much energy as can be generated by renewable sources on an annual basis, developed on-site, or provided nearby. Note that the most current LBC requirements are to be net positive energy and include battery storage systems as a resilience measure.

As the former director of the Solar Energy Research Institute, Denis Hayes advocated for a project that paired extremely low-energy use with on-site solar

PV to achieve NZE. While the scope expanded to include full LBC certification, NZE was a pre-eminent goal due to the integration of on-site solar. To achieve NZE, the design had to bring down building demand to the bare minimum, then deploy as much solar PV on site in the most cost-effective way. Working within the energy budget established by the large sloping array, the design team considered all potential energy uses within the building, and identified how technology, culture, and human behavior could be leveraged in reducing energy use. Many of the systems deployed are defining pieces of the architecture: a high-performing envelope with a triple-glazed curtainwall to minimize heating loads, motorized and automated windows and solar-control blinds to offset cooling loads, thermally massive radiant floors, and an Irresistible Stair that promotes walking over elevator use.

Research has found that the "Irresistible Stair" supports the energy performance as intended. In design, energy analysis revealed that up to 5% of the energy budget could be represented by the elevator. Yet, measured data shows the elevator energy consumption is a mere 2% of the already low building energy demands. In the survey done by the University of Washington's Integrated Design Lab (UW IDL), findings reported that 75% of trips from the second-floor entrance to the top floor of the building use the stair compared to 17%–23% on average in a typical commercial office building (Burpee et al. 2015).

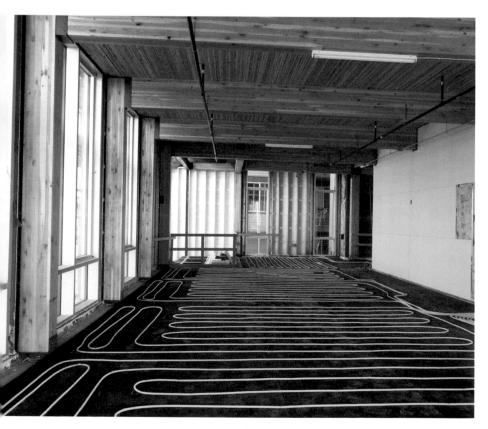

◀ Figure 16.6

Construction phase view of concrete topping slab installation with radiant tubing at perimeter zones for heating and partial cooling.
Source: John Stamets, University of Washington Archives

Steve Doub et al.

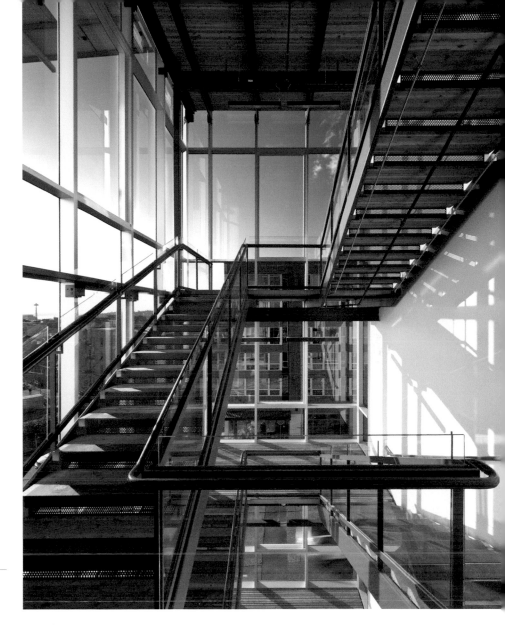

▶ Figure 16.7

Interior view of the
"Irresistible Stair".
Source: Nic Lehoux

Other strategies have proven to be effective at lowering energy demands. The window systems represent a defining feature of the Bullitt Center, both for the exterior aesthetic and for the interior experience. Research performed by the UW IDL (Pena, Meek, and Davis 2017) has shown that the window operations are extremely effective for reducing cooling energy use. They function primarily as a "night flush" strategy where they reduce indoor temperatures and thermal mass temperatures during cooler night time hours, helping to stay comfortable during the subsequent day. The dynamic blinds have not been studied in detail, but anecdotal reports by occupants conclude they perform well in controlling glare in the workspace. Energy use for cooling the space—envisioned to be small amounts of cooling delivered through the radiant floor slab—is shown to be almost nonexistent.

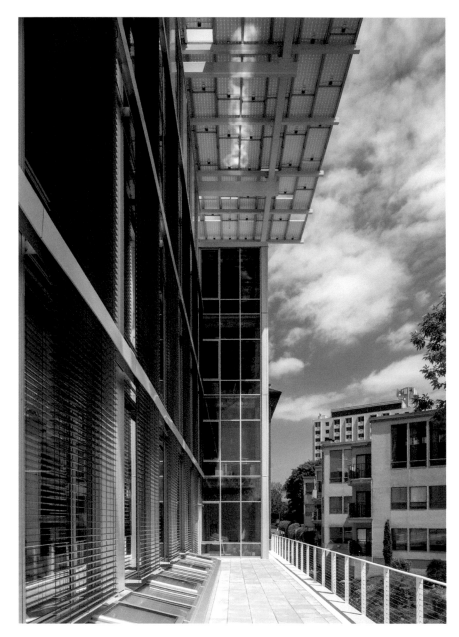

◀ Figure 16.8

View of southeast façade
showing dynamic blinds,
offset from façade to allow
for window operation.
Source: Nic Lehoux

Since the building has been in operation, the Bullitt Center has performed as net positive. The building energy use intensity (EUI) has tracked between 10 and up to 14 kBtu/SF, whereas the solar PV array supports a building EUI of 16 kBtu/SF.

16.4.4 Health and Happiness: Maximizing Physical and Psychological Health and Well-Being

Workers are spending about 90% of their time inside buildings (EPA 2018), and the U.S. population with asthma increased by 4.3 million between 2001 and 2009 (US CDC 2011). According to World Health Organization reports, access to daylight is important for Vitamin D production, sleep cycle regulation, and mood. Furthermore, increase in fresh air exchange reduces the risk of airborne infection transmission since the buildup and exposure to toxic indoor air pollutants, such as mold and dampness, are risk factors for allergies and asthma (WHO 2017).

The Health petal is the one petal where human health is explicit. The LBC imperatives require certified projects to provide operable windows for access to fresh air and daylight within 30 feet of each permanent workspace, and separately ventilated kitchens, toilet rooms, janitor rooms, and copy rooms. It also requires that the building design incorporate biophilic principles into interiors—elements that nurture interactions with natural systems and form connections with the surrounding environment.

Provision of natural daylight was paramount in the design. Through ongoing daylight design studies in cooperation with the University of Washington's Integrated Design Lab, it was determined that extending glazing to the ceiling greatly increased the amount of daylight in the space. Maximizing the scale of each

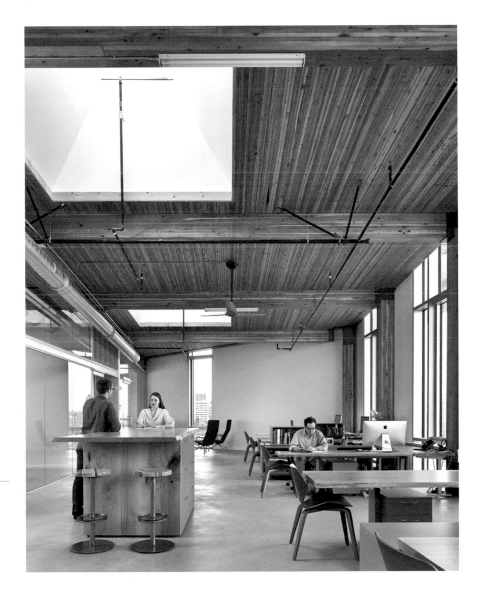

▶ Figure 16.9

Sixth-floor interior view where skylights were introduced to improve daylighting under PV canopy area.
Source: Benjamin Benschneider

uninterrupted unit of glass is solely intended to enhance the transition between the built and natural environment. Narrowing the floor plate and increasing floor-to-floor height (due to a zoning waiver for meeting sustainability goals) further augmented the amount of daylight in the tenant spaces. Skylights were added at the top floor to offset the decrease in daylighting by the overhanging PV array.

Not only does daylight increase physical and psychological well-being, but also it reduces the occupant's reliance on artificial electric light, impacting the overall building energy consumption. In a typical building, lighting accounts for 25% of its annual energy use. With an integrated daylight strategy, 80% of the building is naturally daylit, using only 20% of its annual energy use on lighting.

To be effective, daylighting must balance glare and solar heat gain. This is primarily achieved by automated interior and louvered exterior blinds employed throughout the building. Tuning the ratio of glazing to opaque wall area further helped to balance between daylighting and heat gain.

Similarly, other design strategies meet both energy and experiential goals. Two main features of the building exemplify this biophilic principle—the irresistible stair and the operable windows in the office space. The irresistible stair is fully glazed and is not mechanically heated or cooled, while office space has a combination of manually controlled sliding doors and automatically controlled operable units. This provides natural ventilation for the building, and "preconditions" the concrete floor slabs in the summer to help reduce cooling loads during the day. Each floor has user controls to override the automated system, but automatically reset after 20 minutes. This not only allows users to manage conditions but also has the added psychological benefit of being able to affect the interior environment independent of the automated controls.

16.4.5 Materials: Endorsing Products and Processes That Are Safe for All Species Through Time

The health case for a materials revolution is overwhelming. Manufacturers, designers, and contractors often create or use products with toxic materials that make people and the environment ill. From absorbing chemicals through our skin, or inhaling their emissions once installed, chemicals of concern have a dire impact on the health of everyone who comes in contact with them.

Removing chemicals of concern has wide-reaching effects beyond a building's occupants. The processes to create these harmful substances are toxic to the workers who manufacturer them. The neighborhoods where these chemicals are produced, known as fenceline communities, are also especially vulnerable.

To address the health impacts of materials toxicity and other environmental impacts, the LBC imperatives for the Materials petal require certified projects to use only materials that are free of known harmful chemicals (Red List Free), use materials from local and regionally appropriate sources (Appropriate Sourcing), reduce or eliminate waste during design, construction, and operation (Conservation and Reuse), purchase carbon offsets equal to the carbon generated during construction (Embodied Carbon), and advocate for third-party standards for material extraction and fair labor practices (Responsible Industry). The overall goal is to create new economies and processes that support health at

Steve Doub et al.

all scales. Avoiding Red List materials in construction and reducing the market demand is one of Bullitt Center's most long-lasting impacts. Persistence by the project team and commitment from the manufacturer led to an extensive line of Red List–free products (Thomas 2016).

While there are a number of successful substitutions for less harmful products used in the Bullitt Center, and a range of Red List chemicals avoided, industry change is an important wide-ranging impact. As design began on the Bullitt Center, only a handful of other Living Buildings had been constructed. The concept of a Red List, and even embodied carbon, was just blossoming in the design industry. In the project's early days, the design and construction team had to educate manufacturers about the Red List and teach subcontractors how to recognize and avoid toxins on-site. In 2018, nearly 40 projects are certified with the Materials petal worldwide. Now, we can recognize the impact that the Bullitt Center and the first Living Buildings had on local economic development and on a broader national and global market.

Although the Red List may garner the most attention, there are other imperatives that are equally important for a materials revolution. For example, the Responsible Industry imperative forces projects to use wood from responsibly managed sources. The Bullitt Center team took this on by designing a building framed in Forest Stewardship Council (FSC) timber. Not only did this choice represent a lesser carbon footprint, but also it allowed the team to reduce overall materials by not requiring additional finishes, while also supporting biophilia goals. Using a lower carbon structural material also reduced the amount of carbon offsets needing

▼ Figure 16.10

Example of typical office space interior prior to full tenant improvement, with exposed timber structure, 13-foot ceilings, and expansive glass.
Source: Nic Lehoux

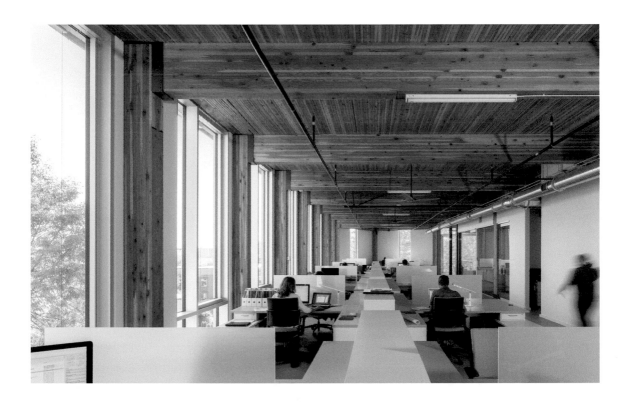

purchase. The ideals of this responsible resource extraction also extend to other raw materials in the Living Building Challenge, including rock, metals, and minerals.

16.4.6 Equity: Supporting a Just, Equitable World

Maslow's hierarchy of needs provides a helpful model to give context to more intangible portions of the built environment. Typically illustrated as a pyramid, a person's physiological needs (air/water/food, protection from the elements) and need for safety (health and well-being) are the lowest two layers of the pyramid, and thus the most basic needs. These requirements are commonly entrusted to design professionals. Continuing up the pyramid, we find psychological needs, such as social belonging, acceptance, and esteem, followed by self-actualization and self-transcendence. The fulfillment of higher needs is beyond basic survival, but still essential to an individual's overall well-being, even though they are less tangible and often difficult to address with specific design solutions. One way the LBC helps address these needs is through the Equity petal.

Admittedly, a single development cannot solve the many complex issues of social and environmental equity in our society, nor should it try. The Equity petal in the LBC is meant to allow designers to address these issues both inside and outside of their buildings. The LBC imperatives for this petal require certified projects to provide human-scaled places that support human interaction (Human Scale and Humane Places), with equal access (Democracy and Social Justice), and must not limit the access by surrounding buildings to nature, fresh air, and daylight (Rights to Nature).

For the Bullitt Center, there are traditional ways the building approaches equity, from fitting contextually within the neighborhood's design to breaking down the building's scale to appeal to pedestrians. But, the true advancements of equity in the Bullitt Center's approach lie in how it was built and how it operates. The core and shell were designed to support democratization of interior space. There are no enclosed offices—all occupants have equal access to daylighting, quality views, and fresh air from the extensive, operable windows. The open office approach is also essential to meeting its low energy consumption through daylighting, natural ventilation, and heating ventilation and air conditioning (HVAC) design.

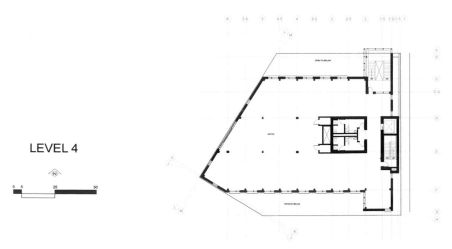

LEVEL 4

◄ Figure 16.11

Typical office floor plan; plan dimension is approximately 70 feet across from the main daylighting facades with center bays developed for support spaces.
Source: The Miller Hull Partnership

Steve Doub et al.

Access to natural amenities extends outside the building as well. The street separating the previously underused park was closed to traffic as part of the project, and the park became a car-free public space contiguous with the building. McGilvra Park meets the LBC requirements.

Similar to the Materials petal, the Equity petal has its own set of goals to provide support for other projects. One of the lasting legacies of the Bullitt Center is the Seattle Living Building Pilot program that was tested on the building. The program allows projects to request departures from zoning codes by providing additional floor area or building heights to meet the high sustainability standards of the LBC.

Since opening, the Bullitt Center has been a laboratory for social experiments. This includes becoming a test case for a utility program that works to overcome the owner/tenant barrier for investing in energy efficiency (Egnor et al. 2016) and the Bullitt Foundation's ultimately successful negotiations with local regulatory agencies to allow using rainwater for potable supply (Bullitt Center 2018). This advocacy seeks to make regenerative development easier for other projects that follow.

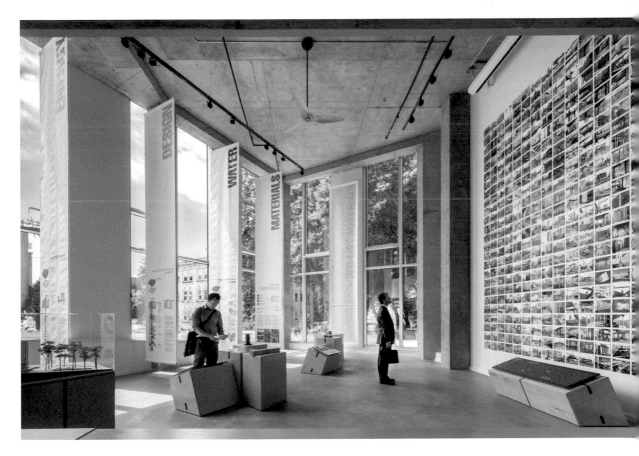

▲ Figure 16.12

First-floor lobby used as educational exhibit area during first several years of operation (now leased office space).
Source: Nic Lehoux

16.4.7 Beauty: Celebrating Design That Creates Transformative Change

Writing to explain the inclusion of beauty as a criteria for the WELL Building Standard, Winer and Keim (2018) summarize conclusions from a range of research studies as ". . . while beauty as an attribute is subjective, it produces a positive emotional experience in building occupants and users by enhancing feelings of happiness and well-being". In further referencing the work of neuroscience researchers at the University of Pennsylvania, they also note "Design with the deliberate intention to incorporate beauty is imperative to human psychological well-being, with positive effects on learning, social behavior, and emotional wellness" (Winer and Keim 2018, referencing Coburn et al. 2017). The increasing body of work in this area tells us that integration of beauty into the built environment should be considered a long-term investment in human health. Unfortunately, many of our built environments are unattractive and uninspiring, and do not engender feelings of well-being in occupants or users.

Environmental performance without beauty is not an acceptable goal because beautiful things are more likely to be learned from, loved, used, maintained, and preserved. To address this, the LBC requires certified projects provide features that are solely for human delight (Beauty and Spirit) and include inspiration and didactic examples for occupants and the public (Inspiration and Education).

The Bullitt Center itself was envisioned as a teaching tool and example for others. The building's core functions, systems, and methods of construction are on display using a mix of existing and new technologies. The simple elegance of the thermal mass concrete floors, along with the presence of the constructed wetland green roof, expose and elevate what are typically "behind the scenes" infrastructure capabilities of heating and storm water management.

In typical commercial spaces, the level of visual interference and noise is frequently called out as an intangible contributor to the general "beauty and feeling of well-being" of occupants. Because of the nature of the LBC, the Bullitt Center is inherently airy, light-filled, and relatively quiet. Given the large expanses of floor-to-ceiling glass, the building's natural light is higher quality than that found in typical office buildings. Traditionally, there would be a solid presence on the overhanging roofline, but carefully placed openings in the rooftop PV array enable dappled light to filter through to offices below and at street level. This creates an uplifting impact for building occupants coming to work and visitors experiencing the space for only a short time.

The Bullitt Center's urban and regional setting leverages adjacent natural features, both borrowed and procured from its surroundings. Perched at the crest of a high hill, the site gives occupants views to nature close by and far away. Floor-to-ceiling operable windows and doors provide them with direct access to 100-year-old sycamore trees in McGilvra Park, a striking sight at any time of year. Although occupying a tight site, the presence of a green roof and a perimeter of native plants provide a beautiful natural buffer to the busy surrounding streetscape. The space between the entrance and sheltering canopy

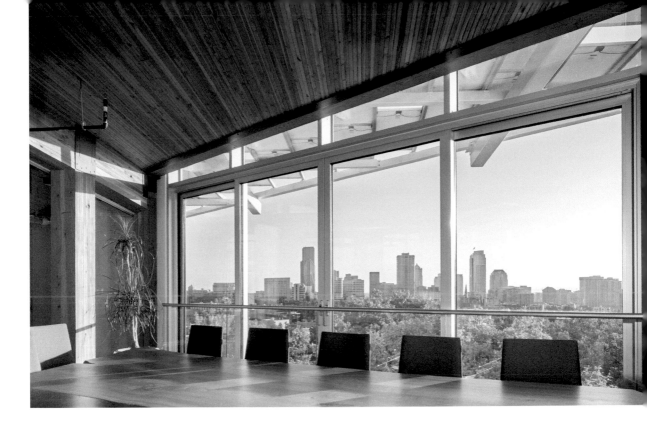

▲ Figure 16.13

View from west-facing conference room on the sixth floor.
Source: Nic Lehoux

of park trees also provides a comfortable place for informal and large group gatherings.

16.5 Conclusions

In terms of human health, the Bullitt Center is delivering at all environmental scales, from the building interiors to regional ecosystems, and planetary impacts. It operates at net positive energy, producing essentially zero carbon emissions. It operates at net-zero water, with no demands on the water supply and wastewater treatment systems. A report funded by the Bullitt Foundation found that over its lifetime, the Bullitt Center will contribute $18 million worth of ecosystem services (in net present value) to the region and community, with all the human health benefits that come from these improved environments (Cowan et al. 2014).

Anecdotal evidence and feedback from the one-year performance period (e.g., the Beauty and Spirit documentation) show that building occupants have high satisfaction with the Bullitt Center, noting that their health and well-being are being thoroughly supported. More importantly, ongoing research studies related to thermal comfort, the active workspace, and lighting studies shows that occupants are engaged in the operation of the building and their spaces (Burpee et al. 2015).

The recent building valuation shows that delivering a regenerative building using a typical commercial development model can be successful in the marketplace, fulfilling the goal of the Bullitt Foundation. It suggests that value can be delivered beyond simple return-on-investment goals. The long-term performance of the building confirms the connection between the occupant experience, building performance, and regional and global health impacts, proving that value can be derived from these connections.

While offering a simple framework for sustainability, the Living Building Challenge is intended to evolve over time. Design and construction of the Bullitt Center began under Version 1.2 and was ultimately certified under Version 2.0. Since the building was completed, the criteria of the LBC have changed even further. For example, the Red List, comprising 14 classes of chemicals representing 362 individual compounds, now lists 22 classes of chemicals representing 777 chemical compounds. Furthermore, net positive energy is now required instead of simple net-zero energy.

While Miller Hull continues to design more LBC projects, the Bullitt Center continues to influence projects across the firm's practice, the profession, and the Living Building Challenge itself. Regionally, nationally, and internationally, there are few projects, if any, that have fully replicated the Bullitt Center. However, its inspiration for future built work has been and will continue to be an invaluable contribution to the profession and will always remain an influential precedent for what is possible.

Acknowledgments

Thank you to Denis Hayes and the Bullitt Foundation for their vision and ongoing leadership as well as the countless people who contributed to the conception, planning, development, and realization of the Bullitt Center.

Bibliography

Architecture 2030. "Why the Building Sector". https://architecture2030.org/buildings_problem_why/. Accessed August 15, 2019.

Boubekri, Mohamed, Ivy N. Cheung, Kathryn J. Reid, Chia-Hui Wang, and Phyllis C. Zee. "Impacts of Windows and Daylight Exposure on Overall Health and Sleep Quality of Office Workers: A Case-control Pilot Study." *Journal of Clinical Sleep Medicine* 10, no. 6 (2014): 603–611.

Bullitt Center. *Rainwater to Potable Water System*. Whitepaper published on Bullitt Center website. November 1, 2018. www.bullittcenter.org/wp-content/uploads/2018/11/Bullitt-Center-Water-System-FINAL.pdf.

Burpee, Heather, Michael Gilbride, Kelly Douglas, David Beck, and John Mesche. *Health Impacts of a Living Building: The Bullitt Center*. Washington, DC: University of Washington, Seattle, June 2015.

Carter, Beth. "In Seattle, a New Office Building Strives for Living Building Status." *ZDNet.com*, November 21, 2011. http://www.bullittcenter.org/2015/04/01/bullitt-center-earns-living-building-certification/. Accessed August 15, 2019.

Coburn, Alex, Oshin Vartanian, and Anjan Chatterjee. "Buildings, Beauty, and the Brain: A Neuroscience of Architectural Experience." *Journal of Cognitive Neuroscience* 29, no. 9 (2017): 1521–1531.

Cowan, Stuart, Brent Davies, David Diaz, Noah Enelow, Kevin Halsey, and Kathryn Langstaff. *Optimizing Urban Ecosystem Services: The Bullitt Center Case Study*, 141. Portland, OR: Ecotrust, 2014.

Egnor, Terry, Denis Hayes, John Jennings, David Rodenhizer, Howard Reichmuth, Kevin Van Den Wymelenberg, and Christopher Meek. "Metered Energy Efficiency Transaction Structure in Net-Zero New Construction: Pay-for-Performance at the Bullitt Center in Seattle, WA." *2016 ACEEE Summer Study on Energy Efficiency in Buildings, Pacific Grove, CA*, 2016.

Hanford, Jim, Marc Brune, Christopher Meek, and Michael Gilbride. "Building Change: The Bullitt Center," *High Performing Buildings*, 24–33. Atlanta, GA: The American Society of Heating, Refrigeration and Air-Conditioning Engineers (ASHRAE), Winter 2016.

Jenkins, Joseph. *The Humanure Book: A Guide to Composting Human Manure*. 3rd ed. White River Junction, VT: Chelsea Green Publishing, 2005.

Living Proof Blog, "Bullitt Center Earns Living Building Certification." April 1, 2015. http://www.bullittcenter.org/2015/04/01/bullitt-center-earns-living-building-certification/.

McLennan, Jason F., and Eden Brukman. "Living Building Challenge 2.0: A Visionary Path to a Restorative Future." *International Living Building Institute*, 47. Seattle, WA: Cascadia Region Green Building Council, 2010.

Peña, Robert, Chris Meek, and Dylan Davis. "The Bullitt Center: A Comparative Analysis between Simulated and Operational Performance." *Technology| Architecture Design* 1, no. 2 (2017): 163–173.

Rider, Traci. R. "How Health Factors into Green Building Rating Systems: Living Building Challenge." *American Institute of Architects*, September 15, 2017.

Thomas, Mary Adam. *The Greenest Building: How the Bullitt Center Changes the Urban Landscape*. Portland, OR: Ecotone Publishing, International Living Future Institute, 2016.

United Nations Intergovernmental Panel on Climate Change (UNIPCC). *Special Report, Global Warming of 1.5 C*. 2018. www.ipcc.ch/sr15/.

United States Center for Disease Control. "Asthma in the US". Last modified May 2011. Atlanta, GA: CDC Vital Signs. www.cdc.gov/vitalsigns/asthma/index.html.

United States Environmental Protection Agency (USEPA). *Report of Environment*. Updated July 16, 2018. www.epa.gov/report-environment/indoor air quality.

United States Environmental Protection Agency (USEPA). *Report to Congress; Impacts and Control of CSOs and SSOs*. Office of Water (4203). Washington, DC: EPA 833-R-04–001, August 2004.

Van Den Wymelenberg, Kevin. "The Benefits of Natural Light." *Architectural Lighting Magazine*, March 19, 2014. www.archlighting.com/technology/the-benefits-of-natural-light_o.

Winer, Rose and Julia Keim. "Why Beautiful Spaces Make Us Healthier," International WELL Building Institute, August 7, 2018. https://resources.wellcertified.com/articles/why-beautiful-spaces-make-us-healthier/.

World Health Organization (WHO). *Health in the Green Economy: Health Co-benefits of Climate Change Mitigation—Housing Sector*. Geneva: World Health Organization, 2011.

World Health Organization (WHO). *How Does Safe Water Impact Global Health*. Geneva: World Health Organization. Online Q&A, June 2008. www.who.int/features/qa/70/en/.

World Health Organization (WHO). *Preventing Noncommunicable Diseases (NCDs) by Reducing Environmental Risk Factors*. Geneva: World Health Organization, 2017 (WHO/FWC/EPE/17.1). License: CC BY-NC-SA 3.0 IGO.

Chapter 17

Regenerative Architecture
Redefining Progress in the Built Environment

Robin Guenther

17.1 Introduction

The greatest challenge facing humanity is the reinvention of the relationship between industrial civilization and the environment that sustains it. The unprecedented scale of human impacts on social and ecological systems threatens health to the extent that current systems, including those that produce the built environment on which human existence depends, are no longer tenable. There is an urgency to create a future where "health is the aim"—its pace quickens with every extinction, extreme weather event, new chronic disease, and generational shift. As economic and social discourse shifts to focus on health and equity, fundamental system changes to support social and ecological restoration and resilience will follow.

Architectural design is entering its own period of radical transformation, fueled by big data and digital practice, population growth and rapid global urbanization, resource scarcity and climate change. As David Orr (2002, p. 30) defines it, "In the century ahead we must chart a course that leads to restoration, healing, and wholeness. The larger challenge is to transform a wasteful society into one that meets human needs with elegant simplicity". This twenty-first-century journey is beginning, influenced by restorative and regenerative thinking. How can design innovation quickly align with the tenets of regenerative design? There is one simple answer: health. Every innovation begins with an inspiration. Health is the catalyst that can transform the built environment—moving from an enterprise that degrades environmental and human health to one that restores and regenerates natural and social capital.

For architects and designers, this requires finding built environment solutions that solve multiple problems without creating unintended negative health consequences—solutions that "do no harm" and in fact "heal" some of the harm that has already been done. Globally, the green building movement is moving beyond conceiving of buildings as resource consumers toward regenerative design, where buildings are designed with inherent capability to be net resource generators. Regenerative design offers a global vision for a resilient and restorative built environment that contributes to a stronger, fairer, and cleaner world economy based on one simple truth: It is impossible to have healthy people on a sick planet.

17.2 Taking Responsibility for Unintended Consequences: Swarm Rules

As industry has expanded to a global scale, it has become impossible to deny the ecological consequences of an over-consuming planetary population. For the first time in human history, the unprecedented impact and reach of human activity on the planet is visible and documented. As a result, ecological concerns are a critical defining issue for this generation. For example, contemporary discussion of health cannot underestimate the looming impacts of continued fossil fuel use and climate change on planetary health. The UK Lancet Commission on health and climate change proclaimed, "The effects of climate change are being felt today, and future projections represent an unacceptably high and potentially catastrophic risk to human health" (Watts et al. 2015, p. 1861). The report also suggests that the effects of climate change threaten to undermine many of the social, economic, and environmental drivers of health that have contributed greatly to human progress, suggesting that climate change has the potential to undo 50 years of global public health gains. What is health in a world with increasing water scarcity and food insecurity? What is health in a world with rising sea levels and increasing extreme weather events? A 2004 cover of *Metropolis* magazine featured rolls of blueprints to suggest the fossil fuel smokestacks of buildings, accompanied by the simple headline "Architects Pollute". Its goal was simple: to get the largest sector contributor to greenhouse gas emissions causing air pollution and climate change to take responsibility and change practice. Why didn't it?

The prevailing narrative has been that these unintended consequences are the inevitable price of "progress". In *The Nature and Etiology of Disease*, Gaydos and Veney (2002, p. 18) state,

> [T]he technological advances that have allowed for increased longevity can also cause an increase in environmental degradation, and these advances arguably lead to new chronic diagnoses. . . . Many of the diseases [today] share common factors related to human adaptation, including diet, activity level, mental stress, behavioral practice, and environmental pollution.

Global warming, ozone depletion, habitat destruction, and toxic chemicals are major global environmental concerns with defined human and ecosystem health impacts. The Lancet Commission on pollution and health (Landrigan et al. 2018) concluded that diseases caused by air pollution were responsible for an estimated 9 million premature deaths in 2015—or 16% of all deaths worldwide. This represents three times more deaths than from AIDS, tuberculosis, and malaria combined, and 15 times more than from all wars and other forms of violence.

Fortunately, big data has made previously invisible impacts clear and measurable, and compels the creators of built environments to gather knowledge, take responsibility, and change practice. Daniel Goleman (2010) refers to this knowledge gathering as "ecological intelligence". This distributed intelligence, akin to a "swarm" of insects, is a system in which individual organizations follow simple "swarm rules" (ibid., p. 49) that work together in countless ways to achieve self-organizing goals. Goleman's three swarm rules are excerpted here; he continues (p. 50):

> Swarm intelligence results in an ongoing upgrade to our ecological intelligence through mindfulness of the true consequences of what we do and buy, the resolve to change for the better, and the spreading of what we know so others can do the same. If each of us in the human swarm follows those three simple rules, then together we might create a force that improves our human systems. No one of us needs to have a master plan or grasp all the essential knowledge. All of us will be pushing toward a continuous improvement of the human impact on nature.

Swarm Rules:

1. Know your impacts.
2. Favor improvements.
3. Share what you learn.

17.2.1 Building Material Transparency: Swarm Rules in Action

The science linking bio-accumulative industrial chemicals with human health impacts continues to provide new information about toxic body burdens, from the effects of low-dose exposures on developing fetuses and children to the cumulative impacts on wildlife. At the same time, resource scarcity and recycling are ushering in building products with more complex chemistry and potential environmental, health, and social justice impacts.

In the construction marketplace, the move toward building product transparency is a key illustration of the power of Goleman's "swarm rules" in action. In 2016, the design industry launched the Health Product Declaration Open Standard, a comprehensive, uniform, open standard that serves as the basis of analysis, evaluation, and comparison of products. The goal: to create a level playing field where project teams can select healthier materials and manufacturers can openly compete on the basis of healthier product chemistry.

Building material sourcing is complex and opaque. Product composition and health profile information is scarce, impossible to locate, and difficult to understand. Research on the ecological and health effects of building material substances is nascent, but the public health community has begun to focus attention on this issue. Many of these substances not only pollute

Robin Guenther

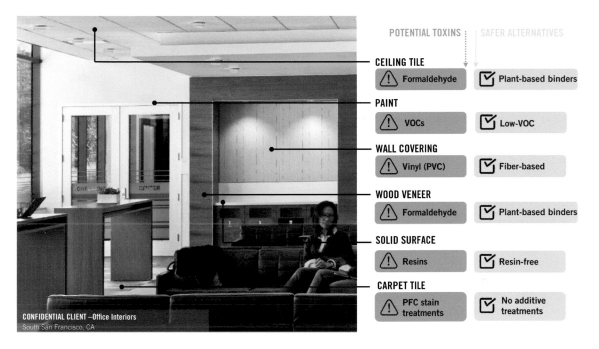

POTENTIAL TOXINS   SAFER ALTERNATIVES

CEILING TILE
⚠ Formaldehyde   ☑ Plant-based binders

PAINT
⚠ VOCs   ☑ Low-VOC

WALL COVERING
⚠ Vinyl (PVC)   ☑ Fiber-based

WOOD VENEER
⚠ Formaldehyde   ☑ Plant-based binders

SOLID SURFACE
⚠ Resins   ☑ Resin-free

CARPET TILE
⚠ PFC stain   ☑ No additive
  treatments   treatments

CONFIDENTIAL CLIENT –Office Interiors
South San Francisco, CA

▲ Figure 17.1

Material health in the workplace. This material application illustration offers a glimpse into the chemical complexity of contemporary building products. An office interior can host materials made from a complex array of synthetic substances with known or suspected negative health impacts, but there exist a range of market-available alternatives.
Source: Perkins and Will

the environment but also have adverse effects on indoor air quality. The U.S. Environment Protection Agency (Wallace 1987) found that indoor environments have pollutant levels of 2–5 times higher, and occasionally more than 100 times higher, than outdoors levels due to occupant activities, building materials, and ambient conditions.

Using the transparency of data unlocked by the Health Product Declaration, the linked movements of "green chemistry", "clean production", and "cradle-to-cradle thinking" are ushering in a materials revolution that is producing a range of alternative healthier products. A dedicated group of owners, designers, and manufacturers is committed to supporting the expansion of voluntary ingredient disclosure. These mutually reinforcing efforts are committed to "sharing what they learn" to drive innovation toward health.

17.3 From Sustainable to Regenerative

The application of swarm rules ultimately looks to define and manifest progress in our built environment. Necessary for making any progress in building with ecological and human health in mind is a cohesive roadmap toward a true sustainable future (a roadmap postulated in Figure 17.2). This diagram suggests that "green" initiatives today, however well intentioned, are focused on

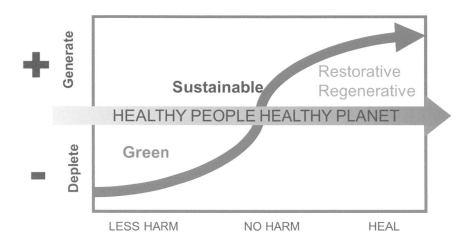

◀ Figure 17.2

Regenerative design
seeks solutions that move
beyond doing "less harm"
to those that do "no harm"
and "heal" the harm that
has already been done.
Health is the catalyst that
will propel current practice
toward regenerative
solutions.
Source: Robin Guenther

reducing negative impacts—using "less" fossil fuel and water. Strategies and systems that "do no harm" are theoretically "sustainable" (i.e., capable of continuing indefinitely with no adverse impacts to human or natural systems over time). On a planet with finite resources where degradation is already threatening the long-term viability of life, "restorative" or "regenerative" systems and initiatives are aimed at both sustaining present status and restoring or regenerating some of what has been lost. Increasingly, planetary survival may depend upon embracing such regenerative systems. This chapter explores the emergence of regenerative design in theory and in practice.

This is not a linear journey. Design strategies that create "less harm" are valuable and important, but they are insufficient to bring about the fundamental change that is needed. The pursuit of health is the catalyst—as solutions seek to shift from delivering unintended health inequities and negative environmental impacts to delivering equitable, cascading health benefits.

17.4 The Theory of Restorative or Regenerative Design

Architects Sim Van der Ryn and Stuart Cowan (2007, p. 33) initially defined ecological design as "any form of design that minimizes environmentally destructive impacts by integrating itself with living processes". Ecological designs, like nature, grow from and reflect the natural systems of a particular place. But Van der Ryn acknowledged that ecological design alone was insufficient—design needed to initiate regenerative processes to replace the degradation resulting from past practices. John Tillman Lyle (1994) first introduced the concept of "regenerative design" to capture a future where human systems create and support natural and social capital. Regenerative design literature is rooted in ecology, living systems theory, and whole-systems thinking.

Mang and Reed further refined the concept of regenerative design by noting that all life engages in four levels of work, "all of which are essential to the system's continuing vitality, viability and capacity for evolution" (2012, p. 27). These are differentiated into two lower levels of work and two upper levels. The first two focus on the current existence of the system itself: "improving the efficiency of its performance and maintaining the effectiveness of its resources respectively" (ibid., p. 27). These levels correspond to the "green design" portion of Figure 17.2, the functions of "doing less harm". The upper two levels "introduce potential life and creativity by asking what the system's unique role is in advancing the whole", or the "restorative" and "healing" portions of Figure 17.2 (ibid., p. 27). It is essential to consider all levels of Figure 17.2 simultaneously. Mang and Reed (2015, p. 8) further suggest that adding value to an ecological system means "increasing its systemic capability to generate, sustain, and evolve increasingly high orders of vitality and viability for the life of a particular place". Pictou Landing Health Centre, the project illustrated in Figure 17.3 and Figure 17.4, demonstrates how a building project can achieve all levels of Figure 17.2 simultaneously.

Regenerative design represents the transition to a built environment that embodies the capability of not only creating the conditions that support

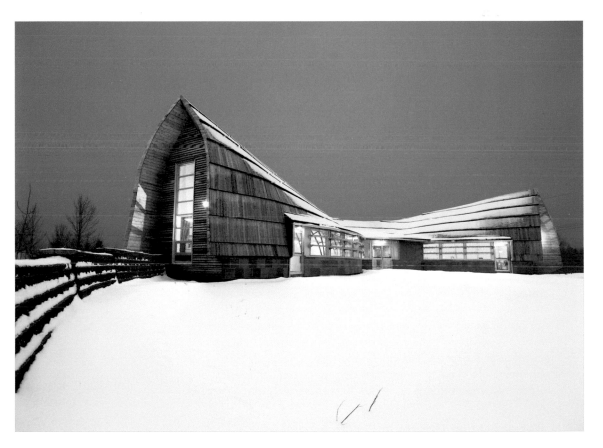

▲ Figure 17.3

Pictou Landing Health Centre, Nova Scotia, Canada, 2004. Richard Kroeker. The community asked that the building serve as a catalyst for social and cultural renewal. Traditional wood use by Algonquian tribes involves local small-diameter trees, bent into arched forms while green and flexible to maximize structural capacity.
Source: Paul Toman

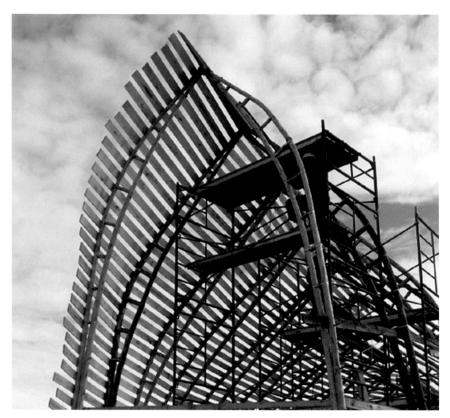

◀ Figure 17.4

The truss system of the Pictou Landing Health Centre was developed after studying traditional Mi'kmaq construction by building traditional lodges and longhouses in collaboration with Mi'kmaq elders, which in turn required training of local Mi'kmaq workers. The building itself is highly insulated, provides shelter from the ocean, and opens up to the sun through its open "arms". This passive design is supplemented through ground-sourced heat pumps and highly efficient heat recovery.
Source: Richard Kroeker

life and health but also repairing or restoring some of what has been degraded or lost. Architect and professor Ray Cole (2012, p. 1) defines regenerative design as

> approaches that support the co-evolution of human and natural systems in a partnered relationship. It is not the building that is "regenerated" in the same sense as the self-healing and self-organizing attributes of a living system, but by the ways that the act of building can be a catalyst for positive change within the unique "place" in which it is situated. Within regenerative development, built projects, stakeholder processes and inhabitation are collectively focused on enhancing life in all its manifestations—human, other species, ecological systems—through an enduring responsibility of stewardship.

17.5 Regenerative Design in Practice

Science writer Janine Benyus, in *Biomimicry: Innovation Inspired by Nature* (1997), points to a future when science will look to nature for inspiration and technology. Likewise, E. O. Wilson (1984), Kellert and Wilson (1995), Stephen Kellert (2005), and multiple authors in this book have reintroduced the human species deep bond with and affinity for nature, captured in "biophilic" design principles, as essential

Robin Guenther

for health and survival. Living Buildings, as defined by architects Bob Berkebile and Jason McLennan (1999) and exemplified in Chapter 16 of this book, offer a glimpse into the state of the industry today in implementing regenerative design principles at a building or neighborhood level.

To date, LEED Platinum–certified buildings and Living Buildings embody individual design strategies and systems that can be viewed as regenerative. For example, the use of green or vegetated roofs, such as the undulating landscape of the VanDusen Botanical Garden (Figure 17.5), demonstrates how a building system can be designed to deliver a series of benefits far beyond weather protection—it manages stormwater, reduces heat island impacts, and continues the natural habitat that might otherwise be disturbed by the placement of the structure. It is a gateway or mediator between the city and the natural habitat of the botanical garden itself. At the recently completed LEED Platinum Unilever Marketplace project (Figure 17.6), the transformation of a 1960s corporate campus arranged around an exterior courtyard includes enclosing the space between existing buildings to create new relationships between corporate divisions, people and nature, interior and exterior, with the express goal of improving culture and health. Started in 2014, "Project Unify" brought together five previously scattered business divisions under a global Sustainable Living plan with a goal of growing the business while dramatically reducing the organization's carbon footprint. The promise of regenerative design is that this creates a cascading series of health and equity benefits that extend through not only the workforce but also the brands and products that Unilever creates.

▼ Figure 17.5

VanDusen Botanical Garden Visitor Centre, Vancouver, British Columbia, Canada, 2011. The VanDusen Botanical Garden Visitor Centre is a Living Building. The green roof provides a rain barrier, harvests rainwater, supports habitat and solar panels, and fundamentally expresses a unified approach to human and natural systems.
Source: Nic Lehoux

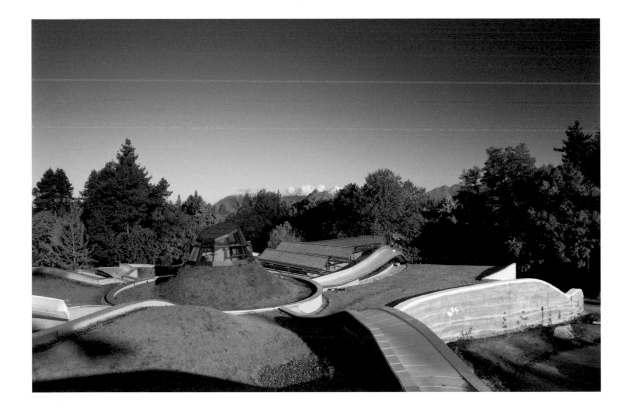

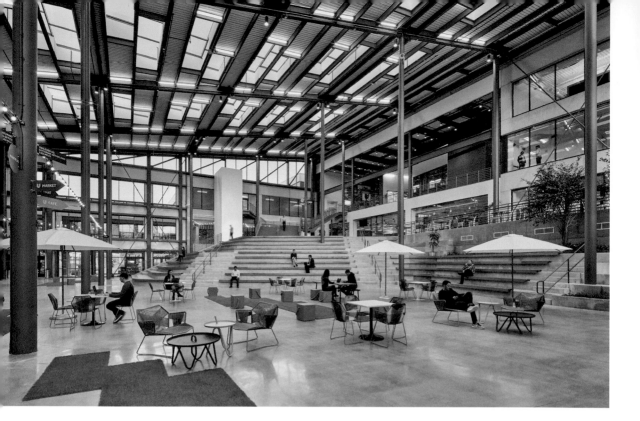

▲ Figure 17.6

Unilever Marketplace and Corporate Headquarters, Englewood Cliffs, New Jersey, 2018. The LEED Platinum Unilever Marketplace, a major renovation of the company's existing headquarters, reduces carbon emissions by 50% while providing a new relationship between building occupants and nature. The goal is to catalyze health and creativity in the workplace that will further drive product innovation toward sustainability and health.

Source: Garrett Rowland Photography

17.5.1 Discovery Health Center

The Discovery Health Center is a 28,000-square-foot ambulatory care building in Harris, New York, and an early example of regenerative design thinking in practice. Completed in 2004 as the first LEED-certified ambulatory building in the U.S., it remains an important example of the concept of building capacity to encourage regeneration of social and natural capital. The Center is a residential treatment facility for adults and children with developmental disabilities, medical frailties, and autism. The client brief for the first campus medical facility was simple:

1. Restore the land, because you won't have healthy people in degraded natural environments.
2. Build the healthiest interior environment possible by examining every component critically.
3. Take responsibility and act.

The selected site was a severely degraded parcel that had been used for industrial chicken farming; the nitrogen runoff was still so intense that the

Robin Guenther

Center's adjacent CSA farm, where they grew food for the residents, was struggling. Through the process of construction, the site was cleaned and the natural water flow to the CSA was restored. To achieve the healthiest building, nontoxic materials were selected that could be maintained with green cleaners. There was no on-site combustion; an electric ground source heat pump system was paired with hydronic heating. Rainwater is harvested from the roof to irrigate the landscape around the building and the adjacent farm.

The building quickly became a metaphor for who the Center wanted to be. Within a year, staff parking lots filled with hybrid cars. In the 10 years since it opened, the Center has installed solar PV to produce much of the electricity needed to run the systems; it has planted an organic orchard on one side of the building and still grazes goats on the other (with edible window sills). Today, its tag line is "food is medicine" and it has adopted a range of health and stewardship practices that further propel its success as an organization and community. Is this a healthcare building? Or is it a structure that builds health? This is the essence of regenerative design in practice: the building as a catalyst for health and stewardship.

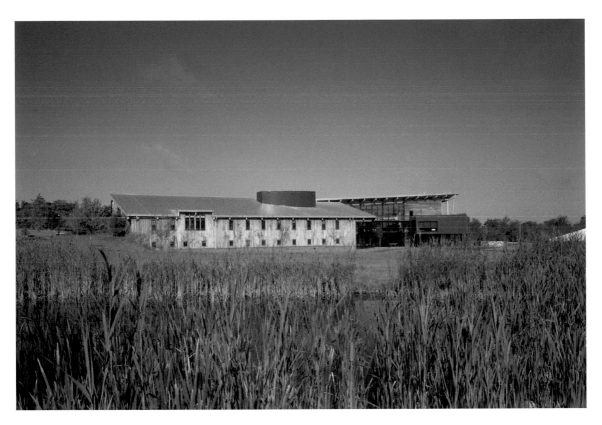

▲ Figure 17.7

Discovery Health Center, Harris, New York, 2003. This health center transformed the Center's approach to environmental stewardship and health promotion.
Source: D. Allee/Perkins and Will

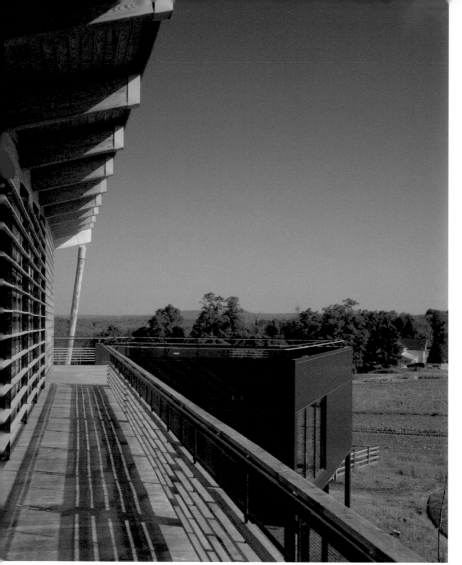

◄ Figure 17.8

Discovery Health Center, Harris, New York, 2003. Connection to nature and the outdoors is central to the experience of the building.
Source: D. Allee/Perkins and Will

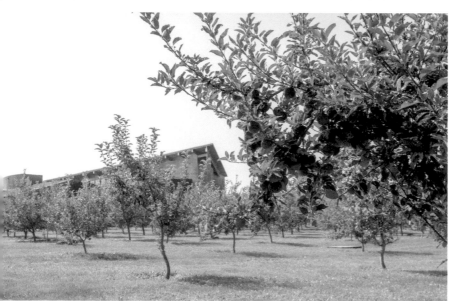

◄ Figure 17.9

Discovery Health Center, Harris, New York, 2003. Today, the building is surrounded by an organic orchard.
Source: Patrick H. Dollard, Discovery Health Center

Robin Guenther

The Center for Discovery Health Clinic is a catalyst for health and stewardship. In the 15 years since its opening, the building has inspired the organization to continue to invest in stewardship of its residents and the land, expanding organic farming and renewable energy investments, and furthering its mission of helping residents expand their capabilities and live their best lives.

17.6 The Future of Restorative and Regenerative Design

Buildings and neighborhoods that restore—that embody many of the principles of restorative or regenerative design—are emerging. All regenerative architecture demonstrates that the built environment can, through design choices, produce a cascading series of benefits instead of externalized harm at every scale. This ethos is made real in the selection of materials used in production, and buildings' overall impact on occupant, community, and global well-being. These goals require a positive feedback loop that implies a continuous progression forward.

In summary, this differs from conventional green or sustainable design thinking, as outlined in Table 17.1. Viewing the building as a catalyst for improving the health and vitality of the whole—well beyond the physical site boundaries and the time of construction—is the essence of future regenerative design thinking.

Regenerative design addresses the fundamental dysfunctional human-nature relationship by viewing the built environment as engaging in a co-creative partnership with nature—with the express goal of restoring and

Table 17.1 Comparing green design to regenerative design

Green design	Regenerative design
Views any system as a collection of individual elements that may or may not be optimized	Creates webs of interconnected dynamic processes that are continually structuring and restructuring
Optimizes effectiveness of individual technologies by eliminating redundancies and focusing on homogenous solutions	Optimizes effectiveness of individual technologies by seeing them as interactive and interdependent elements of an integrated whole
	Turns all strategies into vehicles for regenerating the health and increasing value of humans and ecosystems
Reduces degradation of both human and natural resources	Enhances generative capacities of both human and natural resources
Measurable building performance outcomes	Primacy of process over predetermined outcomes; outcomes realized over time

Source: Robin Guenther

regenerating global socio-ecological systems. Regenerative solutions are inextricably linked to the context and specifics of a place. Regenerative design also requires that we move beyond simply assessing building performance toward a future that is focused on improving the system's state of health—a place where success indicators are not yet developed or widely accepted. Robinson and Cole (2015, p. 135) sum it up this way:

> [R]egenerative approaches are fundamentally about rethinking the role of buildings, the types of questions during the design process, who is asked and how the discussion is guided. . . . It is about the ways that the act of building can be a positive catalyst for positive change within and add value to the unique "place" in which it is situated.

Regenerative design thinking is yielding new exploration in building technologies, such as rethinking tall buildings using timber in lieu of steel and aluminum. The Living Product Challenge, launched in 2014 by the International Living Future Institute, describes a future where a building product's "handprint"—the cascading environmental and health benefits—replaces its current "footprint"— its trail of unintended negative environmental and health consequences (ILFI 2017).

17.6.1 Timber Tower

As a regenerative design strategy, architects are reducing the embodied carbon footprint of tall buildings through the use of sustainably sourced and managed structural timber in order to reduce fossil fuel energy use, reduce the use of nonrenewable building materials, encourage planetary forest rejuvenation, and shift building product markets (Martin 2017). Forests, while growing, sequester carbon dioxide from the atmosphere; when harvested, timber can replace other products whose manufacture creates additional carbon emissions, such as steel and aluminum.

A study by Finnish consulting and engineering company Pöyry and the New England Forestry Foundation (2017) shows that the greatest potential for timber-built structures is in mid-rise (6–14-story) buildings, as it also tends to be more economical to build with timber at that scale. In early 2019, the Council for Tall Buildings and Urban Habitats (CTBUH) named the Norway Mjøstårt mixed-use tower the world's tallest completed timber building. It is 280 feet (85.4 m) tall.

This exploration is accelerating, driven by regenerative design thinking. Multiple looks into the construction capabilities of timber materials have promising findings, including the SOM-developed proposal for a 42-story high-rise as part of its Timber Tower Research Project. In 2016, Perkins and Will worked with Thornton Thomasetti and University of Cambridge to develop a proposal for River Beech Tower, a residential high-rise on the Chicago waterfront that would be taller than any existing timber building.

Robin Guenther

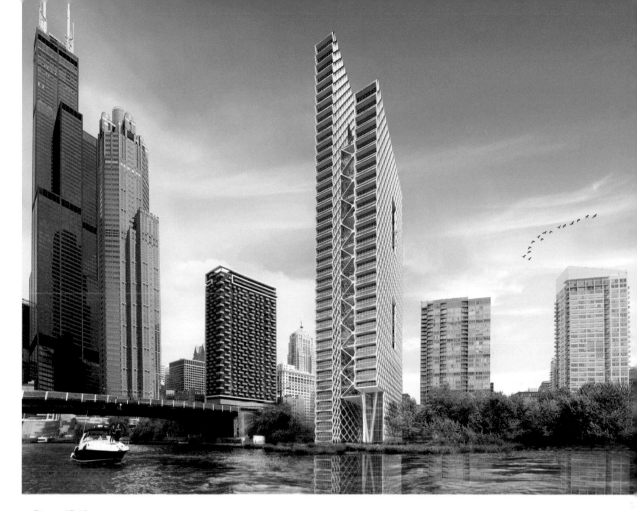

▲ Figure 17.10

River Beech Tower is a proposed 42-story residential building constructed using cross-laminated timber (CLT) technology. This is one exploration of rethinking the construction of contemporary built environments to encourage new relationships with renewable building products that deliver multiple benefits in their life cycle. Timber sequesters carbon and provides habitat; responsible harvesting provides a low-embodied energy building material that is both durable and beautiful.
Source: Perkins and Will

▼ Figure 17.11

River Beech Tower, Chicago, Illinois, unbuilt.
Source: Perkins and Will

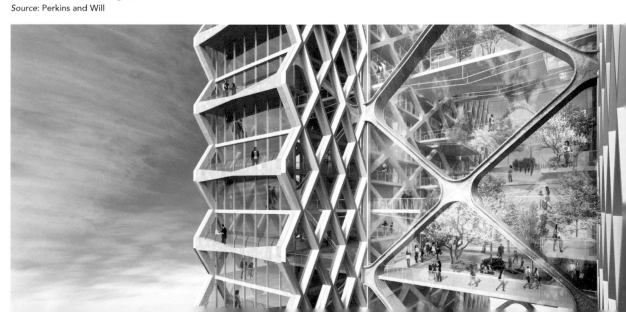

17.7 Conclusions

Unlike green or sustainable design processes, where tools exist to assist designers in understanding and quantifying ecological impact reduction—"less harm"—there are few emerging tools to guide the practice of regenerative design. In 2011, the U.S. Green Building Council began development of REGEN (Svec, Berkebile, and Todd 2012). A framework called LENSES (Living Environments in Natural, Social and Economic Systems), still in active development and refinement, outlines a process to help communities and project teams create places where natural, social, and economic systems can adapt, evolve, and thrive (Plaut et al. 2012; Clear 2019). These tools move well beyond green building tools to consider concepts and elements such as inclusivity, cultural resources, shared authority and governance, and ongoing prosperity. LENSES can be applied at the level of building design and neighborhood development.

As the examples in this chapter demonstrate, this is the leading edge of practice and is an emerging influence on design. Given the scale of the change necessary to realign priorities for greater health and equity and a more balanced interaction with the natural world, this new operating system presents a transformative opportunity to solve for health in the design of the built environment. By fully embracing principles of regenerative design, building designers and owners can demonstrate a commitment to improving health without undermining ecosystems or diminishing the world.

Bibliography

Benyus, Janine M. "Biomimicry." *Innovation Inspired by Nature*. New York, NY: Harper Collins, 1997.

Berkebile, Bob. "Restoring Our Buildings, Restoring Our Health, Restoring the Earth." Essay from Guenther, Robin, and Gail Vittori. *Sustainable Healthcare Architecture*, 17–19. Hoboken, NJ: John Wiley & Sons, 2008.

Berkebile, Robert, and Jason McLennan. "The living building." *The World and I magazine*. Washington, DC: Washington Times Publication, 1999.

Berry, Wendell. "Health Is Membership." *Another Turn of the Crank* 86 (1995): 90. Retrieved from http://home2.btconnect.com/tipiglen/berryhealth.html.

Clear. "Regenerate." (2019). www.clearabundance.org.

Cole, Raymond J. "Regenerative Design and Development: Current Theory and Practice." *Building Research & Information* 40, no. 1 (2012): 1–6.

"Create Better Neighborhoods and Communities." Essay from Guenther, Robin, and Gail Vittori. *Sustainable Healthcare Architecture*. Hoboken, NJ: John Wiley & Sons, 2008.

Gaydos, L. M., and J. E. Veney. "The Nature and Etiology of Disease." In *World Health Systems: Challenges and Perspectives*, edited by Bruce J. Fried and Laura M. Gaydos, 3–24. Chicago, IL: Health Administration Press, 2002.

Goleman, Daniel. *Ecological Intelligence: The Hidden Impacts of What We Buy*. New York, NY: Crown Business, 2010.

Howard Sir, A. *The Soil and Health: A Study of Organic Agriculture*. London: Benediction Classics/Oxford City Press, 2011 (Originally published by Faber & Faber in 1945 as Farming and Gardening for Health or Disease).

International Living Future Institute [ILFI]. *Living Product Challenge 1.1 Guide: Handprinting*. September, 2017. https://living-future.org/wp-content/uploads/2017/10/Handprinting-Guide-Sept-2017.pdf.

Kellert, Stephen R. *Building for Life: Designing and Understanding the Human-Nature Connection*. Washington, DC: Island Press, 2005.

Kellert, Stephen R., and Edward O. Wilson, eds. *The Biophilia Hypothesis*. Washington, DC: Island Press, 1995.

Landrigan, Philip J., Richard Fuller, Nereus Acosta, Olusoji Adeyi, Robert Arnold, Abdoulaye Bibi Baldé, Roberto Bertollini et al. "The Lancet Commission on Pollution and Health." *The Lancet* 391, no. 10119 (2018): 462–512.

Lyle, John Tillman. *Regenerative Design for Sustainable Development*. New York, NY: John Wiley & Sons, 1994.

Mang, Pamela, and Bill Reed. "Designing from Place: A Regenerative Framework and Methodology." *Building Research & Information* 40, no. 1 (2012): 23–38.

Mang, Pamela, and Bill Reed. "The Nature of Positive." *Building Research and Information*, 43, no 1 (2015): 7–10.

Martin, Olivia. "Is Mass Timber Really Sustainable?" *The Architects Newspaper*, November 20, 2017. https://archpaper.com/2017/11/timber-construction-sustainable/.

McDonough, William, and Michael Braungart. *Cradle to Cradle: Remaking the Way We Make Things*. New York, NY: North Point Press, 2010.

Orr, David W. *The Nature of Design: Ecology, Culture, and Human Intention*. New York, NY: Oxford University Press, 2002.

Plaut, Josette M., Brian Dunbar, April Wackerman, and Stephanie Hodgin. "Regenerative Design: The LENSES Framework for Buildings and Communities." *Building Research & Information* 40, no. 1 (2012): 112–122.

Pöyry. *Assessing The Wood Supply and Investment Potential for New England Engineered Wood Products Markets and Mill*. New England Forestry Foundation, July, 2017. Available at: http://newenglandforestry.org/wp-content/uploads/2017/12/CLT-in-New-England-NEFF-report.pdf.

Robinson, John and Raymond Cole. "Theoretical Underpinnings of Regenerative Sustainability." *Building Research & Information* 43, no. 2 (2015): 133–143.

Svec, Phaedra, Robert Berkebile, and Joel Ann Todd. "REGEN: Toward a Tool for Regenerative Thinking." *Building Research & Information* 40, no. 1 (2012): 81–94.

Van der Ryn, Sim, and Stuart Cowan. *Ecological Design*. Washington, DC: Island Press, 2007.

Wallace, Lance A. *Total Exposure Assessment Methodology (TEAM) Study: Summary and Analysis*. Vol. 1. No. PB-88-100060/XAB; EPA-600/6-87/002A. Washington, DC: Environmental Protection Agency Office of Acid Deposition, Environmental Monitoring, and Quality Assurance, 1987.

Walsh, William J. "Design and Stewardship: How the Design of Facilities Helps Create Better Neighborhoods and Communities." Essay in Guenther, R. and G. Vittori, *Sustainable Healthcare Architecture*, 1st ed., 389–391. Hoboken, NJ: Wiley, 2008.

Watts, Nick, W. Neil Adger, Paolo Agnolucci, Jason Blackstock, Peter Byass, Wenjia Cai, Sarah Chaytor et al. "Health and Climate Change: Policy Responses to Protect Public Health." *The Lancet* 386, no. 10006 (2015): 1861–1914.

Wilson, Edward O. *Biophilia: The Human Bond with Other Species*. Cambridge, MA: Harvard University Press, 1984.

World Health Organization. 1948. www.who.int/about/definition/en/print.html.

Chapter 18

A Blueprint for Using Renewable Energies in Remote Locations

Christopher W. Kiss and *Keith Holloway*

18.1 Introduction

Continuously operating a hospital 24 hours a day, 365 days a year consumes an extraordinary amount of energy. Rural hospitals are particularly noticeable within their small communities for their high energy consumption and related environmental impacts. This translates to high operating costs, the determining factor as to whether a health system is able to deliver primary, secondary, and emergency services within remote areas. Rural community hospitals are expensive to operate when considering the need for a diverse range of healthcare services, high facility operating costs, geographic staffing challenges, and low patient volumes when compared to their more urban counterparts. Lowering these operating costs is a tremendous hurdle that must be overcome to provide healthcare in rural communities. Rural hospitals that incorporate renewable energies, like solar, and adopt passive design strategies demonstrate how planning and design decisions can help meet these challenges.

The Military Health System (MHS) is the healthcare delivery system for the Department of Defense (DoD). The MHS has a large portfolio of healthcare facilities, including hospitals, clinics, laboratories, and other building types, located on military installations around the world. Like other communities in the country, military installations have experienced rising hospital operating costs. The continued operation of many small military hospitals has been challenged for their growing costs to the U.S. taxpayer. Military hospitals are located near servicemembers and their families, and some provide the only access to healthcare available to isolated military installation communities.

A portfolio assessment conducted in 2010 revealed that several MHS facilities needed major renewal or replacement. While MHS facilities maintain high-quality standards and accreditations for patient care, many did not support efficient operations and cost more to operate than comparable modern facilities. Consequently, the U.S. Congress approved funding for the replacement of multiple hospitals. To capitalize on this opportunity and improve healthcare settings, the DoD and the MHS modernized federal healthcare design guidelines to incorporate principles of energy conservation and environmental sustainability.

Delivering a new hospital for the military is significantly more expensive than other health systems. Increased federal capital costs are primarily attributed to heightened building security and structural features, acquisition strategy limitations, and building design restrictions related to future adaptability. Despite these design and construction factors, the MHS sought to demonstrate the judicious use of public funds by identifying hospitals with the greatest opportunity for improving operating costs. A project was identified to showcase the new DoD and MHS principles of energy conservation and environmental sustainability and the potential to control hospital operating costs for the military.

This chapter will explore a new small hospital project and how it incorporated principles of energy conservation, environmental sustainability, and economic viability. The design strategies used are applicable to other rural hospital projects, with the potential for greater innovation when federal system requirements are not necessary. The 206,000-square-foot Replacement Weed Army Community Hospital (WACH) is a proof of concept for high-performance healthcare buildings in remote settings.

▼ Figure 18.1

Exterior view of Weed Army Community Hospital in the early evening.
Source: Ken West

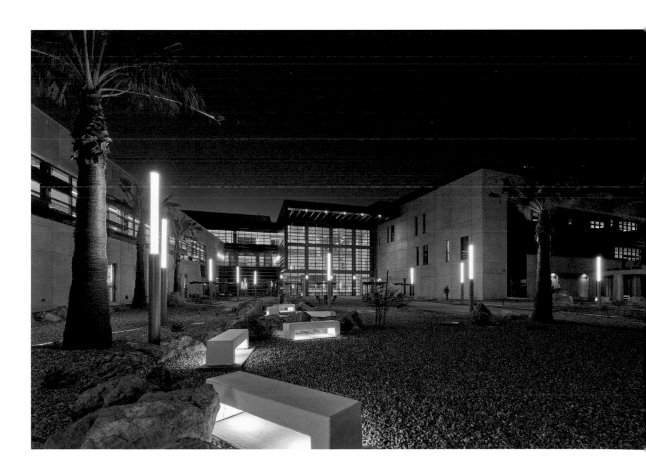

18.2 Building a Remote Hospital

In a remote area of Southern California, a new military community hospital has set new sustainability targets for the resource-intensive hospital building typology. The new hospital's performance objectives were driven by the area's high operating costs and the need for reliable access to healthcare services in this isolated location. The Fort Irwin military installation is located about 37 miles northeast of Barstow, California, within the Mojave Desert. The Mojave is an arid landscape surrounded by mountain ranges that limit rainfall through the rain-shadow effect. The entire military installation covers over 1,000 square miles, while the residential community center where the hospital is located is just slightly larger than 7 square miles.

The WACH supports the primary, secondary, and emergency healthcare needs of more than 8,000 soldiers and their families residing in the Fort Irwin community. This community is home to the National Training Center (NTC). The NTC has the mission to receive and train Battalion Task Force and Brigade-level units (unit sizes range from 4,000 to 6,000 soldiers) in visiting rotations. During these rotations, the hospital has to increase emergency and urgent surgical capabilities to support the shift from community residents to a population that includes soldiers training in the desert. Based on these requirements, the major design considerations were to accommodate the differences in medical needs for the two population types and address the fluctuating needs of an isolated community.

Real-life tactical systems and munitions are used instead of simulations on this military installation because the NTC possesses enough land area to ensure safety during hazardous exercises. While precautions are taken in tactical exercise planning, nearby access to trauma support is a necessity and its absence would be irresponsible. Thus, the WACH hospital program was required to provide emergency and trauma services in support of the military exercises. The next closest trauma center to Fort Irwin is 113 miles away (OSHPD Healthcare Atlas) at Loma Linda University Medical Center, and non-emergency care is 39 miles away at Barstow Community Hospital.

18.3 Establishing Design Goals for the Hospital

The purpose of the new WACH project was to replace an aging facility with a state-of-the-art hospital with surgical care near a high-intensity military training environment. The hospital that was replaced was constructed in the mid-1960s and no longer complied with current structural building codes for the seismic and wind loads of the area. The original hospital had excessive operational costs resulting from outdated mechanical systems, an inefficient building envelope, and significant spatial and operational inefficiencies. Additionally, healthcare services in the former hospital had evolved from an inpatient-centered to outpatient-centered model of care.

Even though Fort Irwin is a relatively small community, it is costly to operate and maintain due to its physical distance from the larger Barstow area. Electrical power is transmitted almost 40 miles to the installation from the closest power provider. Like many small communities, the WACH hospital was the largest single building consumer of electrical power. For the installation to attain its energy conservation goals, the hospital had to be part of the solution.

The goals for the replacement hospital were developed to consider the community's special requirements for the delivery of healthcare. The small, remote community and military training environment required advanced surgical, primary, and specialty care capabilities that had to be fully operational at all times despite the severe climatic conditions. Furthermore, the hospital had to operate efficiently to conserve federal funds, and not significantly alter the power requirements for the installation. These considerations led to the following project goals: to deliver high-quality healthcare in the Mojave Desert; to provide flexibility and future adaptability to the hospital; and to build for sustainability.

18.3.1 Delivering High-Quality Healthcare in the Mojave Desert

The vision of the Weed Army Community Hospital (WACH) replacement project was to optimize facility operations to improve the medical care provided to soldiers, military families, and retirees in the Fort Irwin community. This mission-critical project included the design of a hospital and clinic, central utility plant, ambulance shelter, and helipad.

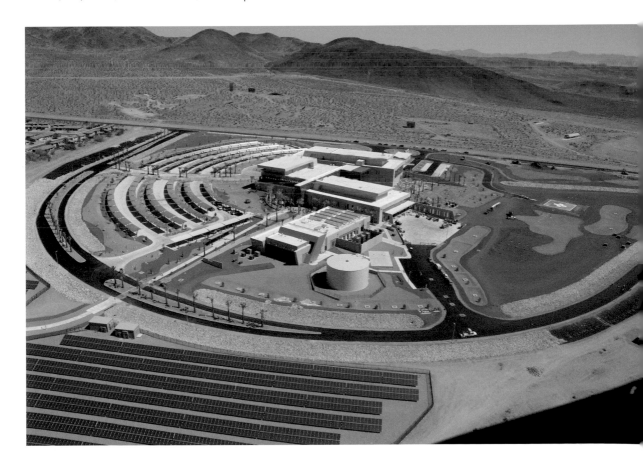

The new hospital's clinical program was determined by assessing the current and future needs of the installation community. Each clinical program element had to have the patient workload necessary to sustain clinical operations and justify staffing requirements. Outpatient clinic services included in the new hospital program are primary care, women's health, behavioral health, surgery, optometry, and occupational health. The diagnostic and treatment services in the clinical program include emergency, pharmacy, radiology, and surgery departments. The inpatient services in the program are a medical/surgical ward and a mother/baby ward. The medical/surgical ward is composed of ten single-bed inpatient rooms and related clinical support areas. The mother/baby ward consists of five single-bed labor, delivery, recovery, and postpartum (LDRP) rooms, one cesarean section (C-section room), and other support areas.

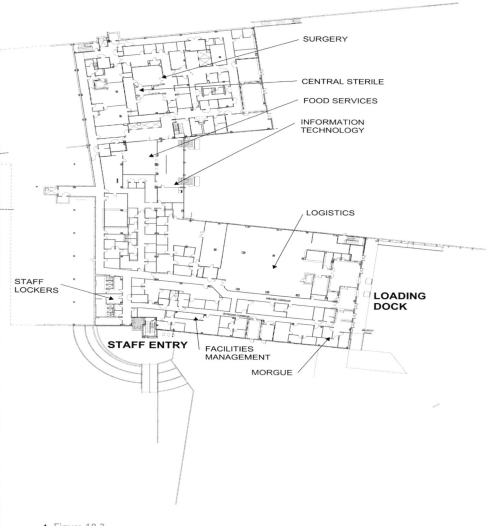

▲ Figure 18.3

Floor plan, first floor.
Source: RLF

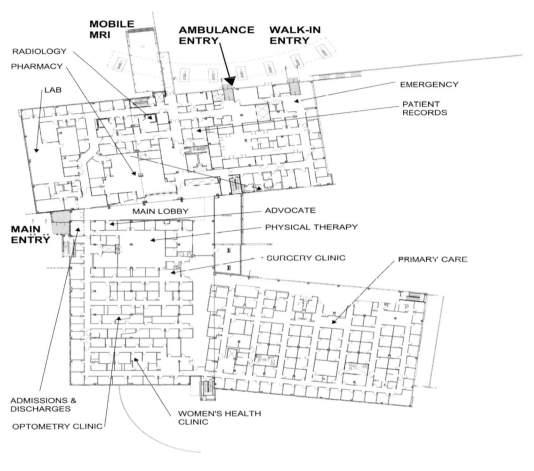

MOBILE MRI

RADIOLOGY

PHARMACY

LAB

AMBULANCE ENTRY

WALK-IN ENTRY

EMERGENCY

PATIENT RECORDS

MAIN LOBBY

ADVOCATE

PHYSICAL THERAPY

MAIN ENTRY

SURGERY CLINIC

PRIMARY CARE

ADMISSIONS & DISCHARGES

OPTOMETRY CLINIC

WOMEN'S HEALTH CLINIC

▲ Figure 18.4

Floor plan, second floor.
Source: RLF

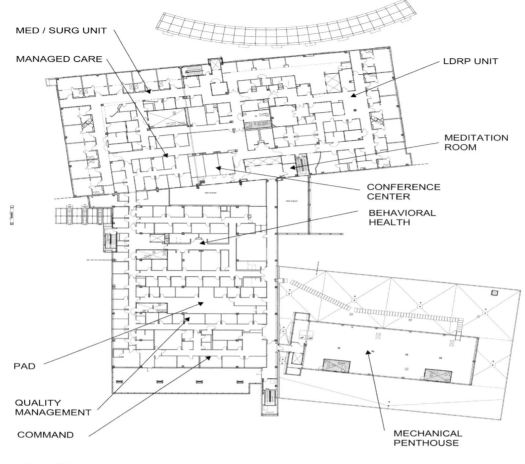

MED / SURG UNIT

MANAGED CARE

LDRP UNIT

MEDITATION
ROOM

CONFERENCE
CENTER

BEHAVIORAL
HEALTH

PAD

QUALITY
MANAGEMENT

COMMAND

MECHANICAL
PENTHOUSE

▲ Figure 18.5

Floor plan, third floor.
Source: RLF

One of the most influential design considerations was the emergency and urgent surgical capabilities of the community hospital. While these capabilities are available for any emergency near the hospital or community, they have been deliberately designed to support the intense training environment of the National Training Center. The emergency department is connected with a restricted urgent elevator to both the inpatient and surgical departments. The emergency department has a trauma room, as well as multiple exam rooms to treat a range of patient types and conditions. The surgical department within the hospital consists of two operating rooms, along with an adjacent central sterilization services department. The WACH hospital design is distinct from other rural hospitals of this size due to the various patient arrival methods and

Christopher W. Kiss and Keith Holloway

the need for advanced imaging systems. Adjacent to the emergency department entrance, a helicopter landing area is constructed to receive either military or civilian medevac aircraft. In addition to general X-ray areas, the radiology department includes a computed tomography (CT) imaging room, specifically for assessing trauma cases.

Access to daylight was essential for energy conservation and indoor environmental quality. Particular attention was made to incorporate windows into the patient areas as well as clinical working spaces. Design discussions detailed work activities of each room type to determine which rooms required daylighting, which should not be daylit for functional reasons, and which could benefit from daylight if it were possible. Inpatient rooms were specifically arranged to receive pristine views of the mountain landscape without overlooking the existing community buildings.

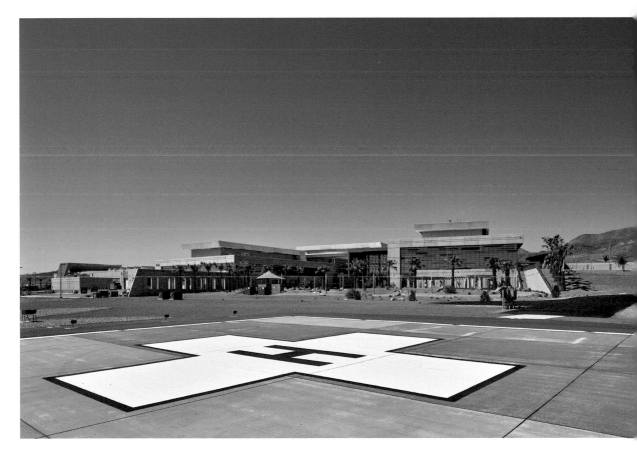

▲ Figure 18.6

Exterior view from helipad.
Source: Ken West

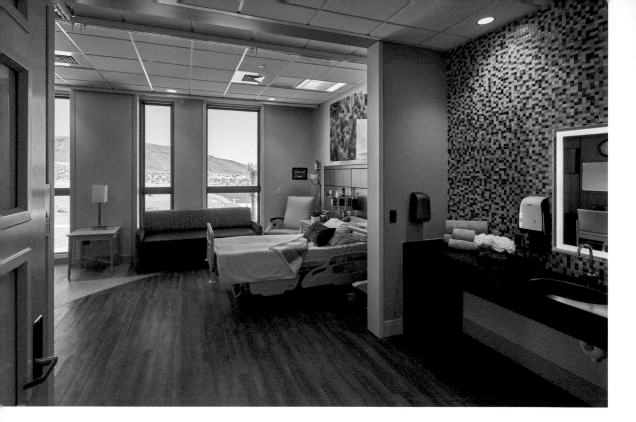

▲ Figure 18.7

Interior view of an inpatient bedroom and its mountain view.
Source: Ken West

18.3.2 Providing Flexibility and Future Adaptability to the Hospital

All modern hospital design should incorporate a strategy to provide flexibility and future adaptability to support changes in healthcare delivery over the building's service life. Rooms or departments that support a variety of different functions without significant alteration are a characteristic of a flexible hospital. Several features were included into the design to provide flexibility for the clinical functions within the hospital. In the inpatient wards, the mother/baby and medical/surgical wards are immediately next to one another. In periods of high-birth workload this adjacency provides the flexibility to utilize the medical/surgical patient rooms for mother/baby patient overflow. Consideration was also given to the inpatient medical/surgical ward to support its use for short-term psychiatric inpatients by locating it nearby the outpatient behavioral health clinic and its providers. In the radiology department, architectural and utility provisions for a mobile magnetic resonance imaging (MRI) unit were provided. Mobile MRI units have been planned for to allow the facility to flex as clinical requirements evolve over time.

Adaptable hospitals are designed to readily allow for the future expansion of services or introduction of new medical technologies. Planning for long-term use and future adaptability is a requirement for all new military hospital construction. Federal requirements for military hospital construction stipulate that an area equal to 25% of the total project area must be planned for future expansion. The requisite planned area for future expansion was divided and allocated to each of the clinical zones to support future growth within any of the clinical areas. Site conditions, such as the direction of medevac helicopter arrival, further refined the shape of the building.

18.3.3 Building for Sustainability

A goal of the new hospital project was to embody the military's emphasis on responsible use of fiscal and environmental resources. Most existing military hospitals were developed under strict guidelines governing first cost of construction, while operating costs were simply addressed by code compliance. Until relatively recent improvements, construction codes did not encourage and incentivize major improvements to energy efficiency of buildings.

Leading up to the design phase of the project, there were several changes in how the military viewed energy and sustainability in hospital construction. The military shifted from certifying its own design and construction to participating in a third-party sustainability assessment. The military chose the Leadership in Energy and Environmental Design (LEED) model to work toward a system-wide improvement in sustainability. In addition, the American Society of Heating, Refrigeration, and Air-conditioning Engineers' (ASHRAE) Standard 90.1 Energy Standard for Buildings Except Low-Rise Residential Buildings prescribed new minimum energy performance criteria and alternative methods of compliance, such as allowing for the use of energy modeling software to simulate the design energy performance.

The first task of the design effort was to create a baseline energy model that met minimal energy efficiency standards to benchmark the energy savings potential of various strategies. During architectural and mechanical systems design, energy modeling and life-cycle cost analysis (LCCA) procedures were used to ensure a healthy, environmentally friendly, and cost-effective facility. The energy model was used to define energy consumption patterns to prioritize design efforts for energy reduction. LCCA was used to compare savings from a proposed design strategy or conservation measure with any added costs, such as maintenance. The combined use of energy modeling and LCCA validated the design decisions adopted.

The next task of the design effort was to identify the most cost-effective passive design strategies and conservation measures to reduce energy use and the carbon footprint of the hospital. Passive design strategies influenced design choices related to massing, orientation, and openings to take advantage of the natural benefits of the site. These strategies impact energy conservation for the life of the building. Hospital massing decisions were made early in the design planning, and reflect the clinical program of inpatient, outpatient, diagnostic, and treatment zones. The energy consumption patterns differ across these three zones while each contributes to the total use pattern. The inpatient zone is continuously operating with artificial lighting and a constant temperature range. The outpatient zone is operated only during normal business hours. The diagnostic and treatment zones have the highest energy loads, due to equipment usage, but have limited operations outside of business hours. With these differences in mind, the outpatient clinics were considered a separate, adjoined building from the inpatient, diagnostic, and treatment zones. This architectural arrangement supported facility operation measures that could shut off artificial lighting and create heating and cooling efficiencies. Arrangement of the major clinical zone building blocks was determined by the comparison of multiple design concept models that were each assessed using energy modeling software. A dozen different configurations were narrowed to four distinct options, all of which supported the clinical program. Energy models of each option were assessed on how well they attained the energy conservation targets of the project.

While outpatient, inpatient, and diagnostic and treatment spaces were divided into separate buildings for energy conservation purposes, these buildings are still adjoined and arranged to create a cohesive clinical operation between them. On the ground-level main entryway there is a large double-height atrium that illuminates the intersection of the hospital's two sections, providing a lobby and waiting area for patients and visitors. Access to daylight is usually increased by decreasing the depth of floor plates or by articulating the building perimeter. Increasing the building perimeter frequently has consequences for both heating and cooling loads, as well as construction cost. Introducing overhead daylight with atria into dense hospital areas can be an effective strategy without increasing building envelope area.

As part of the energy modeling analysis of the hospital design, the building envelope was selected and designed in accordance with insulation ratings and their location. Surprisingly, higher insulation values did not always result in better performance, as shown where lower insulation values allowed heat losses of plug-loads and mechanical systems during the cooling season. Multiple simulations of

▼ Figure 18.8

Interior view of the central atrium and lobby.
Source: Ken West

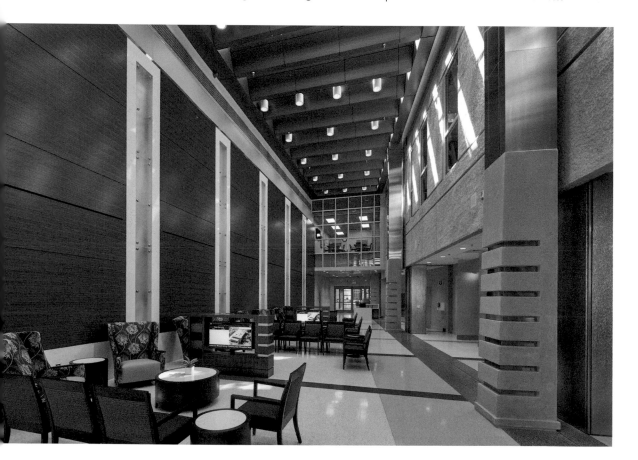

Christopher W. Kiss and Keith Holloway

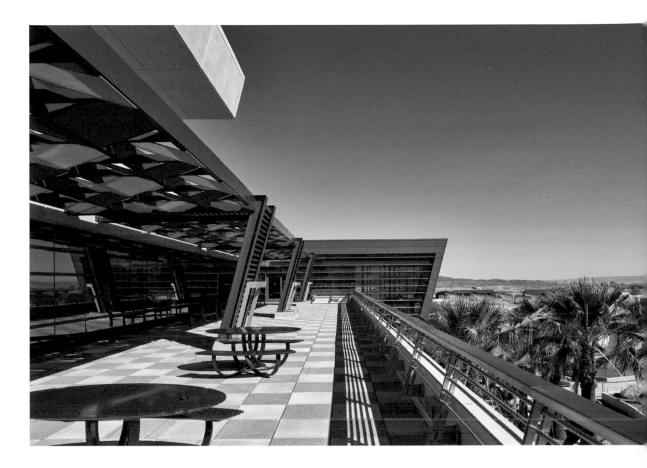

▲ Figure 18.9

Exterior view of third-floor balcony exterior space.
Source: Ken West

glazing choices for the exterior envelope were assessed in the energy models to determine the best transmission of the desired characteristics of the daylighting with the least amount of solar heat gain. Architectural overhangs and window louvers were added features whose arrangements were refined with the modeling. Energy modeling using historical weather data for the area supports the projected best envelope system for the local environmental conditions.

Energy conservation measures of mechanical, electrical, and plumbing (MEP) systems were the most impactful aspect of the hospital design strategy. Lighting strategies to conserve energy were used to specify lighting systems with lower power requirements, such as using LED and compact fluorescent lighting fixtures. Control systems were designed to gain energy savings with both daylighting controls as well as occupied space sensors for artificial lighting. High-efficiency MEP equipment and systems were selected to attain improvements in operational costs. The addition of condensing boilers and high-efficiency chillers and their controls were significant systems investments to attain building performance. The design of the air handling units and overall system was approached with an emphasis on energy performance, with variable zones of operation to support lower levels of operation when not in peak heating, cooling, or off-business hours.

The passive design strategies and conservation measures selected were building separations by occupancy type, massing strategies for building shape and orientation, emphasis on daylighting most occupied spaces, and building envelope and insulation design. These conservation measures were expected to decrease energy use by 33.2% below a minimal code standard design. These conservation measures were expected to have a positive environmental impact by reducing greenhouse gas emissions by over 4,600 metric tons per year below the minimally code-compliant baseline and save over $300,000 a year in energy costs at present rates of inflation. Added costs for these measures amounted to less than 2% of the overall project budget and are projected to have a simple payback of less than five years due to energy savings.

18.4 From Reduction to Production: Net-Zero and Carbon-Neutral

Once the most effective energy reduction strategies were determined, energy production possibilities needed to be considered. The Fort Irwin community would frequently report intermittent electrical brownout conditions, especially during peak usage periods. The most impacted facility was the hospital, which would employ emergency power generators to continue healthcare operations. Surgeries and inpatient care settings both require strict environmental conditions provided by powered mechanical systems that cannot be compromised by the unpredictable brownouts. The emergency generators are diesel powered, which is a logical choice based on the easy availability of diesel fuel on a military installation. However, the use of the generators was more frequent than desired, adding to the negative environmental impacts attributed to the hospital.

Ambitious objectives were proposed to reach the industry energy performance metrics of net-zero and carbon-neutral, both of which provide the functional independence required for remote hospitals. Net-zero energy performance results from the generation of renewable energy on-site greater than the annual energy consumed to operate the facility. Carbon neutrality occurs when the amount of carbon emitted from fossil fuel sources is balanced to the amount of carbon offset by reduction strategies, such as renewable energy sources. For the new hospital to decrease its reliance on the installation and surrounding infrastructure, the addition of power generation was considered. Many potential options were considered for power generation, such as combined heat and power plants. These alternatives use fuel types that were not readily available on the military installation. Renewable sources were discussed because of the geographic location, and solar power generation was an early project consideration.

The outstanding solar irradiance potential of the Fort Irwin geographic region made this an ideal project to include solar energy generation to meet the hospital's power needs. In addition to the previously described conservation measures to decrease the energy intensity of the new hospital, a renewable energy strategy was developed to utilize the tremendous solar potential of the site.

The design team demonstrated a significant return on investment (ROI) to the federal government through a proposal using energy and operational cost models. The large photovoltaic (PV) array addition to the project was a notable benefit to the energy efficiency of the planned medical campus. The PV system designed for this location and climate achieved a surplus of energy for the facility and contributed back to the overall installation power grid. The installation costs of the PV system are projected to be returned within a short period of time.

In addition to the ROI support, several superfluous features of the LEED Silver option were omitted with the LEED Platinum option. The LEED Platinum option was strikingly comparable in cost to the LEED Silver option and was attainable without any additional cost to the government.

The renewable features and systems integrated into the new hospital were the solar photovoltaic (PV) array and the solar thermal water heating systems. The hospital's energy requirements and net-zero objective helped determine the size and location of the 2.3-megawatt array south of the hospital. A solar thermal hot water heating system was designed to complement the hospital's conventional hot water heating system. Solar radiation is used to preheat potable water with relatively basic principles and system components. The new hospital's conventional water heating system receives the preheated water, which significantly reduces the amount of fuel needed to heat the water.

The renewable generation combined with conservation measures allowed the new hospital design to achieve both net-zero and carbon-neutral performance. According to the Environmental Protection Agency's greenhouse gas equivalencies calculator (EPA 2017), the replacement hospital's performance will reduce greenhouse gas emissions by more than 4,600 metric tons per year—the equivalent of the carbon sequestered annually by 990 acres of forest. Over the first 25 years of the hospital's operation, the Army will save more than $23 million in energy costs. The solar photovoltaic will completely offset the electrical usage, and the solar thermal system can provide 65% of the domestic hot water needs for the hospital. This renewable strategy, combined with the conservation measures, will reduce the carbon footprint for the hospital to neutral.

▼ Figure 18.10

Exterior view of the hospital front entryway.
Source: Ken West

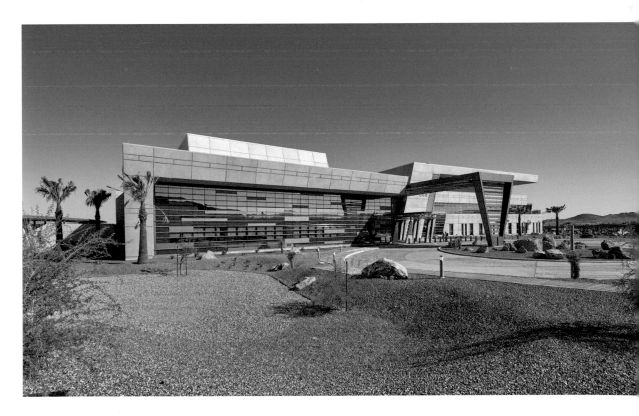

18.5 Conclusions

In the past, the importance of the healthcare delivery mission at Fort Irwin justified the fiscal and environmental drain of community resources. Under new scrutiny, the new hospital sought to change the paradigm that accepted high operating costs in order to deliver world-class care. The new hospital project achieved its goals to create a healthcare environment for a full range of high-quality services in a remote setting; to provide a flexible and adaptable healthcare facility; and to build for energy and environmental sustainability.

The Replacement Weed Army Community Hospital is the first military LEED Platinum, net-zero, and carbon-neutral facility of its kind. As such, it has the potential to set a precedent for future military facilities as well as other remote hospitals across the United States. Lessons learned are that small, remote hospitals can be efficient and add value beyond access to care to their communities. Additionally, energy modeling and life-cycle cost analysis are valuable tools used to inform all phases of hospital design. Finally, major healthcare construction investments are an ideal time to implement ambitious new organizational goals that lead to solutions that are cost effective, reliable, and better for the environment.

In this case study, the MHS, Fort Irwin Community, and the California energy provider were able to agree on a renewable energy grid that will provide significant gain to all three stakeholders for years to come. There are few remaining energy conservation strategies that can be done in the Fort Irwin community that have a potential for impact as significant as the energy sustainability features of the Weed Army Community Hospital replacement.

Critical access hospitals (CAHs) and other small, remotely located hospitals can be self-sufficient and efficiently run facilities that reliably deliver essential healthcare services to rural populations. CAHs receive funding support from the federal government to overcome challenges of delivering healthcare to small populations. The operating costs of inefficiently designed small hospitals are a significant challenge that CAHs must overcome to continue providing their essential services. It is possible to reverse the status quo by positioning the healthcare system as a community leader rather than just a provider of patient care services. Healthcare systems can and should set the example of how to responsibly use environmental resources. Energy modeling techniques, life-cycle cost analysis, and the integration of renewable energies and passive design strategies are all vital to obtain the goals of energy conservation, environmental sustainability, and economic viability.

Bibliography

Beeman, Jeffrey M., and Caitlin McAlpine. "Building the World's 'Greenest' Hospital." *The Military Engineer* 108, no. 705 (2016): 50–53.

Environmental Protection Agency. "Greenhouse Gas Equivalencies Calculator." (2017). www.epa.gov/energy/greenhouse-gas-equivalencies-calculator.

Lavy, Sarel, Christopher W. Kiss, and Jose L. Fernandez-Solis. "Linking Design and Energy Performance in US Military Hospitals." *Architectural Engineering and Design Management* 11, no. 1 (2015): 41–64.

Silvis, Jennifer. "A Solar-Powered Oasis." *Healthcare Design Magazine*, August 20, 2012. www.healthcaredesignmagazine.com.

Chapter 19

Integrating LEED with Biophilic Design Attributes
Toward an Inclusive Rating System

Stephen Verderber and *Terri Peters*

19.1 Introduction

Excessive carbon emissions and the depletion of nonrenewable resources continue to inflict increasingly harmful impacts on human populations and on the planet (Intergovernmental Panel on Climate Change 2014). To meet this global challenge, evaluation systems look to encourage understanding of architecture's role in the health of the environment. These assessments are often governed by a points driven rating system whereby a candidate building and its immediate site and neighborhood are assessed based on energy consumption, building materiality, landscaping, linkages to public transit, water conservation practices, and related "green" characteristics (USGBC 2018a).

Healthcare provider organizations, who typically commission new and renovated healthcare facilities in the public and private sectors of the industry, often value these assessments' seals of approval, regardless of whether they are fully understood. Architects are increasingly using the Leadership in Energy and Environmental Design (LEED) system to denote a building's sustainability, and by proxy its overall architectural design quality in the eyes of its user/occupants. In reality, however, LEED does not seek to directly address, or measure in any way, a given healthcare facility, its campus, or its neighborhood environs from the perspective of its inhabitants' well-being. It is this miscalculation, that sustainability automatically results in user well-being, that must be addressed. Sustainability, while certainly correlated to well-being, needs to be viewed through a broader, more inclusive multidimensional construct than through the measurement of sheer energy conservation (Guenther and Vittori 2013). In short, architecture must no longer view energy-conscious design as existing within a vacuum; instead it must also acknowledge the well-being of its users/occupants.

19.2 Global Rating Systems

Over the past quarter century, numerous rating systems have appeared on the scene, anchored by the four most commonly used rating systems: LEED started in the United States, now used globally, including in Canada (since 2000); BRE Environmental Assessment Method (BREEAM), in the United Kingdom (since 1990); Comprehensive Assessment System for Built Environment Efficiency (CASBEE), in Japan (since 2001); and Green Star, in Australia (since 2003). In tandem, many less frequently used certification standards have gained influence, including HK-BEAM, in Hong Kong (since 1996); Passive House, in Germany (since 1996); Green Mark Scheme, in Singapore (since 2005); the Living Building Challenge, in the United States (since 2006); ASGB, in China (since 2006); DGNB, in Germany (since 2007); Active House, in Denmark (since 2013); and WELL, in the United States (since 2014).

LEED remains the most widely used rating system globally (Say and Wood 2008; Politi and Antonini 2017; USGBC 2018a, 2018b, 2018c), although it does not attempt to address, nor comprehensively evaluate, design excellence from the user/occupant's perspective. LEED is organized in seven categories:

- Sustainable sites: site selection, attributes, and associated infrastructure
- Water efficiency: water retention and conservation measures
- Energy and atmosphere: minimized energy consumption and commissioning protocols
- Materials and resources: ecological construction and materiality practices and building longevity
- Indoor environmental quality: air quality levels, thermal comfort, daylighting, view amenity, and nontoxic material palettes
- Innovation and design process: ecologically attuned design strategies
- Regional priority: applying existing credits for bonus points based on geographic factors

The newest version of LEED is v4 (version 4) and, notably, it now categorizes indoor environmental quality, natural daylighting, and energy-conserving building materials under a "health and human experience" category (USGBC 2018c). LEED buildings, while proven to consume 24% less energy on average compared to their non-LEED-certified counterparts, still remain controversial in their anointment as sustainable. For instance, Newsham, Mancini, and Birt (2009) comparatively analyzed data from 100 LEED commercial and institutional buildings and found, on average, LEED buildings consumed 18%–39% less energy per floor area than their conventional counterparts. However, 28%–35% of these LEED buildings studied consumed more energy. Furthermore, measured building energy performance was found to be only minimally correlated with the LEED certification level bestowed—that is, the number of energy-saving credits awarded (Newsham, Mancini, and Birt 2009; Al-Zubaidy 2015).

With respect to healthcare facilities, one recent study used national cost report data from the U.S. Centers for Medicare and Medicaid Services to develop a benchmarking tool for comparing the operation and maintenance costs of healthcare facilities versus comparable non-health buildings. Thirty-two LEED hospitals were compared to the median cost of non-LEED hospital facilities of comparable type, ownership, and location. The LEED-certified healthcare facilities did not significantly lower annual operation or maintenance costs (Sadatsafavi and Shepley 2016). LEED-certified healthcare facilities are therefore by no means intrinsically associated with positive satisfaction or well-being outcomes for their occupants. This is especially the case as to the therapeutic affordances of engagement with nature, and with perceived indoor human comfort levels as a function of natural daylighting.

19.3 User Well-Being—Beyond Saving Energy

The most rapidly growing age cohort in societies around the globe is the demographic aged 65 and older, and especially the segment aged 85 and older (United Nations 2017). Significantly more attention needs to be devoted to this growing segment of society with respect to the quality of built environments for the provision of long-term care (Verderber and Fine 2000). In the past decade, multiple evidence-based research studies have drawn linkages between environmental design attributes and positive health outcomes among aged populations (Ulrich 1999; Ulrich et al. 2008). However, these developments have yet to find their way into the policies and best practices of healthcare provider organizations whose principal focus is long-term care (Chrysikou, Rabnett, and Tziraki 2016). Four types of 24/7 care facilities for the aged presently qualify for LEED certification: (1) independent living facilities; (2) assisted living (AL) facilities, where residents are provided with autonomous living quarters and can partake in communal spiritual, dining, and social activities; (3) skilled nursing long-term care (LTC) facilities with medical support on-site; and (4) LTC aging-in-place (LTC/AIP) facilities with the option of independent living, assisted living, and skilled nursing supports on-site.

Biophilic theories in architecture and its allied design professions stem from the late 1960s and the proceedings of the Environmental Design Research Association (EDRA). Founded in 1968, EDRA has continuously championed the value of built environments supportive of the functional needs and aspirations of the aged. Specialized offshoots of EDRA gradually appeared, notably the Center for Health Design (CHD). The CHD's Pebble Project, launched in 2000, has been noteworthy in terms of the use of the post-occupancy evaluation as a vehicle to include user/occupant assessment of the case study facility and its campus environs (Anon 2008; Taylor 2012). This area of applied research has gradually spilled over into professional practice, and has become nestled within the more broadly defined salutogenic design movement. The operative assumption here is that biophilic design is an important facet of built healthcare environments for the aged—a constituency that can greatly benefit.

That said, the aim of this investigation is threefold. First, a cross section of North American long-term care settings for the aged is examined by first identifying the criteria upon which a given facility is bestowed LEED certification at the silver, gold, or platinum level. Second, LEED's rating metrics are then examined in direct relation to a set of biophilic design attributes, or affordances. The third aim is to originate a composite LEED-Biophilic score for long-term care facilities and their campus environs based on the assumption this can significantly aid healthcare organizations in the commissioning and operations of higher-quality built environments for their stakeholder constituencies than at the present time. The current LEED metrics do include view quality, window operability, daylighting, and indoor air quality, but these factors are not assessed from the direct perspective of the user/occupant. In short, the basic research question is this: Is it possible to develop a set of facility-campus environ rating metrics that expand beyond LEED's present focus on energy-conscious planning and design attributes to take into account the nature-related satisfaction level and well-being of the user/occupant?

A healthcare provider organization must assess the cost/benefit trade-offs associated with pursuing LEED (Preiser, Hardy, and Schramm 2017). These include the organization's desired image in its community as an environmental steward from a public relations standpoint, its mission statement, its interest in reducing facility operational expenditures, whether LEED will enhance staff recruitment and retention, and whether LEED will result in enhanced status among peers within the industry. Disincentives, on the other hand, can include the considerable upfront cost of LEED registration, the increase in construction costs, and the lack of staff, patient, and family awareness of and experience with LEED or what it represents. At present, if a healthcare provider organization should decide to pursue LEED certification, a process ensues that may (or may not) result in a completed building and campus expressing salient biophilic architectural affordances. LEED alone, in its present configuration, therefore does not directly promote such affordances. The trade-off between LEED certification and non-LEED certification in relation to resident health status and well-being and staff outcomes is summarized in Figure 19.1.

19.4 Methodology

The aim of this investigation was to look closely at the relationship between biophilic design, associated health outcomes, site planning, and architectural attributes. A summary of biophilic design patterns and biological response recently published online in a report by the environmental consulting firm Terrapin/Bright/Green was referenced (2019). This report presents 14 biophilic design patterns variously connected to four health outcomes outlined here:

- Make a positive impact on user/occupant stress reduction and mitigation
- Increase user/occupant cognitive performance levels
- Improve user/occupant psycho-emotional outlook and behavior
- Heighten user/occupant satisfaction, perceived safety, and human comfort levels

This resulted in four site/building attributes, and five common area and resident room attributes, collectively grounded in 10 of the 14 biophilic design

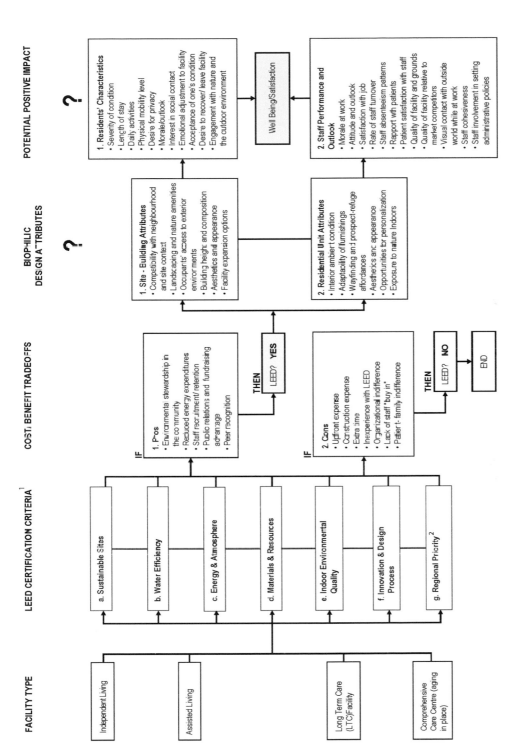

FACILITY TYPE | LEED CERTIFICATION CRITERIA [1] | COST, BENEFIT TRADEOFFS | BIOPHILIC DESIGN ATTRIBUTES | POTENTIAL POSITIVE IMPACT

FACILITY TYPE

- Independent Living
- Assisted Living
- Long Term Care (LTC)Facility
- Comprehensive Care Centre (aging in place)

LEED CERTIFICATION CRITERIA [1]

- a. Sustainable Sites
- b. Water Efficiency
- c. Energy & Atmosphere
- d. Materials & Resources
- e. Indoor Environmental Quality
- f. Innovation & Design Process
- g. Regional Priority [2]

COST, BENEFIT TRADEOFFS

IF
1. Pros
- Environmental stewardship in the community
- Reduced energy expenditures
- Staff recruitment/retention
- Public relations and fundraising advantage
- Peer recognition

THEN LEED? YES

IF
2. Cons
- Upfront expense
- Construction expense
- Extra time
- Inexperience with LEED
- Organizational indifference
- Lack of staff "buy in"
- Patient-family indifference

THEN LEED? NO → END

BIOPHILIC DESIGN ATTRIBUTES ?

1. Site - Building Attributes
- Compatibility with neighbourhood and site context
- Landscaping and nature amenities
- Occupants' access to exterior environments
- Building height and composition
- Aesthetics and appearance
- Facility expansion options

2. Residential Unit Attributes
- Interior ambient condition
- Adaptability of furnishings
- Wayfinding and prospect-refuge affordances
- Aesthetics and appearance
- Opportunities for personalization
- Exposure to nature indoors

POTENTIAL POSITIVE IMPACT ?

1. Residents' Characteristics
- Severity of condition
- Length of stay
- Daily activities
- Physical mobility level
- Desire for privacy
- Morale/outlook
- Interest in social contact
- Emotional adjustment to facility
- Acceptance of one's condition
- Desire to recover/leave facility
- Engagement with nature and the outdoor environment

Well Being/Satisfaction

2. Staff Performance and Outlook
- Morale at work
- Attitude and outlook
- Satisfaction with job
- Rate of staff turnover
- Staff absenteeism patterns
- Rapport with patients
- Patient satisfaction with staff
- Quality of facility and grounds
- Quality of facility relative to market competitors
- Visual contact with outside world while at work
- Staff cohesiveness
- Staff involvement in setting administrative policies

[1] LEED programs currently exist in the areas of health, new construction, renovation and interiors (a seventh category, Reciprocal Priority, constitutes up to 41 points, for a total of 110 maximum points)
[2] LEED version 2009

▲ Figure 19.1

LEED certification and health and well-being in residents and staff..

Source: Stephen Verderber, Terri Peters, Oussama El Assir, and Josh Silver

patterns cited in the aforementioned 2019 report. These nine environmental attributes were defined on the basis of a review of recent literature specifically focused on long-term care architecture and associated site environs within the field of architecture for health (Carstens 1993; Feddersen 2009; Anåker et al. 2017; Regnier 2018). This relationship between the theoretical and applied aspects of the investigational framework is summarized in Figure 19.2.

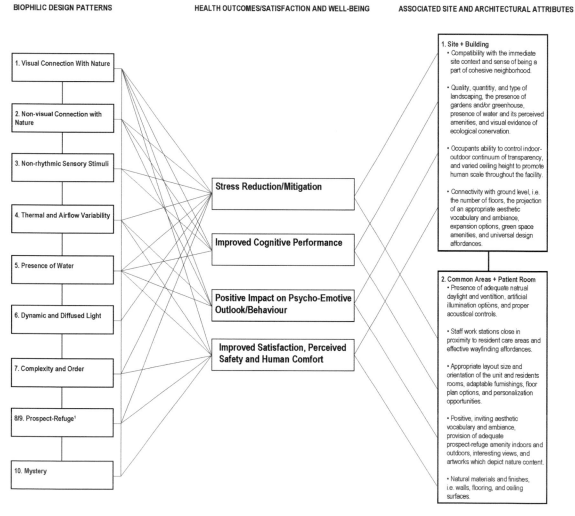

¹Prospect and refuge patterns are combined here as a single construct.

▲ Figure 19.2

Relationships between site and building attributes and biophilic design patterns.
Source: Stephen Verderber, Terri Peters, Lucas Siemucha, and Josh Silver

Stephen Verderber and Terri Peters

The research aims were operationalized using existing built case studies of LEED-certified long-term care facilities for the aged. The purpose was to study the extent to which these facilities—all LEED certified—express biophilic design attributes. This was done through the analysis of site and floor plans, photographs, LEED documentation on its homepage, and written assessments of each facility as provided by its architects. Eighteen North American, LEED-certified case studies were selected for analysis, based on the USGBC's LEED versions 1.0, 2.2, and NC2009. The case studies were drawn from the professional literature in architecture, design awards programs, online sources, including care provider organizations' homepages, and extensive correspondences with the associated architectural firms. These facilities ranged from urban-suburban to rural in locational contexts, varied from one level to seven levels in height, and were examined via floor plans, photographs, written descriptions, and analysis of their LEED project scorecard. Their various site contexts were also assessed via satellite photo imagery together with at-grade photographs of the exterior site and interior building spaces. The LEED scorecard records total points accrued for the case study, vis-à-vis the seven aforementioned assessment categories, and the level of LEED certification bestowed, whether certified, silver, gold, or platinum. Images and site plan drawings of the six case studies with the highest composite scores are presented in Figure 19.3.

Case studies (CS 1–18) are reported in Figure 19.4, ranked from top to bottom based on the number of licensed beds on-site. Three types of facilities are identified: small to moderate-size facilities (20 to 60 beds), moderate-size facilities (64 to 156 beds), and the large facilities (180 to 416 beds). Next, the points awarded for each of the seven LEED scoring categories are reported (Figure 19.4, center column). Each attribute's maximum awardable points are reported in the far-right column of Figure 19.4 (reported in parentheses). Specific points given to a particular variable were driven by the literature review. The case studies were therefore evaluated relative to 15 site and building attributes, and 16 design qualities focused on residential unit common areas and the resident's room.

A team of five evaluators was assembled to assess and score the set of 18 case studies. This was done in four rating sessions that occurred in late 2017 to early 2018. The panel of assessors consisted of the two authors and three well-versed graduate student research assistants in architecture. Each case study was examined in relation to the 31 biophilic variables, and decisions on how many points to score a given case study resulted in lengthy discussions. Photographs, floor plans, sectional drawings, and in some cases video walk-throughs obtained were projected on a large-format video monitor. These rating sessions were conducted as focus groups, each approximately three hours in length. Ultimately a composite LEED-Biophilic (L-B) score was assigned to each case study. The composite score reflected the total LEED points obtained, divided by the LEED points attainable, plus the biophilic points obtained, and then divided by the total maximum biophilic points attainable, multiplied by 100. To summarize, case studies (CS 1–18) were rated based on the 31 biophilic design attributes, providing a basis for subsequent descriptive statistical analyses.

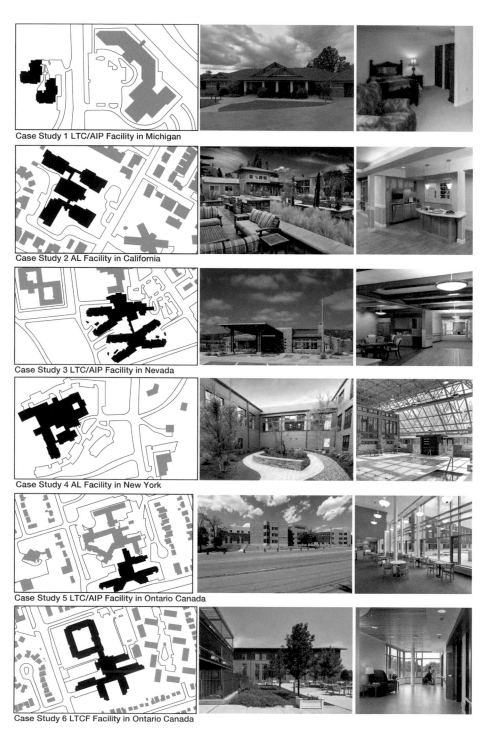

Case Study 1 LTC/AIP Facility in Michigan

Case Study 2 AL Facility in California

Case Study 3 LTC/AIP Facility in Nevada

Case Study 4 AL Facility in New York

Case Study 5 LTC/AIP Facility in Ontario Canada

Case Study 6 LTCF Facility in Ontario Canada

▲ Figure 19.3

The six case studies with the highest composite scores.

Source: Images courtesy of CC Hodgson Architects Group, GGLO Design, Vigil and Associates, MHG Architects PC, MMMC Architects, and Montgomery Sisam; drawings produced by Stephen Verderber, Terri Peters, and Josh Silver

Stephen Verderber and Terri Peters

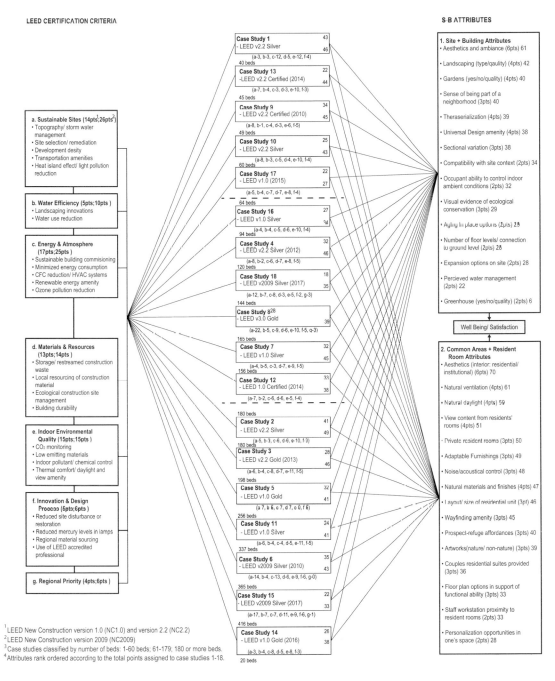

▲ Figure 19.4

Case studies ranked based on number of beds, facility type and score.

Source: Stephen Verderber, Terri Peters, Oussama El Assir, and Josh Silver

19.5 Results

The ranked composite L-B scores for CS 1–18 are reported in Table 19.1. The four assisted living facilities (including Case Study 17, which also houses an LTC unit on-site) had an average bed count of 113.5 licensed beds. The six freestanding LTC case studies had an average bed count of 262 beds, and the eight LTC aging-in-place campuses had an average bed count of 107 beds. The results are of likely interest to healthcare provider organizations, direct care providers, architects, interior designers, and landscape architects. First, the biophilic attributes associated for CS 1–18 were computed, followed by combining the LEED rating score with the biophilic attribute score for each case study. This step yielded a composite LEED-Biophilic score for each case study, referred to ahead as the L-B score.

19.5.1 The Function of Facility Size

The size of a residential long-term care facility, as categorized according to its total bed capacity, is related to its total L-B composite score. First, midsize facilities (from 60–180 beds) were assigned a lower total composite score (N = 6; mean: X = 67.8) compared to either smaller (N = 5; X = 70.2, from a possible 98 maximum points) or larger facilities. The largest case studies—that is, those with 180 or more beds—were most highly scored (N = 7; X = 71.3). These facilities featured the most amenities and tended to have the most expansive sites. An example includes the Case Study 2 assisted living facility in California (180 beds), with its extensively landscaped grounds and courtyard and variety of "outdoor rooms", varied interior space and room configurations, ceiling heights, and adaptable furnishings. A second example is the Case Study 5 LTC/AIP campus in Ontario, Canada (198 beds). This facility features a large dining room with expansive full-height windows overlooking a landscaped courtyard, and residents' bedrooms have interesting views of nature (nearby woods). It also features a variety of interior spaces that provide direct connections to the outdoors, and natural building materials and finishes are visible throughout the interior.

19.5.2 The Function of Facility Type

When these same data were examined based on the type of LTC facility (Table 19.5), it was found that the LTC/aging-in-place campuses garnered the highest total L-B composite scores (N = 8; X = 73.5), followed by assisted living facilities (N = 4; X = 68.3). The lowest composite scores were assigned to the largest facilities—all freestanding LTC facilities (N = 6; X = 66.5). This finding reinforced the pattern that bigger is not better per se as freestanding LTC facilities were by far largest in terms of their bed capacities. This finding is likely attributable to the fact that aging-in-place campuses tend to provide the most varied spaces and amenities among the facility types included in this study. Furthermore, they tend to provide a range of both indoor and exterior spaces perhaps more closely attuned to the broader range of functional capabilities of their residents. Examples ranged

Stephen Verderber and Terri Peters

Table 19.5 Case studies analyzed and scored resulting in a composite LEED-Biophilic score

Case Studies 1–18	Facility Type	Scoring Terminology	a-Sustainable Sites	b-Water Efficiency	c-Energy & Atmosphere	d-Materials & Resources	e-Indoor Environmental Quality	f-Innovation & Design Process	g-Regional Priority	Total Points Awarded + Composite Score
1. LTC/AIP Facility in Michigan LEED v2.2 Silver	LTC/AIP[1]	L[2] B[3](C[4])	3(14)	3(5)	12(17)	5(13)	12(15)	4(5)	--	39(70) 89(147)
2. AL Facility in California LEED v2.2 Silver	AL[5]	L B(C)	5(14)	3(5)	6(17)	6(13)	10(15)	3(5)	--	33(69) 90(140)
3. LTC/AIP Facility in Nevada LEED v2.2Gold	LTC/AIP	L B(C)	6(14)	4(5)	8(17)	7(13)	11(15)	5(5)	--	41(69) 74(135)
4. AL Facility in New York LEED v2.2 Silver	AL	L B(C)	8(14)	2(5)	6(17)	7(13)	8(15)	5(5)	--	36(69) 78(132)
5. LTC/AIP Facility in Ontario, Canada LEED v1.0 Gold	LTC/AIP	L B(C)	7(14)	5(5)	7(17)	7(14)	9(15)	5(5)	--	40(70) 73(132)
6. LTCF Facility in Ontario, Canada LEED v2009 Silver	LTCF[6]	L B(C)	14(26)	4(10)	13(35)	6(14)	9(15)	6(6)	0(4)	52(110) 78(127)
7. LTC/AIP Facility in Ontario, Canada LEED v1.0 Silver	LTC/AIP	L B(C)	5(14)	5(5)	3(17)	7(14)	9(15)	5(5)	--	34(70) 77(127)
8. LTC/AIP Facility in Florida LEED v3.0 Gold	LTC/AIP	L B(C)	22(26)	5(10)	9(35)	6(14)	10(15)	5(6)	3(4)	60(110) 67(123)
9. LTC/AIP Facility in Maryland LEED v2.2 Certified	LTC/AIP	L B(C)	8(14)	1(5)	4(17)	3(13)	6(15)	5(5)	--	27(69) 79(120)
10. LTC/AIP Facility in Maryland LEED v2.2 Silver	LTC/AIP	L B(C)	8(14)	3(5)	5(17)	4(13)	10(15)	4(5)	--	34(69) 68(119)
11. LTCF Facility in Ontario, Canada LEED v1.0 Silver	LTCF	L B(C)	6(14)	4(5)	4(17)	5(14)	11(15)	5(5)	--	35(70) 65(116)
12. LTCF Facility in Nova Scotia, Canada LEED 1.0 Certified	LTCF	L B(C)	7(14)	2(5)	6(17)	6(14)	5(15)	4(5)	--	30(70) 71(115)
13. LTCF Facility in Minnesota LEED v2.2 Certified	LTCF	L B(C)	7(14)	4(5)	3(17)	3(13)	10(15)	3(5)	--	30(69) 66(111)
14. LTCF Facility in Ontario, Canada LEED v1.0 Gold	LTCF	L B(C)	3(14)	4(5)	8(17)	5(14)	8(15)	3(5)	--	31(70) 64(110)
15. LTCF Facility in New York LEED v2009 Silver	LTCF	L B(C)	17(27)	7(10)	7(35)	11(14)	9(15)	6(6)	1(4)	58(110) 55(109)
16. LTC/AIP Facility in Ontario, Canada LEED v1.0 Silver	LTC/AIP	L B(C)	4(14)	4(5)	5(17)	6(14)	10(15)	4(5)	--	33(70) 61(109)
17. AL/LTC Facility in Ontario, Canada LEED v1.0	AL/LTC[7]	L B(C)	5(14)	4(5)	7(17)	7(14)	8(15)	4(5)	--	35(70) 49(100)
18. AL Facility in Illinois LEED v1.0 Silver	AL	L B(C)	12(27)	7(10)	8(35)	3(14)	5(15)	2(6)	3(4)	40(110) 53(90)

1 Long Term Care/Aging in Place Campus
2 Total awarded LEED points by category. Number in paranthases denotes total attainable LEED points
3 Biophillic points (total attained)
4 Composite score [(L points attained divided by L total + B points divided by B total) × 100] with L total points correspoding to that case study's version of LEED and its assessed B points total (in relation to the maximum 98 B points allowed)
5 Assisted Living Facility
6 Long Term Care-Freestanding Facility
7 Assisted Living with LTC unit on sitet

Source: Stephen Verderber, Terri Peters, Oussama El Assir, and Josh Silver

from the Case Study 1, in Michigan (20 beds), to the Case Study 5, in Ontario (198 beds).

This finding, however, invites closer scrutiny particularly with respect to the highest-rated facilities in terms of their composite L-B score. The top rated 50% of the case studies averaged 150.4 beds, which placed them in the midrange in terms of overall facility size, yet this does not mean all that much when viewed more broadly. This is because the top 50% of facilities spanned all three facility types represented—assisted living, freestanding long-term care nursing facilities, and the more comprehensive LTC/aging-in-place campuses. Restated, the quality of biophilic design attributes is more important than the sheer physical size of a facility—that is, a facility's architectural design quality takes precedence over the amount of space provided per se.

A second pattern revealed concerned the relative usefulness of the biophilic design attributes as individual metrics in rating healthcare facilities for the aged. These items were rank-ordered (Figure 19.4, far-right column) in terms of the total number of points assigned to each item: items 1–15 for site and building attributes, and items 16–31 for the common areas and resident bedroom attributes. This ranking reflected the cumulative score assigned to each of the 18 case studies.

19.6 Toward the Establishment of an Inclusive Rating System

As for the research methods used in this pilot investigation, it would have been preferable to conduct on-site post-occupancy evaluations at each of the 18 case study sites. However, funds to do this were unavailable at the time. In the future, this step is recommended as there is no substitute for direct observation versus a reliance on correspondence and archival data sources, such as drawings, photographs, and Skype interviews with the architects and firms that worked on the 18 case studies. For these reasons, while this study provides a useful introduction to the core issues, and a platform for further research and applications to professional practice, it is best appreciated as a pilot study. With that said, the following minimum recommendations are hereby put forth in order to create a more inclusive points-based rating system that embraces ecological and sustainability concerns with biophilic design patterns and principles:

For the USGBC:

1. Establish an internally consistent LEED rating system: First and foremost, if LEED is to remain a leading source of "green" certification, the rating system is in need of streamlining. All project profiles in the USGBC homepage database need to include site plans, photographs, client, design team information, and project narratives. A single, unified points rating system is needed for healthcare. For example, current LEED versions BD+C, LEED Interiors, LEED Existing Buildings, LEED Homes are all being used to evaluate 24/7 residential care environments for the aged. Inconsistencies between these various versions remain problematic. As an example, a project certified under LEED BD+C New Construction v2.2 can earn a maximum of 69 points. By contrast, another of the 18 case studies was rated using LEED BD+C New Construction version 2009 and its score

totaled 110. Case study 18's score was 40/110, thereby meeting LEED v1.0 Silver certification status.

2. Create interdisciplinary partnerships and a more inclusive rating system: After this internal standardization process has been completed, next, the USGBC should seek out collaborative partnerships with organizations that actively promote the topic of biophilic and salutogenic research and its applications in professional design practice. The USGBC has become, in this respect, rather complacent. While many organizational improvements have been made over the past 19 years, it is time for a thorough internal reassessment—one that bridges its core mission with salutogenic and biophilic design patterns/principles. This will itself fuel further innovations in the future, including joint conferences, awards programs, and interdisciplinary journals.

For the environmental design research community:

3. Lobby to integrate biophilic design in professional practice: Healthcare provider organizations need to place high value on the development of widely recognized best practices in ecological and life-affirming design. One way to achieve this is through a single, unified, more inclusive LEED rating system. The integration of these two currently independent knowledge bases provides a unified platform for significantly higher-quality 24/7 healthcare built environments than at present. Unfortunately, the current LEED program remains lacking in this regard (Fitzgerald and Spaccarotella 2009). Similarly, the concept of "total facility performance" is in urgent need of redefinition (Peters 2017).

4. Establish an equivalent professional organization to collaborate with the USGBC: At present there is no clear-cut "point organization" specifically devoted to biophilic research and design activities nor any professional organization with this as its specific charge. This area of research and its applications to professional practice currently most closely rest within the broad manifold of concerns addressed by the EDRA.

For architects and allied design and planning professionals:

5. Establish ecohumanist, evidence-based organizational policies: Promote the establishment of new research opportunities—that is, grants, internships, and fellowships—in order to generate new ecohumanist knowledge in the planning, design, and daily operation of care settings. Similarly, any such evidence-based design awards programs should recognize and honor ecological sustainability as equal in merit with other metrics used in evaluation (Verderber et al. 2014; Peters and Verderber 2017).

6. Work with clients to broaden their vision of design excellence: At present LEED is viewed in North America by most healthcare provider clients as the preeminent gold standard for architectural sustainability, yet this investigation has shown it is noticeably lacking in terms of its autonomy from the experiential, everyday aspects of built environments for healthcare. The LEED rating system, however, continues to be presented to client organizations by their architects as the most respected vehicle for a client organization to proclaim its ecological "greenness" and present itself as a bona fide environmental steward in its local community.

19.7 Conclusions

Eighteen LEED-certified 24/7 residential care environments for the aged were examined for their ecological and energy conservation merits in direct relation to their biophilic design affordances. The highest composite-scored case studies were found to express what might be defined as an "ecohumanist" design perspective—an aesthetic vocabulary expressing ecological principles together with a significant degree of person-nature connectivity (Verderber 2010). A facility's size, as measured by the number of licensed beds and type of facility, was found to have an impact on the presence (or absence) of such biophilic design attributes in 24/7 long-term care residential settings for the aged.

Healthcare provider organizations and their architects, interior designers, and landscape architects are ideal advocates to promote research that promotes environmental design excellence (Moffat 2006). Innovative thinking, combined with coordinated advocacy efforts, will result in greater inclusivity. Architects can lead the way as advocates in this regard for a rating system that unifies ecological sustainability with person-nature patterns and principles. In light of these findings, a single rating system fusing the current LEED system with biophilic design affordance appears to be warranted.

Non-convergence—or what more aptly might be defined as mutual exclusivity—continues to prevail between the sustainable healthcare design and biophilic design movements. This investigation has been the first to systematically compare the LEED certification system in direct relation to the expression of biophilic design attributes in architecture for health. The overarching finding was that LEED certification in and of itself neither guarantees nor predicts a high level of ecohumanist architectural design excellence. It is the client's and designer's responsibility, therefore, to recognize that rating systems should never distract from the end goal—total user wellness and satisfaction.

Bibliography

Adams, Annmarie, and Sally Chivers. "There's no Place Like Home: Designing for Long-Term Residential Care in Canada." *Journal of Canadian Studies* 50, no. 2 (2017): 273–298.

Al-Zubaidy, Mehdi S. Kaddory. "A Literature Evaluation of the Energy Efficiency of Leadership in Energy and Environmental Design (LEED)-Certified Buildings." *American Journal of Civil Engineering Architecture* 3 (2015): 1–7.

Anåker, Anna, Ann Heylighen, Susanna Nordin, and Marie Elf. "Design Quality in the Context of Healthcare Environments: A Scoping Review." *HERD: Health Environments Research & Design Journal* 10, no. 4 (2017): 136–150.

Anon. "The Pebble Project Defined." *Healthcare Design*, 2008. Online. www.http//healthcaredesignmagazine.com/architecture/pebble-project-defined/htp.

Antonovsky, Anton. *Health, Stress and Coping.* San Francisco, CA: Jossey-Bass Publishers, 1979.

Antonovsky, Aaron. "The Salutogenic Model as A Theory to Guide Health Promotion." *Health Promotion International* 11, no. 1 (1996): 11–18.

Berry, L. D. Parker, R. Coile, D. K. Hamilton, D. O'Neill, and B. Sadler. "The Business Case for Better Buildings." *Frontiers in Health Services Management*, 21, no. 1 (2004): 3–21.

Billings, Jenny R., and Ferhana Hashem. "Salutogenesis and the Promotion of Positive Mental Health in Older People." In *Proceedings of the EU Thematic Conference "Mental Health and Well-Being in Older People—Making It Happen"*. Madrid, Spain: European Commission, April 2010.

BREEAM. "Explore BREEM, Explore the Data Behind Breem Projects." 2018. www. http://tools.breeam.com/projects/explore/index.jsp.

Carstens, Diane Y. *Site Planning and Design for the Elderly: Issues, Guidelines, and Alternatives*. New York, NY: John Wiley & Sons, 1993.

Chrysikou, Evangelia, Richard Rabnett, and Chariklia Tziraki. "Perspectives on the Role and Synergies of Architecture and Social and Built Environment in Enabling Active Healthy Aging." *Journal of Aging Research* 2016, no. 1 (2016): 1–7.

De Fátima Castro, Maria Ricardo Mateus, and Luís Bragança. "A Critical Analysis of Building Sustainability Assessment Methods for Healthcare Buildings." *Environment, Development and Sustainability* 17, no. 6 (2015): 1381–1412.

Feddersen, Eckhard, and Insa Ludtke. *Living for the Elderly: A Design Manual*. Basel, Switzerland: Birkhauser Verlag AG, 2009.

Fitzgerald, Nurgul, and Kim Spaccarotella. "Barriers to a Healthy Lifestyle: from Individuals to Public Policy—An Ecological Perspective." *Journal of Extension* 47, no. 1 (2009): 1–8.

Frankel, Cathy Turner Mark. *Energy Performance of LEED for New Construction Buildings—Final Report*. White Salmon, WA: New Buildings Institute, 2008.

Golembiewski, Jan A. "Psychiatric Design: Using a Salutogenic Model for the Development and Management of Mental Health Facilities." *World Health Design: Architecture, Culture, Technology* 5, no. 2 (2012): 74–79.

Golembiewski, Jan A. "Start Making Sense: Applying a Salutogenic Model to Architectural Design for Psychiatric Care." *Facilities* 28, no. 3–4 (2010): 100–117.

Guenther, Robin, and Gail Vittori. *Sustainable Healthcare Architecture*, 2nd ed. Hoboken, NJ: John Wiley & Sons, 2013.

Kellert, Stephen R., Judith Heerwagen, and Martin Mador. *Biophilic Design: The Theory, Science and Practice of Bringing Buildings to Life*. Hoboken, NJ: John Wiley & Sons, 2011.

Memmott, Mark. "'Oldest Old' Are the World's Fastest Growing Age group." *National Public Radio*, 20 July 2009. Online www.npr.org/sections/thetwo-way/2009/07/oldest_old_are_worlds_fastest.html.

Moffat, David. "Compassion in Architecture-Evidence-Based Design for Health in Louisiana by Stephen Verderber [EDRA/Places Awards 2006--Research]." *Places* 18, no. 3 (2006).

Newsham, Guy R., Sandra Mancini, and Benjamin J. Birt. "Do LEED-Certified Buildings Save Energy? Yes, but . . ." *Energy and Buildings* 41, no. 8 (2009): 897–905.

Pachauri, Rajendra K., Myles R. Allen, Vicente R. Barros, John Broome, Wolfgang Cramer, Renate Christ, John A. Church et al. *Climate Change 2014: Synthesis Report. Contribution of Working Groups I, II and III to the Fifth Assessment Report of the Intergovernmental Panel on Climate Change*. Geneva, Switzerland: IPCC, 2014.

Peri Bader, Aya. "A Model for Everyday Experience of the Built Environment: The Embodied Perception of Architecture." *The Journal of Architecture* 20, no. 2 (2015): 244–267.

Peters, Terri, "Design for Health: Sustainable Approaches to Therapeutic Architecture." In *Architectural Design*, edited by Terri Peters, vol. 246, 6–15. Hoboken, NJ: John Wiley & Sons, March 2017.

Peters, Terri, and Stephen Verderber. "Territories of Engagement in the Design of Ecohumanist Healthcare Environments." *HERD: Health Environments Research & Design Journal* 10, no. 2 (2017): 104–123.

Politi, Stefano, and Ernesto Antonini. "An Expeditious Method for Comparing Sustainable Rating Systems for Residential Buildings." *Energy Procedia* 111 (2017): 41–50.

Preiser, Wolfgang F. E., Andrea E. Hardy, and Ulrich Schramm, eds. *Building Performance Evaluation: From Delivery Process to Life Cycle Phases*. Cham, Switzerland: Springer, 2017.

Regnier, Victor. *Housing Design for an Increasingly Older Population: Redefining Assisted Living for the Mentally and Physically Frail*. Hoboken, NJ: John Wiley & Sons, 2018.

Sadatsafavi, Hessam, and Mardelle M. Shepley. "Performance Evaluation of 32 LEED Hospitals on Operation Costs." *Procedia Engineering* 145 (2016): 1234–1241.

Sadler, Blair L., Leonard L. Berry, Robin Guenther, D. Kirk Hamilton, Frederick A. Hessler, Clayton Merritt, and Derek Parker. "Fable Hospital 2.0: The Business Case for Building Better Health Care Facilities." *Hastings Center Report* 41, no. 1 (2011): 13–23.

Say, Candace, and Antony Wood. "Sustainable Rating Systems Around the World." *Council on Tall Buildings and Urban Habitat Journal* (CTBUH Review) 2 (2008): 18–29.

Taylor, Ellen. "Evidence-Based Design and the Pebble Project: 12 Years Later." *Healthcare Design*, September 6, 2012. www.healthcaredesignmagazine.com/trends/architecture/evidence-based-design-and-pebble-project-12-years/.

Terrapin, Bright, Green. "14 Patterns of Biophilic Design." 2019 Online. www.terrapinbrightgreen.com/report/14-patterns/pdf.

Ulrich, Roger S., Craig Zimring, Xuemei Zhu, Jennifer DuBose, Hyun-Bo Seo, Young-Seon Choi, Xiaobo Quan, and Anjali Joseph. "A Review of the Research Literature on Evidence-Based Healthcare Design." *HERD: Health Environments Research & Design Journal* 1, no. 3 (2008): 61–125.

Ulrich, Roger S. "Effects of Gardens on Health Outcomes: Theory and Research." In *Healing Gardens: Therapeutic Benefits and Design Recommendations*, edited by Clare Cooper Marcus and Marni Barnes, 27–86. New York: John Wiley, 1999.

United Nations. "Demographic Profile of the Older Population." *World Population Ageing, 1950–2050*. Geneva: World Health Organization, 2017.

United States Green Building Council (USGBC). "Buildings and Climate Change." 2018 Online. www.documents.dgs.ca.gov/dgs/pio/facts/LA%20workshop/climate.pdf.

United States Green Building Council (USGBC). "LEED Is Green Building." 2018a Online. http://new.usgbc.org/leed.

United States Green Building Council (USGBC). "LEED Numbers: 16 Years of Steady Growth." 2018b Online. http//usgbc.org/articles/leed-numbers-16-years-steady-growth.

United States Green Building Council (USGBC). "LEED: Challenges and Opportunities." 2018c Online. www.usgbc.org/articles/part-3-challenges-and-opportunities-2010-present.

United States Green Building Council (USGBC). "LEED v.4." 2018d Online. http//new.usgbc.org/leed-v4.

United States Green Building Council (USGBC). "LEED V.4.1." 2018e Online. https://new.usgbc.org/leed-v41.

Van Malderen, Lien, Tony Mets, Patricia De Vriendt, and Ellen Gorus. "The Active Ageing—Concept Translated to the Residential Long-Term Care." *Quality of Life Research* 22, no. 5 (2013): 929–937.

Verderber, Stephen. *Innovations in Behavioural Health Architecture*. Abingdon, Oxon and New York, NY: Routledge, 2018.

Verderber, Stephen. *Innovations in Hospital Architecture*. Abingdon, Oxon and New York, NY: Routledge, 2010.

Verderber, Stephen. *Sprawling Cities and Our Endangered Public Health*. Abingdon, Oxon and New York, NY: Routledge, 2012.

Verderber, Stephen, and David J. Fine. *Healthcare Architecture in an Era of Radical Transformation.* New Haven, CT: Yale University Press, 2000.

Verderber, Stephen, Shan Jiang, George Hughes, and Yanwen Xiao. "The Evolving Role of Evidence-Based Research in Healthcare Facility Design Competitions." *Frontiers of Architectural Research* 3, no. 3 (2014): 238–249.

Verderber, Stephen, and Cabrenia M. Thomas. "Rebuilding A Statewide Network of Community Health Centers for the Medically Underserved: A Longitudinal Assessment." *Journal of Public Health Management and Practice* 19, no. 5 (2013): E10–E22.

Wilson, Edward O. *Biophilia.* Cambridge, MA: President and Fellows of Harvard College, 1984.

Chapter 20

Connecting to Context
Place-Based Approaches to Biophilic Healthcare Design

Mara Baum

20.1 Introduction

The first "modern" healthcare facilities of the eighteenth and nineteenth centuries relied heavily on a connection to the natural environment. Sanatoria, derived from the Latin word *sana* ("to heal"), were constructed in pastoral settings well beyond the city wall. Large windows, exterior verandahs, and expansive grounds were integral to this healing environment, where patients could breathe fresh air, eat nourishing food, and rest without disturbance, allowing the body to recuperate naturally. The discovery of antibiotics and more effective surgical procedures in the early twentieth century ushered in a new approach to healthcare that is reflected in more recent hospital design. While this model has proven efficient for enabling hospital staff to advance medicine and treatment, it has often done so with limited regard to the restorative benefits of nature that had once been critical to sanatoria design.

20.2 The Case for Biophilic Design

20.2.1 Our Innate Connection to Nature

Today, healthcare designers and health professionals are increasingly seeking ways to balance the complex technology of modern medicine with the body's inherent need for a restorative environment that supports rest, reduces stress, and restores health from within. Opportunities to interact with nature, however, are no longer always readily accessible. While there is a recognized value of both views to nature and healing gardens (Boehland 2005; Cooper, Marcus, and Barnes 1999; Cooper Marcus and Sachs 2014; Therapeutic Landscapes 2018; Guenther and Vittori 2013), they are neither universally available nor always successful in achieving their goals—particularly for patients with limited mobility and staff with limited break opportunities (Nejati et al. 2016).

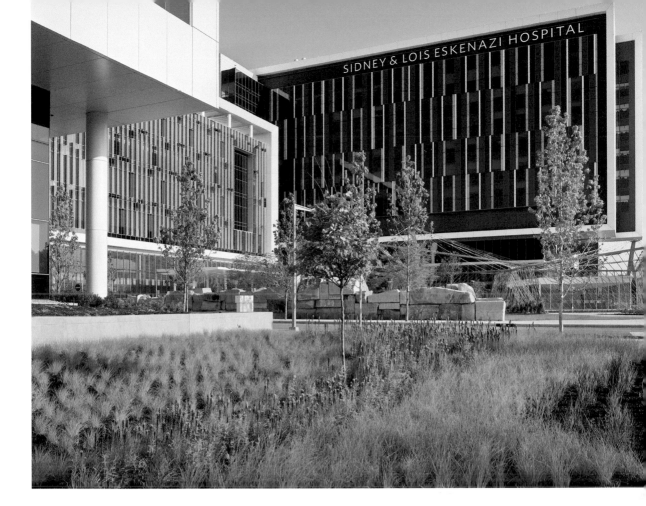

▲ Figure 20.1

With local, natural construction materials and native and adapted plantings, outdoor spaces at Eskenazi Health are unique to its Indiana setting.
Source: Timothy Hursley

Naturalist and author Edward O. Wilson (1984,1993) introduced the concept of "biophilia" to address the "missing link in sustainable design" that ties people to the natural world. In its simplest form, biophilia is the "innately emotional affiliation of human beings to other living organisms". In more complex terms, biophilia can refer to the psychological connection to the natural world—including but not limited to flora and fauna—that humans developed with over millennia. Like other animals, Homo sapiens evolved in an outdoor world. This predisposed us to specific reactions to elements such as daylight, water, plant life, breezes/natural ventilation, certain spatial relationships, and more (Wilson 1984).

It is not surprising that these same elements would support our overall health and well-being. With the average American spending over 85% of the day indoors (Klepeis et al. 2001), however, it is clear humans' relationship with the natural world is much different in present time than that of our ancestors. Consequently, our physiological need for nature requires a conduit through the built environment more than ever before.

20.2.2 The Case for Biophilia in Modern Healthcare

In 1984, environmental psychologist Roger Ulrich identified a potential link between nature and health outcomes when he published a study in the journal *Science* comparing two sets of patients recovering from gallbladder surgery. Those patients whose beds had views of trees required less pain medication and recovered faster than those whose view was limited to a brick wall. Ulrich's study was the first to clearly document the relationship between the natural world and clinical outcomes. Numerous follow-up studies have further quantified the positive impact that contact with nature can have on our health and well-being, addressing issues such as stress reduction, improved sleep, reduced blood pressure, and more (Kellert and Wilson 1995; Ulrich 1984, 2008; Van den Berg et al. 2015). Researchers and practitioners developed several theories to help explain these circumstances, including attention restoration theory, stress recovery theory, restorative environments theory, prospect/refuge theory, and more. In every case, human interaction or connection with a specific aspect of nature is considered to lead to improved healing, cognitive performance, or other benefits (Bergman, Jonides, and Kaplan 2008; Hartig, Mang, and Evans 1991; Heerwagen and Orians 1995; Joye and van den Berg 2012; Kaplan 1992, 1995; Pati and Barach 2010).

There is no "one-size-fits-all" approach to biophilic design; its rich array of strategies and opportunities is as diverse as the climates and cultures they are implemented within. Design strategies range from providing vegetation directly within a space to incorporating natural materials, to mimicking spatial relationships commonly found in nature. Direct physical contact with nature—through sight, touch, smell, and sound—is at the core of biophilic design, but is not the only available approach. Metaphoric connections to nature incorporate patterns, textures, and cycles from nature, such as stochastic patterns, fractal patterns, the diurnal cycle, and familiar natural materials. Humans also experience a physiological response to spatial relationships or elements commonly found in nature, such as those that provide a sense of prospect and refuge, mystery or adventure, or a mild sense of danger (Kellert 2005). Several texts offer detailed discussion on the implementation of various biophilic design strategies, such as *Building for Life* (Kellert 2005) and *14 Patterns of Biophilic Design* (Browning, Ryan, and Clancy 2014); a summary of these strategies is provided in Table 20.1.

A multitude of factors influence the determination of the best biophilic design strategies for any given building. Four strategy areas are discussed in this chapter that look to establish a strong sense of "place", or context, with biophilia in mind: climate, ecosystems, culture, and interiors. These starting points influence all building types, and can be excavated for opportunities to create unique and context-sensitive design. The infection prevention requirements, medical planning conventions, and local or national code requirements that all provide an added layer of complexity to hospital design must be considered along with these interventions, but do not automatically disqualify a project from attaining biophilic results.

Two recently completed hospitals, located on opposite sides of the world, demonstrate two contrasting approaches to biophilic design. Eskenazi Health Main Campus in Indianapolis, Indiana, and the Ng Teng Fong General Hospital and Jurong Community Hospital (NTFGH-JCH) campus in Singapore are both public hospitals that provide care to the full spectrum of disease groups and patient populations. Yet given the unique challenges and opportunities of their locations, culture, and medical approaches, the two hospitals offer designers two vastly distinct ways in which to incorporate the natural world into medical facilities.

Table 20.1

The following design elements represent a selection of biophilic design strategies that can be integrated into healthcare facilities. Not every strategy will be appropriate for a given building, region, or local culture.

- *Direct contact with nature through the senses:*
  - *Views, e.g. verdant vegetation, water features, or movement of clouds in the sky*
  - *Sounds, e.g. rain falling, birds chirping, or a bubbling brook*
  - *Smells, e.g. herbs or fruits, such as mint or lemon, or smells of plants and earth*
  - *Touch, e.g. the feel of breezes or direct sun on our skin*

- *Metaphoric connections with nature: forms, patterns, and cycles.*
  - *Experience of natural systems, e.g. rainfall or the changing of seasons*
  - *Experience of natural cycles; e.g. connection to the diurnal cycle through dynamic daylight patterns*
  - *Patterns from nature, e.g. fractals or stochastic patterns*
  - *Natural materials, e.g. wood or stone*

- *Spatial relationships or elements*
  - *A blurring of the interior/exterior edge*
  - *Duality of prospect and refuge*
  - *A sense of mystery, peril, and excitement*

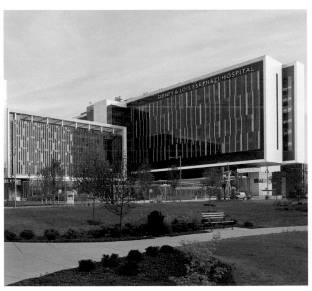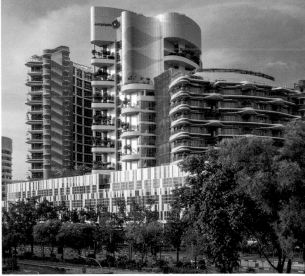

▲ Figure 20.2

A half a world apart, Eskenazi Health Main Campus (left) and Ng Teng Fong General Hospital and Jurong General Hospital (right) represent different place-based approaches to biophilic healthcare design.
Source: Timothy Hursley and Rory Daniel

20.3 Eskenazi Health Main Campus and Ng Teng Fong General Hospital and Jurong Community Hospital: Different Approaches to Similar Goals

Located in an urban medical corridor just west of downtown Indianapolis, Eskenazi Health Main Campus replaces a nearby hospital from the early 1900s. Opened in 2013, the LEED Gold certified, 1.2 million-square-foot Eskenazi Health Main Campus includes one of the state's only Level 1 trauma centers, an emergency department, a burn unit, 315 acuity adaptable beds, and over 200 exam rooms.

Also located in an urban setting, the Ng Teng Fong General Hospital and Jurong Community Hospital campus lies approximately ten miles west of downtown Singapore in a part of the city that 200 years ago had been a mangrove swamp. As a public hospital, NTFGH-JCH was designed as a prototype for the Singapore Ministry of Health's effort to provide high-quality, affordable care to all Singaporeans. Early in the design phase, the hospital's CEO issued another challenge: to build a "hospital without walls", or one that seamlessly connects to the environment. Completed in 2015, the facility's two most striking architectural elements are its vegetative balconies and undulating floorplates—both of which serve to blend indoor and outdoor spaces. Like Eskenazi, NTFGH-JCH was also designed to meet significant sustainability criteria, earning it the Green Mark Platinum certification and recognition as an AIA Cote Top Ten winner.

20.3.1 Climate

Although the two hospitals share commonalities in terms of urban settings, commitment to public health, and sustainability goals, they are vastly different in other ways. Singapore lies just one and a half degrees north of the equator, providing it an average daytime temperature of 81 degrees Fahrenheit (27°C) and an even amount of daylight (approximately 12 hours) throughout the year. While most sites farther from the equator must negotiate a wide range of sun angles that change throughout the day and year, sun position in the sky is relatively consistent from day to day, allowing for the design to mitigate nearly all direct sun entering the building through the use of fixed sun shades and vertical vegetation. Limiting direct sun penetration into a space also limits the need for blinds, which in turn protects patients' views of greenery that are often shielded when the blinds are drawn. Research has found that once blinds are pulled, they are rarely put back up (Schleib et al. 2013). Relatively even temperatures across the day and year, and regular rainfall, mean that vegetation remains green year-round.

These consistent temperatures and hours of daylight allowed designers to incorporate nature in NTFGH-JCH in ways that they could not at Eskenazi Health, where average daytime temperatures in Indianapolis fluctuate greatly with the seasons—from 35 degrees Fahrenheit (2°C) in January to 85 degrees in July (29°C)—and daylight can range from 9 hours in winter to 15 in summer. While Eskenazi Health Main Campus's outdoor spaces are comfortable during many parts of the year—and water features can help to improve thermal comfort in the warmer months—the campus also relies heavily on views to the outdoors, to view gardens, including the adjacent Ball Gardens.

Mara Baum

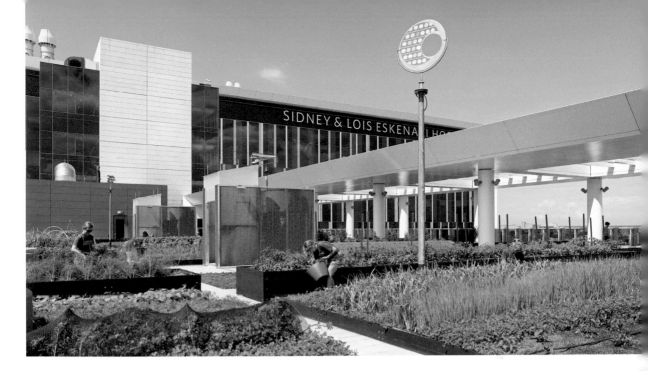

▲ Figure 20.3

Eskenazi Health's rooftop Sky Farm produces thousands of pounds of produce to be served inside the hospital.
Source: Timothy Hursley

Eskenazi Health Main Campus leverages design to accentuate seasonal changes, further connecting occupants to natural patterns and cycles. A central entry plaza known as the Commonground provides seating, community gathering space, a place for a farmer's market, and two different water features. The Pavilion Restaurant, located within the Commonground, evolves throughout the year; its living canopy of vines grows and changes from month to month, conveying the passing of time. The restaurant serves "slow fast food" that emphasizes seasonal and locally produced foods. Atop Eskenazi Health Main Campus's Outpatient Care Center lies the 5,000-square-feet "Sky Farm". Weather permitting, patients, staff and visitors can relax within the rooftop vegetable garden that yields thousands of pounds of fresh produce per year, providing healthy dining options for the hospital. Seasonal produce provides an experiential, place-based way to connect with the natural world.

20.3.2 Ecosystems

The ecosystems native to the two hospital campuses are also starkly different. The island city-state of Singapore encompasses just 278 square miles of land that was once largely mangrove swamps and lowland forests. Although 95% of Singapore today is urbanized, pockets of nature—such as the Bukit Timah Nature Reserve—still display the nation's unique biodiversity, which includes a variety of palm, rattan, fern, and fig species. This set of flora informs the biophilic design of NTFGH-JCH, and can be seen in features such as planted rooftops, gardens at ground level, and balconies that provide patients and staff with immediate and proximate views of similar plant life that can be found in native, undeveloped Singapore.

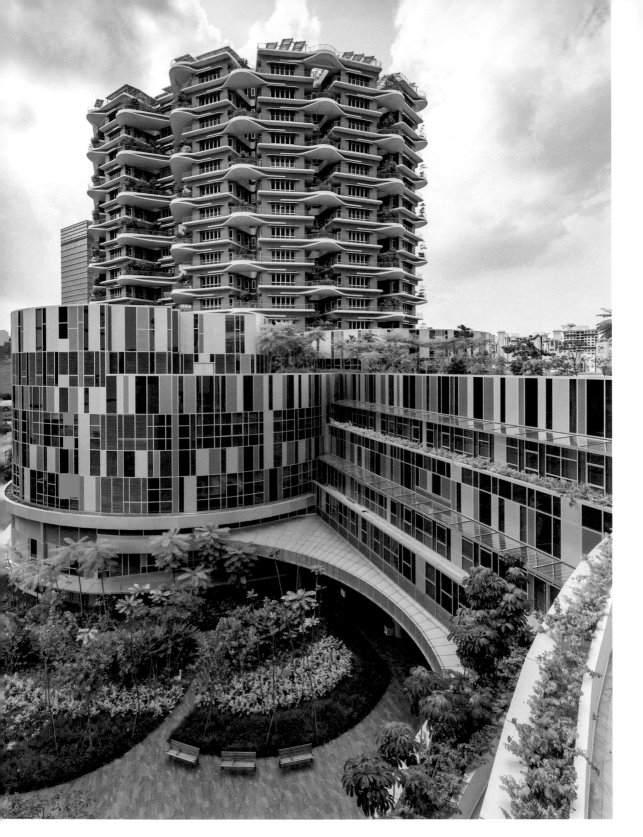

▲ Figure 20.4

Ng Teng Fong General Hospital and Jurong Community Hospital take full advantage of the lush vegetation native to Singapore.
Source: Rory Daniel

Mara Baum

Unhindered by seasonal weather changes, NTFGH-JCH takes full advantage of its tropical locale with plantings on, within, and up the sides of buildings. Like an oasis within a dense city, the site features a large public garden and additional gardens designated for patients and staff at all levels throughout the campus. The patient tower facades incorporate exterior platforms with planter beds. These are positioned to give nearly every patient direct views of vegetation, regardless of how high they are within the building. In addition to potential benefits that can come with views of vegetation (Wilson 1984), plants also can improve air quality, reduce ambient temperatures, and provide exterior sun shading. Incorporating native species and local materials builds on an individual's personal familiarity and comfort with the environment. Use of native and adaptive species can also be less expensive and easier to maintain over time.

A wholly distinct geography informs the design of Eskenazi Health Main Campus, which lies in the rolling limestone hills of central Indiana that (historically) have been home to both temperate grasslands and forests. As such, designers chose Indiana limestone, native wildflowers, and deciduous trees to landscape the grounds of Eskenazi Health Main Campus and to serve as inspiration throughout the hospital grounds. Indiana limestone is used throughout the site, and is one of the focal points of the Commonground. A large art piece assembled of limestone boulders lines the plaza's western edge and features a cascading waterfall that runs year-round and can freeze over in winter. Tables and chairs extend along the length of the waterfall, offering a space for staff and visitors to linger and listen to the white noise of the water flow. Water elements have been shown to have both an energizing and calming effect on people and can help to reduce stress (Mador 2008), and recall the natural lakes and streams of the Indiana landscape. A second water feature at the opposite end of the Commonground resembles a shallow spring. Water bubbles up from the ground, inviting visitors to touch and play in it during warm weather. Visitors experience this differently throughout the year, as water flows only in warm months. When dry, winding stone ripples at the base of the water feature become visible, evoking a gently rolling landscape.

20.3.3 Culture

Culture also plays a significant role in biophilic design. In hospital design, culture may include medical regulations and philosophies as well as patient expectations, particularly when it comes to building systems. For example, operable windows and natural ventilation are standard in all Singaporean public medical/surgical units. While a non-air-conditioned space in an 80-plus-degree climate may create significant discomfort among Americans, Singaporeans, who typically live and work in non-air-conditioned environments, can prefer higher indoor temperatures than their U.S. counterparts—and can become uncomfortable when the temperature drops to set points common in the U.S. (Chen and Chang 2012; Schiavon et al. 2016).

Typical public hospital wards in Singapore can have up to nine patients per room—most of whom have limited access to much-needed daylight and ventilation when patients adjacent to the windows pull their privacy curtains. NTFGH-JCH eliminates that problem with its unique sawtooth-pattern floor

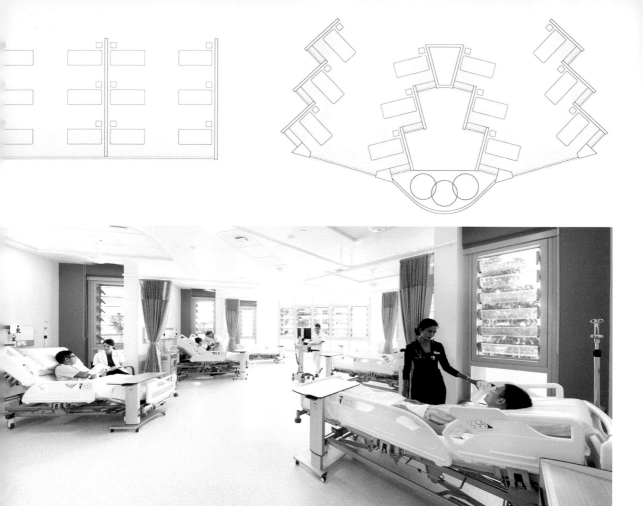

▲ Figure 20.5

The typical Singaporean patient room (upper left) provides access to daylight, views, and natural ventilation only to the two patients closer to the windows. The unique sawtooth pattern of the Ng Teng Fong General Hospital patient room (upper right and bottom), by comparison, provides each patient with a window.
Source: Rory Daniel

plate that provides every patient with a window positioned only a few feet from the bed. With numerous studies citing a wide range of health benefits associated with daylight, this immediate proximity can have a positive impact on patients (Aries, Aarts, and Van Hoof 2015; Beute and de Kort 2014).

Not only does the design give patients access to daylight and views but also the windows located at each bed are fully operable—providing patients direct control of their immediate environment. The towers' floor plates were configured directly in response to the position of the sun and the prevailing breezes, intended first to maximize ventilation rates and then to offer solar shading and acoustical protection. Extensive computational fluid dynamics modeling demonstrated that the patient ward fenestration creates a small wind tunnel effect, with pressure differentials that increase ventilation rates at the patient bed. This modeling played a critical role in shaping the floor plan of the patient towers.

Mara Baum

Most of the facility is primarily passively cooled and naturally ventilated, with air conditioning reserved largely for operating suites, imaging, isolation, and intensive care rooms. Single-loaded corridors allow for outside air to pass over just one patient bed before crossing the ward and exiting the building. The jalousie windows at the patient beds are structured so that part of the window always remains open, guaranteeing a minimum air flow. Thermal mass, ceiling fans, cross ventilation, and exterior shading ensure comfortable temperatures throughout the day.

The single-loaded corridor design, while implemented for ventilation-related infection prevention purposes, also brings daylight and views to staff spaces that would conventionally fall deep within a floor plate. Daylight has been shown to reduce stress, improve mood, increase alertness, reduce medical errors, and benefit health outcomes (Joseph 2006). Direct access to daylight and views to the outdoors also have been shown to increase staff alertness and reduce medical errors when compared with spaces that offer daylight but no views, or neither daylight or views (Zadeh et al. 2014). A majority of NTFGH-JCH staff have daylight and views to the outdoors from their work spaces, including all nurse stations. Natural ventilation and extensive daylighting also provide a secondary benefit of cost savings through reduced energy consumption.

Conventional American medical planning practices, meanwhile, can at times lead to deep floor plates with limited fenestration and no potential for natural ventilation. Code also prevents the use of natural ventilation in many space types. Eskenazi Health Main Campus circumvents this problem by incorporating several light wells and interior courtyards, bringing natural light into the heart of the facility. The emergency department's "Well of Wishes" is one such interior courtyard and aims to calm ill, injured, and otherwise stressed patients and families. The Well of Wishes is a view garden—offering emergency room visitors the direct opportunity for views of vegetation while they remain in a secure and conditioned environment. Views of vegetation have been found to reduce heart rates and help to mitigate perception of pain (Ulrich 2008).

20.3.4 Interiors

While gardens offer a beneficial direct connection with nature, elements like interior finish selection and artwork can help to create metaphoric connections to nature. These furnishings can be readily scaled for inclusion in any budget, are often easily updated, and can help reinforce the identity of a given project. Eskenazi Health Main Campus's extensive public art program helps to create year-round metaphoric, sensory, and spatial connections to nature. The program dates to the early twentieth century, when art in hospitals was not yet commonplace, and includes historic Indiana landscapes by the locally renowned painter T. C. Steele. Eskenazi's newest art pieces are modern interpretations of nature-inspired art, incorporating images, patterns, and textures found in the outdoors. These types of metaphoric connections have been repeatedly shown to mitigate stress reactions and support health and well-being. Ulrich's ongoing research indicates that patients and staff benefit from both active and passive interactions with nature (Browning, Ryan, and Clancy 2014; Kellert 2005; Ulrich 2008).

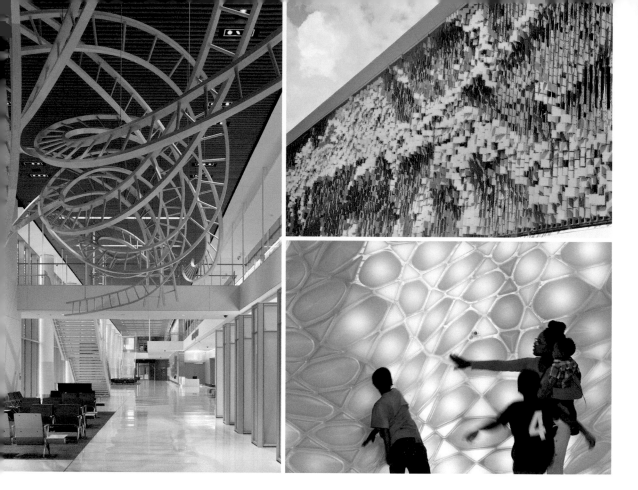

▲ Figure 20.6

The Eskenazi Health art program, including *Paths Crossed* (left) and *May/September* (upper right), leverages metaphoric connections with nature, regardless of the weather conditions.
Source: Timothy Hursley

The massive art piece *May/September* by artist Rob Ley dominates the southern edge of the site, encompassing one side of a seven-story parking garage. Comprised of nearly 7,000 angled, colored metal panels, the art installation appears to shift and change as visitors move past it. Although physically static, this appearance of movement creates the perception of an evolving stochastic pattern. Stochastic patterns are commonly found in nature. Like clouds moving in the sky or the chirping of birds, they can be analyzed statistically but cannot be precisely predicted. Stochastic patterns and other non-rhythmic movements have the effect of simultaneously stimulating and relaxing our brains; even brief contact provides us with the opportunity for rejuvenation (Browning, Ryan, and Clancy 2014; Kellert 2005).

May/September is one of several Eskenazi Health Main Campus art pieces that provide a sense of movement and transformation. Others incorporate changing colors, light, wind, materiality, and other dynamic elements. At the upper levels of the Outpatient Care Center, for example, patterned sun shades and dichroic glass accentuate the movement of the sun throughout the day and

Mara Baum

year by generating changing shadows, colors, and patterns. These natural cycles and systems offer ephemeral movement and visual and/or auditory stochastic patterns that support both distraction and restoration.

Inside the Eskenazi Health Main Campus's Outpatient Care Center lobby, the signature *Paths Crossed* installation by Aaron Stephan floats above the concourse. An abstracted metaphor of the double helix of our DNA, it is composed of six spiraled ladders made of local Indiana maple. It creates a sense of excitement and demonstrates a balance of simplicity and complexity that is commonly found in natural patterns and systems. At first glance the piece appears to be highly complex, but upon further examination, the pattern is easily discernable. As humans we are drawn to these types of patterns—our minds do not like boredom, yet we also want to understand the pattern behind complexity (Van den Berg, Joye, and Koole 2016; Salingaros and Masden 2008).

20.4 Conclusions

There is no correct single way to approach biophilic design. Each healthcare facility should identify the palette of strategies that best meets its needs based on its unique climate, location, culture, and other factors. Yet, when integrated holistically throughout a building or campus, biophilic design can positively impact the health, well-being, and overall experience of all who enter a space. Our brains thrive on the complex visual and auditory experiences found in nature, and we become bored and mentally drained by wholly artificial and visually sterile environments (Salingaros and Masden 2008).

Despite its benefits, many facilities still face challenges to biophilic design. Budget constraints and concerns about infection prevention may prohibit the incorporation of some types of art pieces, natural materials, or decorative elements that infuse biophilia into spaces. If a limitation prevents specific biophilic strategies, other approaches can be considered. Although there may be a value to lush, vegetated landscapes, simple natural finish materials or nature imagery showing both prospect and refuge are arguably better than nothing at all (Sachs 2017).

Apart from its individual health benefits, biophilic design could aid public health on the global scale. People who have greater contact with natural environments are more likely to have a greater conservation ethic (Kellert and Wilson 1995; Kellert 2005). Climate change is considered by many to be the greatest public health threat of the twenty-first century, and conservation-related actions that can be taken now may be able to help offset some of the impacts to be felt in years to come (Frumkin et al. 2008; Younger et al. 2008). While it may be a mental leap to suggest that biophilic design will help to stave off climate change, there is a measurable connection between biophilia and environmentalism (Baum 2005; Orr 1993; Wilson 1993). Understanding its limits, the incorporation of natural elements—both direct and indirect—into the design of the built environment can have a profound impact on human health and well-being.

Bibliography

Aries, Myriam B. C., Mariëlle P. J Aarts, and Joost van Hoof. "Daylight and Health: A Review of the Evidence and Consequences for the Built Environment." *Lighting Research & Technology* 47, no. 1 (2015): 6–27.

Baum, M. L. *Biomimetic and Biophilic Design as a Model for Regenerative Redevelopment of the Post-industrial San Francisco Bay Edge.* Berkeley, CA: University of California, 2005.

Berman, Marc G., John Jonides, and Stephen Kaplan. "The Cognitive Benefits of Interacting with Nature." *Psychological Science* 19, no. 12 (2008): 1207–1212.

Beute, Femke, and Yvonne A. W de Kort. "Salutogenic Effects of the Environment: Review of Health Protective Effects of Nature and Daylight." *Applied Psychology: Health and Well-Being* 6, no. 1 (2014): 67–95.

Boehland, J. "Hospital, Heal Thyself: Greening the Design and Construction of Healthcare Facilities." *Environmental Building News* 14, no. 6 (2005).

Browning, William, Catherine Ryan, and Joseph Clancy. *14 Patterns of Biophilic Design.* New York: Terrapin Bright Green, LLC, 2014. www.terrapinbrightgreen.com/reports/14-patterns/#.

Chen, Ailu, and Victor W-C. Chang. "Human Health and Thermal Comfort of Office Workers in Singapore." *Building and Environment* 58 (2012): 172–178.

Cooper Marcus, C., and Marni Barnes, eds. *Healing Gardens: Therapeutic Benefits and Design Recommendations.* Vol. 4. Hoboken, NJ: John Wiley & Sons, 1999.

Cooper Marcus, C., and N. A. Sachs. *Therapeutic Landscapes.* Hoboken, NJ: John Wiley & Sons, 2014.

Frumkin, Howard, Jeremy Hess, George Luber, Josephine Malilay, and Michael McGeehin. "Climate Change: The Public Health Response." *American Journal of Public Health* 98, no. 3 (2008): 435–445.

Guenther, Robin, and Gail Vittori. *Sustainable Healthcare Architecture*, 2nd ed. Hoboken, NJ: John Wiley & Sons, 2013.

Hartig, Terry, Marlis Mang, and Gary W. Evans. "Restorative Effects of Natural Environment Experiences." *Environment and Behavior* 23, no. 1 (1991): 3–26.

Heerwagen, Judith. H., and Gordon H. Orians. "Humans, Habitats, and Aesthetics." In *The Biophilia Hypothesis*, edited by R. Stephen Kellert and Edward O. Wilson. Washington, DC: Island Press, 1995.

Joseph, Anjali. *The Impact of Light on Outcomes in Healthcare Settings.* Concord, CA: Center for Health Design, 2006.

Joye, Yannick, and Agnes Van den Berg. "Restorative Environments." In *Environmental Psychology: An introduction*, edited by Linda Steg, Van den Berg, E. Agnes, and Judith De Groot, 57–66. London: Wiley-Blackwell, 2012. www.agnesvandenberg.nl/EPc06.pdf.

Kaplan, Stephen. "The Restorative Benefits of Nature: Toward an Integrative Framework." *Journal of Environmental Psychology* 15, no. 3 (1995): 169–182.

Kaplan, Stephen. "The Restorative Environment: Nature and Human Experience." *The Role of Horticulture in Human Well-Being and Social Development* (1992): 134–142.

Kellert, Stephen R. "The Biological Basis for Human Values of Nature." In *The Biophilia Hypothesis*, edited by S. R. Kellert and E. O. Wilson, 42–69. Washington, DC: Island Press, 1993.

Kellert, S. R. *Building for Life: Designing and Understanding the Human-Nature Connection.* Washington, DC: Island Press, 2005.

Kellert, Stephen R. "Kinship to Mastery." *Biophilia in Human Evolution and Development.* Washington, DC: Island Press, 2003.

Kellert, Stephen R., Judith Heerwagen, and Martin Mador. *Biophilic Design: The Theory, Science and Practice of Bringing Buildings to Life*. Hoboken, NJ: John Wiley & Sons, 2008.

Kellert, Stephen R., and Edward O. Wilson, eds. *The Biophilia Hypothesis*. Washington, DC: Island Press, 1995.

Klepeis, Neil E., William C. Nelson, Wayne R. Ott, John P. Robinson, Andy M. Tsang, Paul Switzer, Joseph V. Behar, Stephen C. Horn, and William H. Engelmann. "The National Human Activity Pattern Survey (NHAPS): A Resource for Assessing Exposure to Environmental Pollutants." *Journal of Exposure Science and Environmental Epidemiology* 11, no. 3 (2001): 231.

Loftness, Vivian, and Megan Snyder. "Where Windows Become Doors." *Biophilic Design: The Theory, Science and Practice of Bringing Buildings to Life*. New York: John Wiley (2008): 119–131.

Mador, Martin L. "Water, Biophilic Design, and the Built Environment." *Biophilic Design: The Theory, Science and Practice of Bringing Buildings to Life*, 43–57. New York: John Wiley & Sons, 2008.

Nejati, Adeleh, Susan Rodiek, and Mardelle Shepley. "Using Visual Simulation to Evaluate Restorative Qualities of Access to Nature in Hospital Staff Break Areas." *Landscape and Urban Planning* 148 (2016): 132–138.

Orr, David W. "Love It or Lose It: The Coming Biophilia Revolution." In *The Biophilia Hypothesis*, edited by S. R. Kellert and E. O. Wilson, 415–440. Washington, DC: Island Press, 1993.

Pati, Debajyoti, and Paul Barach. "Application of Environmental Psychology Theories and Frameworks to Evidence-Based Healthcare Design." *Environmental Psychology: New Developments* (2010): 1–36.

Sachs, Naomi A. "The Case for Nature or Nature-ish." *Health Environments Research & Design Journal* 10, no. 5 (2017): 157 161.

Salingaros, N., and K. Masden. "Neuroscience, the Natural Environment, and Building Design." *Biophilic Design: The Theory, Science and Practice of Bringing Buildings to Life*, 59–83. New York: John Wiley & Sons, 2008.

Schiavon, Stefano, Bin Yang, Yoni Donner, V. W-C. Chang, and William W. Nazaroff. "Thermal Comfort, Perceived Air Quality, and Cognitive Performance When Personally Controlled Air Movement is Used by Tropically Acclimatized Persons." *Indoor Air* 27, no. 3 (2016): 690 702.

Schleib, Jonah C., Russell Unger, Richard Leigh, Christina Anjesky, Jamie Kleinberg, Shannon Mcullough, and Erin Mulberg. *Seduced by the View: A Closer Look at All – Glass Buildings*. New York, NY: Urban Green Building Council, 2013. https://issuu.com/urbangreen/docs/seduced_by_the_view.

Therapeutics Landscapes Network. 2018. www.healinglandscapes.org.

Ulrich, Roger S. "Biophilic Theory and Research for Healthcare Design." *Biophilic Design: The Theory, Science and Practice of Bringing Buildings to Life*, 87–106. New York: John Wiley, 2008.

Ulrich, Roger S. "View Through A Window May Influence Recovery from Surgery." *Science* 224, no. 4647 (1984): 420–421.

Van den Berg, Agnes E., Yannick Joye, and Sander L. Koole. "Why Viewing Nature Is More Fascinating and Restorative than Viewing Buildings: A Closer Look at Perceived Complexity." *Urban Forestry & Urban Greening* 20 (2016): 397–401.

Van den Berg, Magdalena, Jolanda Maas, Rianne Muller, Anoek Braun, Wendy Kaandorp, René van Lien, Mireille van Poppel, Willem van Mechelen, and Agnes van den Berg. "Autonomic Nervous System Responses to Viewing Green and Built Settings: Differentiating Between Sympathetic and Parasympathetic Activity." *International Journal of Environmental Research and Public Health* 12, no. 12 (2015): 15860–15874.

Vincent, Ellen, Dina Battisto, Larry Grimes, and James McCubbin. "The Effects of Nature Images on Pain in a Simulated Hospital Patient Room." *HERD: Health Environments Research & Design Journal* 3, no. 3 (2010): 42–55.

Wilson, Edward O. *Biophilia*. Cambridge, MA: President and Fellows of Harvard College, 1984.

Wilson, Edward O. "Biophilia and the Conservation Ethic." In *Evolutionary Perspectives on Environmental Problems*, 263–272. Abingdon, Oxon and New York, NY: Routledge, 1993.

Younger, Margalit, Heather R. Morrow-Almeida, Stephen M. Vindigni, and Andrew L. Dannenberg. "The Built Environment, Climate Change, and Health: Opportunities for Co-Benefits." *American Journal of Preventive Medicine* 35, no. 5 (2008): 517–526.

Zadeh, Rana Sagha, Mardelle McCuskey Shepley, Gary Williams, and Susan Sung Eun Chung. "The Impact of Windows and Daylight on Acute-Care Nurses' Physiological, Psychological, and Behavioral Health." *HERD: Health Environments Research & Design Journal* 7, no. 4 (2014): 35–61.

Chapter 21

The Anti-Prototype
Why Community Health Requires Local Solutions

Michael Murphy, *Amie Shao*, and *Jeffrey Mansfield*

21.1 Introduction

Global health challenges are vast and innumerable, warranting prototypical solutions that are scalable, replicable, and cost-effective. The prototype formula works for drugs, practice methods, and technology, and has saved countless lives while mitigating costs. However, in the face of large problems, including healthcare access, disease outbreak, and natural disasters, architectural prototypes are rarely successful. Although intended to be agile and adaptable, applications of prototypes generally favor technocratic replicability over contextuality. In place of a contextual solution, the universally applicable prototype offers an off-the-shelf solution to global crises. The unfortunate result is that the "universal prototype" downplays the root causes of the crises, focusing on a reaction to disasters rather than creating the conditions that would minimize them. Preventative infrastructural measures are de-prioritized and healthcare infrastructure becomes reliant on international aid and technology. In this essay, we examine the historical foundation and attraction to the "universal" prototype and question the wisdom of a one-size-fits-all approach to global health. We then explore how contextual and locally informed architecture can promote health, equity, economy, and environment.

21.2 The Colonial Prototype

When Maison Tropicale, Jean Prouvé's 1949–1951 prefabricated and flat-packed residential prototype for tropical climates, exhibited in New York and London in 2007 and 2008, respectively, it was presented as the built manifestation of modernism itself: its form and materiality spoke of lightweight structural integrity, rapid deployability and assembly, and industrial supply chains, all at once.

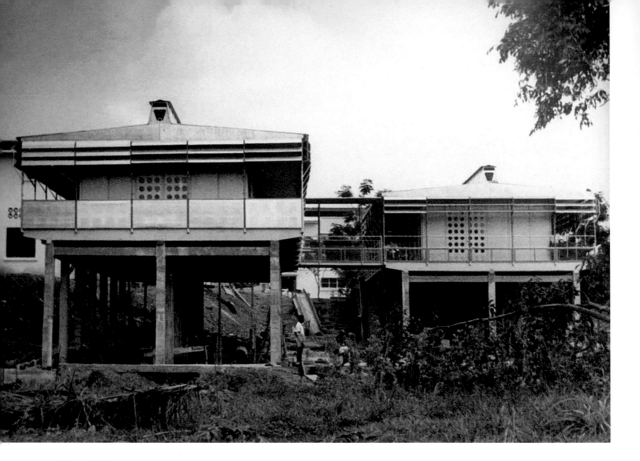

▲ Figure 21.1

Jean Prouvé's Maison Tropicale assembled in Brazzaville, Congo. Jean Prouvé, c. 1951.
Source: Wikiarquitectura

First erected in 1951 as a complementary pair in Brazzaville, Republic of Congo, Les Maisons Tropicales were Prouvé's response to a shortage of housing in the French colonies of West Africa. Light, flat-packed, and designed for mass production, Maison Tropicale was a precursor to contemporary prefabricated construction methods. Its components, fabricated off-site in French factories, could be transported via air and ground freight and assembled by a small team on the ground without much construction expertise. Each aluminum wall panel measured four meters wide, corresponding to the width of rolling machines at the factory, and could be rapidly assembled onto a folded sheet steel portal frame. Its cooling strategy consisted of a mix of fixed and moveable panels to support cross ventilation, an outer skin of adjustable and reflective aluminum louvers, a double roof that hung over a verandah to facilitate natural ventilation and minimize solar heat gain, and blue glass porthole windows designed to protect against ultraviolet rays (Balazs 2008). In terms of material processes, Maison Tropicale is colonialism manifest: raw materials to produce Maison Tropicale's aluminum components were extracted from the West African colonies, shipped to the company's factories in France, refined into aluminum components, and eventually transported back to the colonies, to be used in a project that promised to bring about "social transformation" (Rossen 2013). Maison Tropicale, through its synthesis of health, wellness, and technocratic efficiency, symbolized the "civilizing mission" of its colonial vanguards. But if Maison Tropicale exemplified a

Michael Murphy et al.

technocratic solution to a problem, it also exposed its ignorance, or inability to engage local knowledge, customs, and practices in dwelling and settlement.

Ostensibly a universally applicable prototype that could be rapidly erected to mitigate the building crisis in the colonies, only three Maisons Tropicales were assembled—the pair in Brazzaville at the company's offices, and another erected in Niamey, Niger, in 1949—well short of its grand promise and that of the French colonial project. An expensive transplant that appealed neither to the local aesthetic nor to conservative French bureaucrats, and incompatible with its evolving functionality, the experimental status of Maison Tropicale frames the tropics as a design laboratory and begs the question of whether architecture ought to be prototyped in the factory at all. Is it possible for architecture to be universally applicable, or does this come at the cost of a building's ability to engage with its local context?

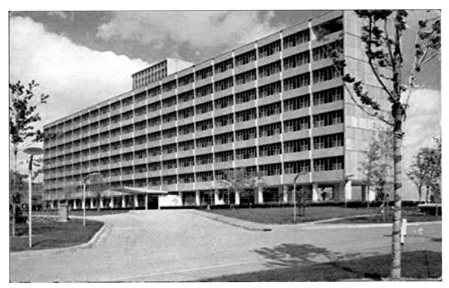

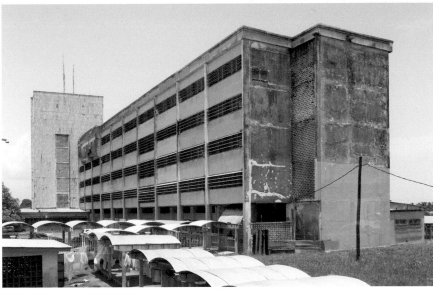

▶ Figure 21.2

John Kane Hospital, Pittsburgh, PA, USA, 1958 (top), and Litchfield Whiting Bowne and Associates, John F. Kennedy Medical Center, Monrovia, Liberia, 1971 (bottom).
Source: Top photo: Michael Merante; bottom photo: MASS Design Group

21.3 The Postcolonial Development Prototype

The end of the Second World War brought a new global coalition organized around the ideals of peacekeeping, social and economic development, humanitarian aid, and disaster relief. The United Nations and its host of affiliated bilateral organizations (including the World Bank, International Monetary Fund, UNESCO, and the World Health Organization [WHO], as well as fledging agencies like USAID) stepped in to help as newly formed African countries struggled to establish political rule and economic stability during the postwar years.

In the context of the Cold War, a gripping fear by the superpowers that poor, developing, and third-world countries would be sympathetic to democratic, first-world or communist, second-world regimes drove tropical medicine, and global health campaigns. Undertaken by international aid organizations and foreign governments, these campaigns offered financing, logistical support, and healthcare infrastructure, effectively turning hospitals into instruments of foreign policy. During the Cold War, a dizzying amount of healthcare facilities were funded and built within Africa by external Western powers, such as the United States and Great Britain, expropriating preexisting Western prototypes into African contexts—not dissimilar from Maison Tropicale.

21.3.1 John F. Kennedy Medical Center

In 1971 the John F. Kennedy Medical Center appeared in Monrovia, Liberia, as a close facsimile of Mitchell & Ritchie's John Kane Hospital of Pittsburgh from 13 years prior (Pade 1953). Part of a plan by the Liberian government to implement a new healthcare system in the 1960s, the project to construct a new hospital in Monrovia found an eager supporter in President Kennedy. Kennedy, who had personally stewarded international development efforts as a senator and who, in his new capacity as president, had proclaimed the 1960s the "Decade of Development", quickly pledged American funding toward the construction of the hospital. In the form of a $6.8 million loan and $9.2 million in grants from USAID to supplement $1 million in contributions from the Liberian government, the funding was seen, by the president and by Congress, as an opportunity to generate support for American politics in Africa. Designed by the New York firm Litchfield Whiting Bowne and Associates, construction began on the hospital in 1965, and the John F. Kennedy Medical Center was opened in July 1971.

It did not take long for the infrastructural shortcomings of the facility to reveal themselves. The "monument to American inefficiency", as Secretary of State William Rogers called it (Horan 1998, p. 13), incurred astronomical operating costs: by the 1980s, maintaining and operating the 500-bed JFK Medical Center accounted for more than 40% of the Liberian government's total recurring costs for its national healthcare system. Being the only hospital in the country, and one fitted with sophisticated but inflexible systems, much of the costs were related to operational maintenance of the facility and its equipment. A report by the U.S. State Department in 1980, in language that can be described as colonial and patronizing, centered on such contradictions: the modern medical facility, with its up-to-date medical supplies and technocratic systems, was

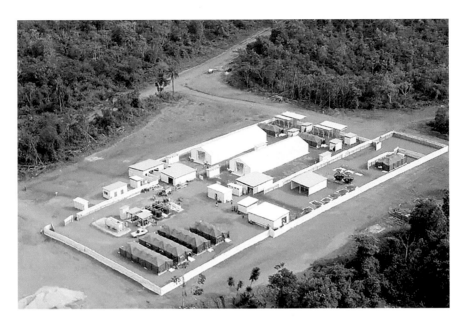

▲ Figure 21.3

Aerial photograph of an Ebola treatment unit, assembled by the U.S. Army in Barclayville, Liberia (2015).
Source: U.S. Army

too "sophisticated" for its context. It described the building as "an American transplant to African society", whose "building design and layout, although correct for a modern hospital, are said not to conform to African cultural patterns" (US Department of State 1980, p. 10).

Although the hospital garnered a reputation centered on its pitfalls, it was also an internationally excellent hospital to which people migrated from around West Africa for healthcare. Its architecture, while an import from the West, contained thoughtful climatic interventions, including the orientation of the tower to maximize the consistent ocean breeze through small six-bed naturally ventilated wards, concrete block screens that gave shelter from the rain but allowed natural ventilation to pass through open corridors, and floor-to-ceiling jalousie windows to maximize natural daylighting and ventilation. If one looked closely, the horizontal louvers were similar to the Maison Tropicale. However, the hospital was anomalous. In the absence of a strong healthcare system around it to provide primary and secondary care it was doomed to ultimately fail. Among the tallest structures in Monrovia, the hospital was occupied by rebel forces and used as a machine gun perch during the ensuing 14-year Liberian civil war, sustaining heavy damage and acquiring a reputation for death in place of health. The hospital suffered heavy damage, doctors fled the country during the conflict, and the facility has not been fully repaired or maintained since.

Today it suffers from a lack of coordination in planning, maintenance, and care, with various international aid groups undertaking piecemeal renovation projects and operating small zones within the hospital. While their services are crucial, they do not represent a holistic view of the medical needs of the community. Such buildings, inadequate in their services, minimally adapted to the local built environment and cultural practices, and whose legacies are intertwined with complex and often violent postcolonial nation-building processes, were fodder for a brewing discontent over modern architecture's utopian fixation. The inauspicious outcomes of the JFK Medical Center project contributed to an abandonment of long-form, permanent construction projects. Intragovernmental agencies dismissed the demands of engineers and infrastructure experts in favor of privatizing foreign investment, healthcare, and construction delivery to NGOs, private foundations, and international corporations. In this operational shift, USAID, along with other Western, bilateral coalitions, focused efforts on humanitarian aid and disaster relief. Rapid response, prefabricated prototypes, medical tents, and bags of rice gained relevance as agents of Western international diplomacy.

21.3.2 Tappita Regional Referral Hospital

Nearly half a century after JFK Medical Center opened its doors, global health delivery is still repeating past missteps. The 100-bed, $10 million Tappita Jackson F. Doe Regional Referral Hospital in Nimba County, Liberia, built in 2011 by the Chinese as a gift to Liberia, is the most advanced tertiary-level hospital in the country (Sirleaf 2011). But its location, in the middle of a remote jungle, and its premise make little sense. Though geographically not far from the capital, inadequate road infrastructure makes it a seven-hour trip to Tappita, out of reach for most Liberians. In the rainy season, simply reaching the hospital—to receive treatment or deliver prescription drugs—has proven difficult if not impossible (Front Page Africa 25 May 2018). Even the idea that the hospital has a catchment area including all of Liberia and West Africa seems far-fetched: the surrounding area lacks infrastructure, like hotels, housing, and food, to support people traveling for care. It is located near a small village, where people need basic primary care, but the hospital, with its focus on specialty care (it holds Liberia's only CT scanner), offers only major surgery and brain scans. It is not aligned with the needs of the people and its context.

Like the JFK Medical Center and Prouvé's prototype, the Tappita facility demonstrates some thoughtful solutions: to attract high-quality doctors, the design integrates doctors' housing on campus and the hospital is a teaching facility. Locally informed design adaptations include semi-enclosed exterior corridors that, like at JFK, facilitate natural ventilation while offering shelter from torrential rain. The layout of buildings creates courtyard spaces where patients and doctors can relax or quickly walk to other parts of the hospital. However, the facility hasn't been designed for long-term impact: three massive on-site generators and fuel to operate these generators make up as much as 40% of the hospital's operating budget. Simply keeping the hospital running burdens the hospital's bottom line, and frequent intentional power outages are necessary to keep these costs down (Front Page Africa 23 May 2018). Because the hospital is outfitted with Chinese equipment, maintaining the hospital requires Chinese labor and Chinese parts, a form of technocratic control that makes routine maintenance overly complicated, expensive, and dependent on external powers. With its CT scan, mammogram, chemistry, and blood machines no longer functioning due to the astronomical costs associated with their maintenance, the hospital constantly teeters on the edge of turning into a graveyard of expensive medical equipment (Front Page Africa 7 April 2018).

Emblematic of many monolithic hospitals built in Africa by foreign interests, Tappita represents a focus on specialty/tertiary care in imbalance with an urgent need for basic primary care services. The hospital, like other facilities throughout Liberia and Africa at large, evokes the truism "The poor get sick, and the sick get poorer", and underlines the concept that the health of a community is often an economic problem (Farmer 2005). This "gift" of tertiary care comes at the expense of roads, sewage, and primary care, which the society desperately needs. Built with imported materials and foreign labor, such facilities symbolize a transactional gift from a foreign government seeking to gain a long-term economic foothold on the resources of a given country.

21.4 Prototype Clinics

The civil war that sieged Liberia from 1989 to 2003 decimated the nation's health system, destroying over 80% of the country's public health infrastructure (Kruk et al. 2010). JFK Medical Center, one of Liberia's leading hospitals, was left in various stages of disrepair with highly unrealistic maintenance costs, hampering the nation's recovery.

Recognizing an urgent need to update its healthcare infrastructure with basic services, the Liberian government in 2006 began the process of reforming its healthcare system based around improved healthcare facilities (Gwenigale 2011). The resulting ten year, comprehensive national health policy, issued in 2010, prioritized distributing medical care from Monrovia, the capital, into a decentralized care network of specialized rural referral centers. Once again, prototypes were employed to provide a solution. A U.S. architectural firm drew up a set of simple plans and elevations for each prototype. The prototype was the same regardless of site, climate, and context. Predictably, the results were improperly oriented buildings that failed to maximize the benefits of wind and natural light. Poor construction quality, coupled with limited basic amenities, like running water and electricity, led to catastrophic system failures. After much investment, doctors still delivered babies at night with headlamps, and buildings stood in visible disrepair with crumbling walls and collapsing ceiling panels. Other buildings remained unoccupied. Had these simple designs responded to site and context, they could have worked. What went wrong was an overall lack of standards and coordination in the planning, design, and construction of these prototypes.

Each of the foregoing scenarios, like Maison Tropicale, illuminates how the practice of transplanting architecture to ill-suited foreign contexts fails to understand local conditions and is ultimately unsuccessful. The most common results are substandard and damaged infrastructure, equipment, and spaces, lack of investment in infrastructure and primary care services, and chronically reactive measures. These conditions left Liberia wholly unprepared for a disaster that would ultimately amount to one of the worst health disasters of the century.

21.5 Acute on Chronic: The Emergency Prototype

When Ebola struck in 2014, Liberia had only 50 physicians in the entire country, or 1 for every 70,000 citizens—a public health crisis in itself (Shah 2016). The Ebola outbreak illustrated a new kind of global health crisis, which Dr. Paul Farmer describes as "acute on chronic" (Farmer 2010, p. 4). In medical parlance, the term is used to describe an acute exacerbation of a chronic condition; in Liberia the chronic lack of infrastructure, upstream investment, and capacity magnified the acuity of the outbreak.

As Ebola threatened to become a global pandemic, the international healthcare community responded with a fleet of prefabricated emergency tents and shelters that served as pop-up Ebola treatment units (ETUs), an army of doctors and medical professionals, injections of funding and aid, and other short-term strategies designed to stem the epidemic. But this influx of aid didn't come overnight, and for several weeks, the number of patients outpaced the number of beds. The situation was so dire that ambulances had to return patients to their homes without getting treatment, and hospitals, many of which were already stretched beyond capacity, shuttered their doors over the fear of spreading the virus (Verderber 2016). Emergency response, while lauded for its ready-and-waiting rapid deployability and easy assembly, clouded a grimmer reality: lack of investment in long-term infrastructure in favor of reactive prototypical solutions made the 2014 Ebola outbreak exponentially more severe.

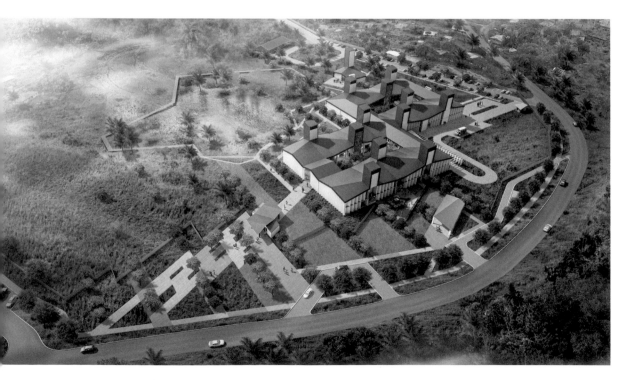

▲ Figure 21.4

Aerial rendering of Redemption Hospital, Caldwell, Liberia. Under construction.
Source: MASS Design Group

Michael Murphy et al.

21.6 Preventative Architecture for Preventative Healthcare

There is an alternative to the largely inefficient investment in global prototypes—and one that is committed to creating locally informed, contextually tailored solutions to community health. What emergency responses failed to tap into was local knowledge and priorities established by the Liberian government's 2010 National Health Infrastructure Standards. Prior to the outbreak, the Liberian government and its Ministry of Health had been developing this document, proactively working to assess needs, identify priorities, and plan national health infrastructure guidelines and strategies. Although Ebola interrupted progress, the Ministry of Health, recognizing that preventative healthcare requires preventative architecture, quickly asked MASS Design Group to revisit these priorities following the outbreak.

21.7 Case Study 1: Redemption Hospital, Caldwell, Liberia

▼ Figure 21.5

Rendering showing the restored wetlands along the southern edge of the new Redemption Hospital site, which offers doctors and patients rejuvenating walking trails and easy access to nature.
Source: MASS Design Group

Reeling from the catastrophic panic around the Ebola outbreak, the spectacular failures of Tappita, and the inefficiency of rigidly standardized prototype clinics, the Liberian Ministry of Health is working to rebuild community trust in its national healthcare system. Through participation in community engagement activities, several community-informed strategies have emerged to inform the design process for new facilities. The new Redemption Hospital in Caldwell (located approximately 30 kilometers from the original Redemption Hospital in Monrovia) embodies Liberia's renewed drive to build an optimized system that will not only avert future epidemics but also deliver comprehensive services to a growing population.

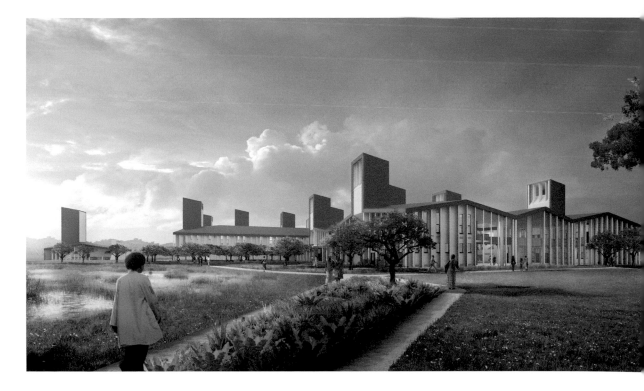

21.7.1 Contextual Response

The design of the new Redemption Hospital seeks to create a more welcoming threshold by integrating a parklike public space at the entry of the hospital campus. Rather than providing security with an uninviting fence, as at the JFK Medical Center, MASS Design Group sought to avoid triggering trauma associated with militarized spaces, and instead introduced a visually transparent yet secure edge around the hospital. This boundary condition allows patients and doctors to connect with the community. At existing facilities in Monrovia, informal markets with a variety of vendors routinely spring up around entrances, creating congested motorcycle parking and complex ambulance routes. Rather than preventing these natural informal activities from occurring, our new design plans for these activities and introduces generous pedestrian entrances with integrated seating and shading areas. Additionally, the design creates more efficient and separated vehicular flows to decongest ambulance routes and reduce chaos around the hospital.

The outdoor landscape further supports the project's mission to renew trust in Liberia's healthcare system. The organization of the campus as a complex of three communal courtyards promotes outdoor gathering spaces to improve the patient experience. Integrating the hospital with a restored wetland, the design leverages the natural landscape with walking trails meant for use by both patients and the community. Adjacent to the maternal ward, the restored wetland offers expectant mothers an environment that encourages outdoor activities while reducing mosquito-borne diseases by increasing water circulation and creating healthy habitats for bird, fish, and amphibian species that feed on mosquitoes.

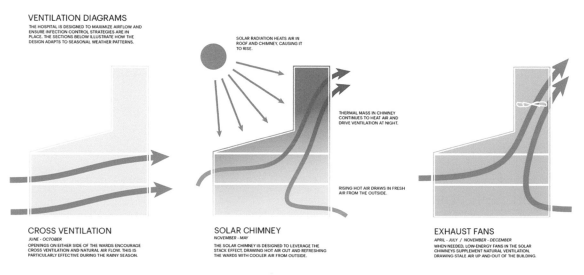

▲ Figure 21.6

Ventilation diagrams illustrating the stack effect ventilation system at the Redemption Hospital, which pairs passive ventilation techniques with low-energy fans.

Source: MASS Design Group

21.7.2 Environmental Strategies for User Comfort and Durability

Phase 1, currently under construction, is a two-story, 155-bed facility for pediatric and maternity services. It will integrate two forms of fail-safe passive ventilation for safety and comfort. In the hot dry season, when there is little wind, the hospital utilizes solar chimneys to ventilate the spaces by pulling air up and out through the stack effect. During Liberia's rainy season, passive cross ventilation, supplemented with mechanical ventilation in the form of low-cost, low-maintenance fans, cools the humid air.

These strategies not only minimize energy use and reduce operational costs but also ensure effective infection control through consistent air changes.

Each component of the design takes lessons from local practices and innovative global hospitals, as well as considers the challenges of healthcare delivery in Liberia. Utilizing local knowledge and responding to context, the design creates a healthy and resilient campus that supports the safety and well-being of patients, staff, and visitors, and provides durability to Liberian's health infrastructure.

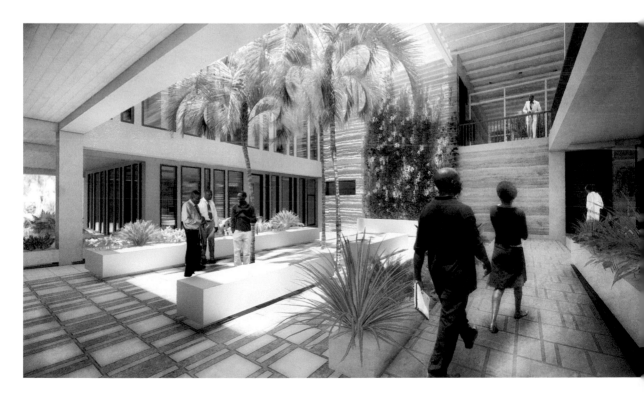

▲ Figure 21.7

The design of the ACEGID facility creates courtyards that foster collaboration between scientists.
Source: MASS Design Group

21.8 Case Study 2: African Center for Excellence in Infectious Diseases (ACEGID), Ede, Nigeria

During the West African Ebola crisis, a lack of specialized laboratories and highly trained scientists in the region hindered critical progress in monitoring emergent pathogens. Genomic sequencing underpins the diagnostic, treatment, and vaccine development required to stop outbreaks, and is needed to monitor the changes pathogens accrue over time. In sequencing, patient samples are analyzed by highly trained scientists with specialized equipment in safe and secure labs—conditions absent in much of Africa. Without regional facilities equipped for this work, blood samples from the Ebola outbreak were sent to the U.S. and Europe, drastically delaying progress.

In 2014, as part of a $150 million World Bank grant in the aftermath of the Ebola epidemic, the African Center of Excellence for Genomics of Infectious Diseases (ACEGID) at Redeemer's University was formed in partnership with academic, clinical, and research institutions in Nigeria, Sierra Leone, and Senegal. ACEGID, in partnership with the Broad Institute and MASS Design Group, proposes a means of stopping the next epidemic more quickly by constructing and equipping a 1300-square-meter genomics lab in Ede, Nigeria. The lab is designed to support genomic sequencing, accelerate vaccine development, monitor microbial outbreaks, promote knowledge transfer, build local as well as international capacity through training, and contribute to community and global health. The intent is to anticipate rather than react. The design of the two-story research center co-locates offices, classrooms, a gallery, communal spaces, and courtyards on the ground floor to facilitate causal interactions and the exchange of ideas between scientists and visitors.

▼ Figure 21.8

A trellis roof superstructure supplements native plantings to offer ample shading from the harsh Nigerian sun while also helping to define outdoor spaces.
Source: MASS Design Group

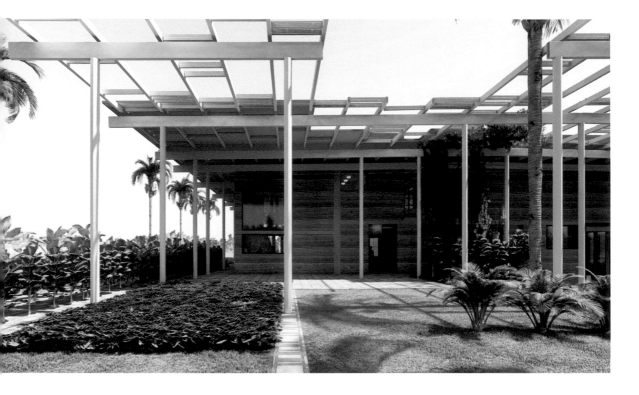

Michael Murphy et al.

21.8.1 Contextual Response

Aesthetically, leveraging locally sourced labor and materials, drawing connections to vernacular building methods with rammed-earth walls, and showcasing the beautiful Nigerian landscape, the goal was to create an internationally recognized yet highly contextualized facility that the community can take pride in.

Instead of the "prototype", if we focus on the opportunities to invest in local and contextual solutions, buildings themselves will evolve organically to their context, and the architecture will engender positive change.

21.8.2 Environmental Strategies for User Comfort and Durability

To mitigate the effects of the harsh Nigerian climate, which alternates between a hot and arid dry season and a hot and humid wet season, buildings in Nigeria typically rely on extensive air conditioning to create hermetic indoor environments. The design of the center does the opposite: It capitalizes on the beauty of the Nigerian landscape with endemic trees and shrubs and a large vine-planted trellis roof superstructure that provides ample shading over courtyards and outdoor decks.

The orientation of the building to prevailing winds, coupled with slow-moving fans, helps mitigate the hot temperatures and ensures constant air circulation throughout the courtyards, decks, and interior spaces. Rammed-earth walls, constructed by local laborers trained during the building process with a mixture of local earth and a waterproofing admixture, make the building impervious to extreme weather conditions. These 300mm-thick walls offer a high

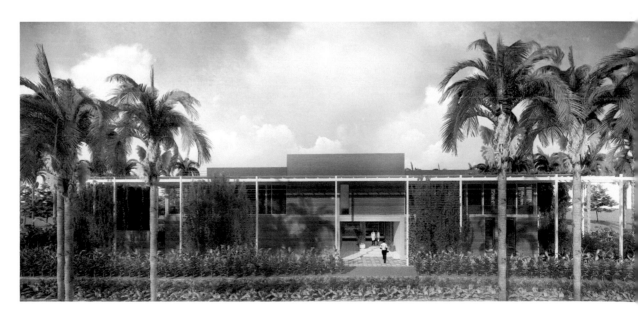

▲ Figure 21.9

Rammed-earth walls and native landscaping connect the ACEGID to the local Nigerian context.
Source: MASS Design Group

thermal mass, absorbing heat during the day and releasing it throughout the night, thus reducing the building's mechanical energy load. These passive strategies, beyond reducing the facility's carbon footprint, also reduce its dependence on frequently unreliable and unaffordable electrical power.

The environmental strategies and corresponding goals related to user comfort and durability for the two case studies presented earlier are summarized in Table 21.1.

Table 21.1 Environmental strategies to address user comfort and durability for the two case studies

	Case Study 1: Redemption Hospital	Case Study 2: African Centre of Excellence for Genomics of Infectious Diseases (ACEGID)
Goal 1	Promote cultural sensitivity and appropriateness to make users feel connected to the facility and rebuild trust in medical institutions	
	• Inviting, non-institutional, park-like approach with generous integrated seating and shading areas • Allocate space for impromptu public gatherings and markets that would otherwise block the entrance or ambulance access • Efficient and separated vehicular flows to decongest ambulance routes and reduce chaos around the hospital entry	• Using local, familiar, and native trees and landscaping • Leveraging locally sourced materials and labor to construct rammed-earth walls using an ancient technique
Goal 2	Create contextual buildings that respond to local climate, weather, and ecosystems to ensure user comfort and safety	

	• Fail-safe passive ventilation
	  ▪ Orientation captures prevailing winds
	  ▪ Solar chimneys to ventilate the space by pulling air up and out through the stack effect
	  ▪ Frequent air changes ensure infection control
	• Leverage the landscape design to improve patient experience:
	  ▪ Complex of communal courtyards, walking trails
	  ▪ Integrating the hospital with a restored wetland to create a relaxing environment for expectant mothers
	  ▪ Siting buildings and circulation to mitigate mosquitoes while increasing water circulation and creating healthy plant habitats that promote mosquito-eating bird, fish, and amphibian species
		• Consider the demands of the climate, weather, and ecosystems, as well as operational requirements
		• Orientation captures prevailing winds and encourages natural ventilation through the building's exterior courtyards and decks
		• Trellis structure provides additional exterior shading around courtyards and decks and help mitigate the hot and humid temperatures of Nigeria

- Minimize energy use and reduce operational costs through passive cross-ventilation strategies
- Supplement passive ventilation with mechanical ventilation in the form of low-cost, low-maintenance fans to cool humid air during Liberia's intense rainy seasons

- 300mm-thick rammed-earth walls offer a high thermal mass, absorbing heat during the day and releasing it at night, thus reducing mechanical energy required
- Lower the cost of mechanical systems through passive ventilation
- Programming to support genomic sequencing, accelerate vaccine development, monitor microbial outbreaks, promote knowledge transfer, and build local and international capacity
  - Optimize the ground floor for offices, classrooms, galleries, communal spaces, and courtyards to facilitate casual interactions and the exchange of ideas between scientists and visitors

21.9 Conclusions

Maison Tropicale, JFK Medical Center, prototype clinics, Tappita Hospital, and the emergency tents and ETUs that sprang up during the Ebola outbreak are all examples of the same problem. Whether in Brazzaville, Monrovia, or the Liberian forest, and whether during the colonial, postcolonial, neoliberal, or modern period, prototypes seek to find scalable solutions for the most pressing problems of their time and geography. These problems, vast in scale and untethered to a specific site, appear to require an approach independent of site. Imaging this intractable problem, it is common and understandable that architects, engineers, and global health experts think about "replicable" solutions that can be widely applied. Unfortunately, these solutions tend to fail, and create as many, if not more, problems as they solve. While Prouvé's Maison Tropicale is interesting as a piece of furniture, it is a failure as architecture and infrastructure.

Great architecture is singular but driven by universal ideas. Bad architecture is universal and specific to none. Governments such as Liberia's seek to offer scalable, replicable strategies, and not just solicit international aid. Prototypes in Liberia make sense for fabricators, but not for Liberians. Buildings based on the climactic and contextual demands of its environs, not on predetermined markets created by vendors, are an anti-technocratic strategy that seeks to produce replicable outcomes, not just replicable widgets. The effects of late industrial capitalism and its means of production have over-engineered our built environment to be designed through reductive cost and labor strategies rather than considering the needs of people and communities. In this reality, another truism is revealed: Technocratic control is another form of colonial control. Instead of returning to where Prouvé began with good intentions in 1949, can architecture chart a new path forward?

When fully embraced, building contextual, customizable solutions promotes an ethos that can outline a global strategy for better, more equitable
building. Sometimes the "local" solution is the only solution. If we work toward
a locally informed, customizable design process, we will produce better health
outcomes and create the conditions for positive economic, educational, environmental, and emotional growth. It is not simply a social architecture, moral
imperative, or sustainable approach, but a mind-set that seeks to create emerging markets that fundamentally challenge the market structure paradigm.

Bibliography

André Balazs Properties. "La Maison Tropicale: The House." www.lamaisontropicale.com/
www/. 2008.

Embassy of the People's Republic of China in the Republic of Liberia. "China-aided
Tappita Hospital in Liberia Officially Opens." http://lr.china-embassy.org/eng/
sghdhzxxx/t795008.htm. 2011.

Farmer, Paul. *Pathologies of Power: Health, Human Rights, and the New War on the
Poor*, 140. Berkeley, CA: University of California Press, 2005.

Farmer, Paul. *Testimony to the US Senate Committee on Foreign Relations*. Report from
United States Senate, January 27, 2010.

Front Page Africa. "Jackson Doe Hospital in Nimba County Faces Imminent Collapse."
April 7, 2018. https://frontpageafricaonline.com/health/jackson-doe-hospital-in-
nimba-county-faces-imminent-collapse/.

Front Page Africa. "Liberia: Bad Road Hampers Access to Tappita Hospital in Nimba
County." May 25, 2018. https://frontpageafricaonline.com/health/bad-road-hampers-
access-to-tappita-hospital-in-nimba-county/.

Front Page Africa. "Liberia's Second Largest Referral Hospital Turns to Agriculture for
Sustenance." May 23, 2018. https://frontpageafricaonline.com/health/liberias-
second-largest-referral-hospital-turns-to-agriculture-for-sustenance/.

Gwenigale, Walter. "'Foreword' in Republic of Liberia, Ministry of Health and Social
Welfare." *National Health and Social Welfare Policy and Plan, 2011–2021*, no. 1.
Monrovia: Ministry of Health and Social Welfare, 2011.

Horan, Harold E. *Association for Diplomatic Studies and Training Foreign Affairs Oral
History Project*, edited by Charles Stuart Kennedy. Washington, DC: Association for
Diplomatic Studies and Training, 1998.

Kruk, Margaret, Peter Rockers, et al. "Availability of Essential Health Services in Post-
Conflict Liberia." *Bulletin of the World Health Organization* 88: 527–534. Doi:
10.2471/BLT.09.071068, 2010.

Pade, William. *New County-Home Hospital Is Acclaimed by Architects as Model*.
Pittsburgh, PA: The Pittsburgh Press, May 10, 1953, p. 9. https://www.newspapers.
com/clip/6337891/john_j_kane_hospital_in_scott_township/.

Rossen, Isabella. "La Maison Tropicale: From Failure in Niamey to Masterpiece in New
York." *Failed Architecture*. https://failedarchitecture.com/la-maison-tropicale-from-
failure-in-niamey-to-masterpiece-in-new-york/. 2013.

Shah, Sonia. *Pandemic*. New York: Farrar, Straus and Giroux, 2016.

Sirleaf, Ellen Johnson. "Annual Message to the Legislature January 25, 2010 (2009
Message)." *The Annual Messages of the Presidents of Liberia 1848–2010*, edited by
D. Elwood Dunn. Berlin: De Gruyter, 2011.

United States Department of State. "Liberia Impact Study: John F. Kennedy Medical
Center." *669–0054*. Report. Monrovia, March 1980.

Verderber, Stephen. *Innovations in Transportable Healthcare Architecture*, 137–138. New
York: Routledge, 2016.

Chapter 22

Epilogue
The Future of an Architecture for Health

David Allison, *Eva Henrich*, and *Edzard Schultz*

22.1 Introduction

Predicting the future is inherently challenging, especially in healthcare. Many forces influence the way we deliver care, and they are in a state of permanently accelerating transformation. Political and economic pressures, the science of medicine, evolving care practices, technological innovations, consciousness raising of individuals, availability of information, and demographic patterns all influence the uncertain reality of how health will be addressed in the future. One certainty is that change, often evolutionary and incremental, but at times revolutionary, is inevitable. The other certainty is that the rate and scope of change in healthcare are increasing. If one looks back at healthcare that was delivered 50 years ago, what we have today would be unimaginable—an observation that will likely be equally mystifying 50 years from now. To make it more complicated, architecture for health in the future will be unique for different geographic and sociopolitical contexts.

Despite cofounding factors, most health organizations share similar goals: improve health outcomes, enhance human experiences, optimize efficiency, and reduce costs. Especially in the developed world with its aging population, we are seeing a dramatic shift from addressing acute illnesses, injuries, and communicable diseases to treating chronic conditions that are the result of lifestyle and environmental factors, like cancer, heart disease, diabetes, obesity, and psychological diseases. Healthcare providers, organizations, and systems are increasingly recognizing that they can no longer simply focus on reactively treating diseases and injuries, but must play a larger role in protecting, promoting, and sustaining the health of the populations they serve. As a result, a paradigm shift is underway where healthcare is moving beyond the walls of hospitals and toward a more coherent, connected, and coordinated health management network that provides traditional health services in addition to education, prevention, rehabilitation, and wellness programs.

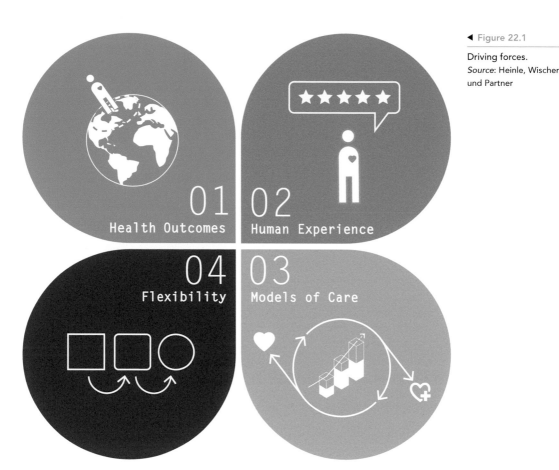

22.2 Forces That Drive the Future of an Architecture for Health

Not knowing exactly where healthcare is heading makes it difficult to know what and how to design. Despite a multitude of uncertainties, there are drivers that seem to be universal. They can provide fundamental guidance for those of us creating architectural settings for health. While each driver must be met with the nuance of its geographical and sociopolitical context, the following themes must be addressed in some way to achieve environments that support health. Four overarching directives need to be acted on to support health and healthcare activities. These directives, or goals influenced by multiple drivers, have existed since the advent of what we understand as modern medicine and will likely continue to be relevant in the future.

- Designed settings should optimize health and health outcomes at the level of the individual and community, and globally. In healthcare settings, this would naturally include improving health outcomes for individuals seeking care, in

David Allison et al.

addition to protecting both patient and staff safety. Beyond healthcare facilities, this would include protecting the workforce and public safety, optimizing the health status of individuals and populations, and protecting the micro, meso, and macro environments.

- Designed settings should support and enhance human experiences in general, especially those related to health and healthcare delivery. In healthcare, this includes optimizing the healthcare experience for patients and families and optimizing the work experience for staff and employees. In other settings, such as schools, this may include creating classrooms with functional layouts that support learning, providing access to daylight and nature, and comfortable furniture scaled to the populations served. At the community scale, this would include providing safe, well-lit, and walkable streets, mixed-use districts, and equitably distributed civic and public green spaces, to name a few.

- Designed settings should support efficient and effective care models for the ever-present purpose of doing "more with less". In healthcare, there are ever increasing financial and regulatory pressures to do more, better, with fewer human and material resources. Care providers are increasingly expected to see more patients, provide higher-quality care, and demonstrate better outcomes. Hospitals and medical centers are often the largest economic engines and employers in their communities and have the greatest local environmental impact. It is critical that care environments are designed to optimize care delivery and minimize waste in all forms.

- Designed settings should not only address the needs of today but also be able to adapt to ever-changing needs, whether expected and unexpected. There are at least three timeframes important for the consideration of changing needs. They are immediate (changes driven by patient acuity or status), cyclical (changes driven by evolving care models or census variations), and life cycle (changes throughout the building life cycle). The first includes the need for the environment to accommodate changing needs over the duration of a patient encounter or stay. Examples of this would include adaptable patient rooms and nursing units designed to allow patients to remain in one setting as they progress from intensive care to acute care to discharge. Another example would be a preoperative and postoperative care unit where the unit flexes from all preop patients in the morning to all postoperative patients at the day's end.

    The second is over a set cycle, such as a day, week, or year. Changing care needs and staffing patterns may change over multiple shifts each day. Alternatively, census changes in the needs of the community and the addition of new service lines would drive changes in the ebb and flow of patients over weeks or years.

    Changes that must be accommodated over the 30- to 50-year (or more) life of a building might be driven by evolving patient demographics; patient and population health needs and expectations; reimbursement, regulation, and medical science; care processes; and other technological advances. Some of these can be envisioned and anticipated, while others cannot.

22.3 Scalar Domains of Consideration for an Architecture for Health

Creating architectural settings in the future must address the health of individuals, organizations, communities, and ecosystems efficiently and effectively. Each domain of health correlates to specific spatial conditions within different scales of the built environment. Individual well-being is impacted at the smallest scale (micro) by one's immediate "life space", or places inhabited routinely, and the activities that occur within them. Although we humans are highly adaptable to our environments, we can reasonably conclude that those places where individuals spend the greatest amount of time will have the greatest impacts on their health. It can also be assumed that vulnerable individuals who are already stressed by other factors in their lives may be more susceptible to additional stressors from the environment. Research in a variety of settings, including healthcare, the workplace, and schools, has shown that environmental conditions, such as light, sound, thermal conditions, privacy, security, indoor air quality, and the ability to control the environment, can all impact human stress, health, and well-being in immediate and long-term ways.

At the organization, social group, or community scale, the design of specific buildings, campuses, neighborhoods, and other related places can impact health. For communities, this includes viable infrastructure, access to a diverse range of public and retail services, safe communities, a healthful environment, walkability, transportation options, economic opportunities, and social cohesiveness. Organizations are seen in the form of large national health systems, geographically dispersed private systems (like Kaiser Permanente), regionally integrated health systems, education providers and systems, private businesses, and nonprofit groups, to name a few. These organizations have a significant impact on the economic and environmental health of the locales where they exist. The design of the facilities in these organizations should reflect their overall mission, clarify their identity, and optimize their ability to promote and support health across the populations they serve.

Finally, at the global scale, built environment decisions and interventions made at smaller scales collectively have a cumulative impact that is not frequently understood, considered, or valued at the local scale. These impacts include climate change, natural resource depletion, habitat destruction, and social/economic impacts in other parts of the world. The decisions and actions associated with creating built environments in the future must consider global and ecological health more broadly.

22.4 The Influence of Geographic and Sociopolitical Context

There are several distinct and significant contexts that potentially influence the future of human and ecological health and healthcare delivery. The challenge in the developed world will likely continue as more people are living longer and aging with chronic diseases. The pressing issue for the developing world will be creating an adequate and accessible public health infrastructure for rapidly growing and inherently younger populations, often with limited resources.

David Allison et al.

22.4.1 The United States

The United States stands out in many ways as an economically prosperous nation without an accessible public universal healthcare system. Compared to other industrialized Western nations, the United States prioritizes individual autonomy and personal responsibility on issues like healthcare. This results in inequity of access to healthcare services, with a significant portion of the poor and lower middle class either underinsured or uninsured. The U.S. is also composed of a geographically large and dispersed population distributed over a combination of immense rural areas, vast suburban landscapes, and urban centers with growing ex-urban peripheries.

In the U.S., there are vast distinctions of access (physical and economic) to healthcare depending on where you live. Healthcare services tend to be concentrated in wealthier, denser, and more mobile populations. Lower population densities in rural, suburban, and ex-urban areas make delivering healthcare to these populations more challenging and inherently less efficient. This is compounded by the reality that people in rural areas are inherently older, have lower incomes, and are less likely to work for companies that provide health insurance as a benefit. Access to care in these areas for the elderly and poor is compounded by limited access to public transit.

22.4.2 Social Democracies

The dominant context for healthcare among economically developed countries involves social democracies where healthcare is a right with some form of universal coverage and government control over its delivery. These countries generally represent a greater political will and cultural commitment to community and the common good. They also tend to be geographically smaller countries where populations are more densely concentrated in urban communities with diverse and comprehensive transportation infrastructure. These conditions inherently enable greater equity in access to healthcare, greater coordination in the delivery of healthcare, and improved physical connectivity to services for all populations. However, progress can also be slow because authorities are reluctant to set precedent.

22.4.3 China

China represents another unique context due to the immense size of its population and the fact that it is a rapidly growing economic power with a unique mix of socialism and capitalism. Its population has been migrating from rural to ultra-dense urban areas for some time, and its middle and upper classes are growing rapidly. As a result, it is experiencing a significant building boom in healthcare, as in many other sectors. Healthcare delivery, to a greater degree than in the U.S., remains concentrated in very large hospitals and medical centers. It is also characterized by a rapidly aging population that gave birth to fewer children and whose young people have moved away from their parents to pursue economic opportunities. As a result, there are fewer young adults to take care of their parents. So, the biggest challenge faced in China is providing care for rapidly expanding urban populations and managing care for the elderly.

22.4.4 Developing Countries

Most of the world's population lives in developing countries where healthcare services, settings, and systems must in many cases be built virtually from scratch. They typically have severely medically underserved populations and suffer from struggling or emerging economies. They often lack comprehensive access to state-of-the-art healthcare, primary care services, and fundamental public health infrastructure. The challenges these countries face include a relative lack of technical, human, and economic capacity to deliver, maintain, and support sophisticated healthcare services, technologies, and, at times, basic public health resources.

22.5 Trends for an Architecture for Health Moving Forward

Geographic and sociopolitical contexts impact the way and degree to which emerging trends in the delivery of healthcare and health-supportive settings will or will not be relevant. This chapter outlines only a small subset of trends that may be most relevant in more mature and established contexts, but they may also apply in different ways for rapidly evolving societies. These trends are inspired by and draw from the work and case studies included earlier in this book. The selected trends include the following:

1. Ubiquitous healthcare
2. Hospitals without walls
3. Resilience and sustainability
4. Ability to accommodate change
5. Pretest design

22.5.1 Ubiquitous Healthcare

Healthcare in the mid-twentieth century was characterized in large part by hospitals that existed like isolated fortresses of medical science and acute clinical care. By the turn of the millennium, various forces in both the U.S. and elsewhere increasingly drove the growth of more comprehensive and integrated national or regional health networks and geographically distributed systems. The twenty-first century will continue to see increasing ubiquitous access to health resources and services in a vast array of settings, from home to hospital and throughout the community—anywhere and anytime. Instead of the focus on the hospital as the center of this universe, the system will be organized to allow the individual to be the focus. Individuals will increasingly be tethered digitally to a vast array of resources and will draw on services as needed, when needed, and where most convenient, cost effective, and appropriate. The most complex healthcare will continue to be specialized in nature, concentrated at "super hospitals" with core

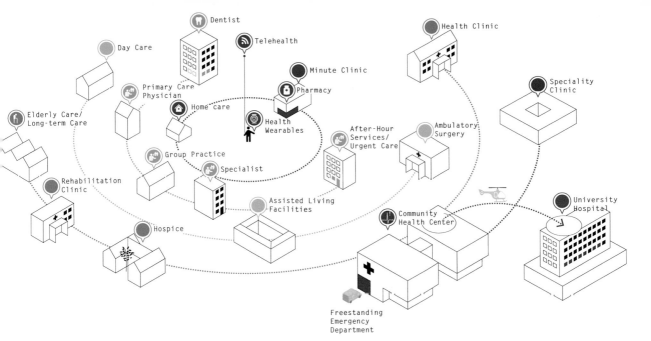

▲ Figure 22.2

Ubiquitous healthcare.
Source: Heinle, Wischer und
Partner

medical departments focusing on care for the critically and chronically ill. Hospitals as we think of them today will increasingly be places for the sickest patients, almost exclusively for trauma, complex medical interventions, and critical care.

At the other end of the spectrum, healthcare will continue to be pushed toward less intensive but more cost-effective and accessible venues. What was once inpatient care delivered in hospitals is increasingly moving to outpatient settings, while outpatient care is transitioning to home and community-based care. It will be crucial in this expanding universe of touch points that patient records are shared efficiently, securely, and timely across a network of sites and modalities. The delivery of healthcare is transitioning from episodic moments of care in hospitals to individuals with access to a physical and virtual continuum of care services and resources.

- Health maintenance and prevention/wellness will occur through mobile devices, at home, at work, and/or in the community.
- Long-term care will increasingly be represented by "aging in place", with care delivered at home and in the community, group homes, and assisted living centers, and only when necessary in skilled nursing facilities.
- Primary care will be delivered both virtually and physically by a collaborative team of physicians and physician extenders. When needing to see a care provider in person, this might occur in a variety of settings, from group medical practices to minute clinics and urgent care centers.
- Specialty care will be delivered in a variety of ambulatory and inpatient settings to disease and need-specific populations.
- Emergency, trauma, intensive, and acute inpatient care will still occur in the hospital, either within the community or at regional tertiary care hospitals.
- Tertiary and quaternary care will be delivered in university hospitals and academic medical centers. This care is the most complex, equipment- and expertise-focused care, and relies on cutting-edge medical technology and science.

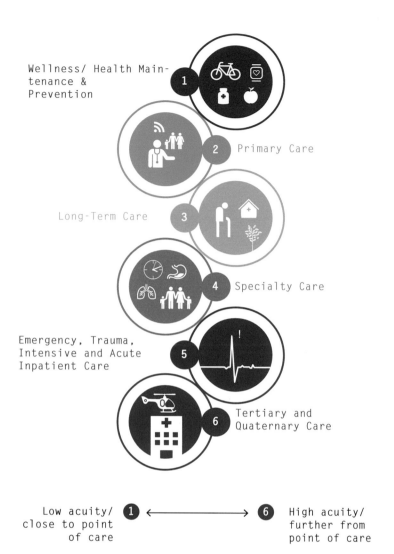

Wellness/ Health Main-
tenance &
Prevention

1

Primary Care

2

Long-Term Care

3

Specialty Care

4

Emergency, Trauma,
Intensive and Acute
Inpatient Care

5

Tertiary and
Quaternary Care

6

Low acuity/ **1** ⟷ **6** High acuity/
close to point   further from
of care   point of care

◀ Figure 22.3

Continuum of health intensity.
Source: Heinle, Wischer und
Partner

22.5.1.1 Primary Drivers

There are several forces driving this trend. Economic pressures are driving care
to less expensive and intensive settings. Meanwhile, advances in science and
technology are enabling things like minimally invasive and facility-specific medical interventions, improved connectivity, and coordination of care between
multiple providers and settings. At the same time, an increasingly educated
and health-conscious consumer of healthcare is expecting better quality, con-
venience, access to information, and greater participation and control over his
or her health. The goal is to promote health and, when healthcare is needed,
to provide the right care, at the right time, in the most appropriate and cost-
effective settings.

22.5.1.2 Design Considerations

Ubiquitous healthcare will occur through an expanding constellation of settings and access points distributed throughout communities. At one end of the continuum, specialty care centers will remain, including tertiary or quaternary care superhospitals and disease- or condition-specific treatment centers. Freestanding emergency and urgent care centers, along with a variety of ambulatory care centers, primary care services, and minute clinics, will be located closer to home. Proactive involvement in maintaining one's health and preventing illness will become increasingly enabled by technology in everyday life: The individual will become more of an active agent in managing his or her own health and healthcare. This will include earlier and more targeted treatment to avoid hospitalization by using digital solutions for home monitoring. Telemedicine will enable receiving health services without physically seeing a clinician or visiting a healthcare facility. An example for such a program is the "my digital doctor" initiative from Sweden.

While design professionals will still need to address hospitals and other conventional healthcare settings, a greater focus will be addressing health in the array of settings that impact health. This includes providing better opportunities to promote, protect, and sustain health in the home, school, workplace, and community. There will need to be a greater emphasis on healthy community planning and design: places that are safe, equitable, walkable, transit-oriented, mixed use, vibrant, therapeutic, and sustainable.

An increasing focus on population health and wellness will also drive the design of communities to optimize rapid and efficient access to, and delivery of, care that cannot be provided virtually. Density, mixed uses, and diverse transportation options will be required to create enriching and health-supporting communities. Workplaces and schools will need to be designed to promote and maintain health by including greater access to daylight and connections to nature, supporting better working conditions, improving indoor air quality, and promoting amenities that encourage exercise and healthy lifestyles.

The home environment will need to be barrier free and support recovery, home care, rehabilitation, and aging in place. Architects had very little impact on the design of suburban single-family homes in the U.S. throughout the mid- to late twentieth century. However, an increasing migration back to cities in the U.S. and urban migration globally mean that an increasing amount of new housing will be located in cities. Larger-scale and denser urban development will necessitate a greater role and responsibility on the part of design professionals to create safe, healthy, sustainable housing that will enable aging and healthcare in place.

22.5.2 Hospitals Without Walls

Within a ubiquitous healthcare milieu, hospitals and academic medical centers will increasingly be envisioned and designed both conceptually and physically as hospitals without walls. The hospital as an isolated fortress exclusively for the episodic delivery of acute medical treatment is a relic of the past. Services traditionally delivered in the hospital will increasingly be distributed and delivered

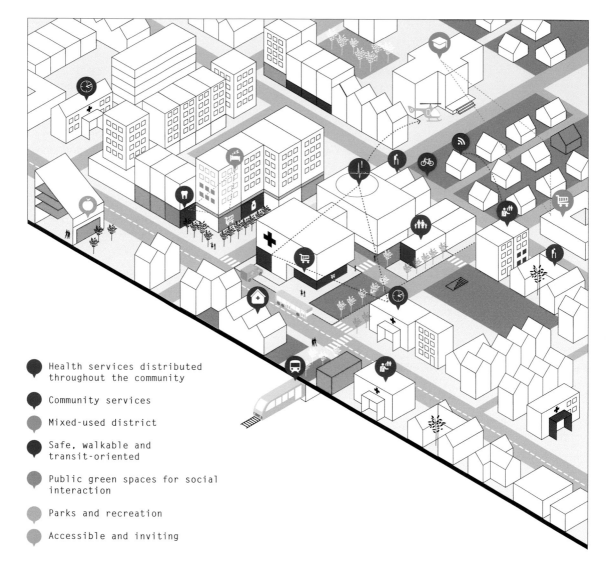

Health services distributed throughout the community

Community services

Mixed-used district

Safe, walkable and transit-oriented

Public green spaces for social interaction

Parks and recreation

Accessible and inviting

throughout the community, and community services will be brought onto the campus and into the walls of the hospital. Services that will need to be accommodated on campus must include health-promoting activities, community services, and a variety of activities of daily life. Hospital buildings and campuses will need to be more accessible and inviting, bringing in visitors in times of wellness and sickness alike.

▲ Figure 22.4

Hospital without walls.
Source: Heinle, Wischer und Partner

22.5.2.1 Primary Drivers

Hospitals are inherently significant institutions in their communities. They are places where most significant life events occur, including births, illnesses, and death. They are places of work, learning, exchange, social engagement, and spiritual moments. They are typically the largest, or one of the largest, economic engines and employers in their communities, and they often have a significant physical and environmental impact on their communities. As such, they should be more integrated with the daily life of their communities. It is becoming increasingly recognized that simply treating disease, injury, and illness is not an effective way to maintain and support healthy populations. Yet hospitals have historically been located at the periphery of the community or have evolved as imposing, unfriendly, single-use campuses for acute medical care in the urban core. The hospital and healthcare campus should become more of a civic resource and serve as a role model for health promotion.

22.5.2.2 Design Considerations

Health campuses and wellness districts should be conceived as mixed-use districts and include public spaces for healthful recreation and social interaction. The campus should include public green spaces and tree-lined green streets, parks and plazas, public art, and recreational activities and events. The campus should be designed for a variety of uses that extend beyond traditional healthcare to include a wide range of activities of daily life, including retail, daycare, housing, and civic spaces. They should be safe, walkable, and transit-oriented developments. The impact of parking should be tempered by placing it underground, or when surface parking is necessary it should be designed as "parking in the park", with trees, dark sky compliant lighting, and bioswales. Campus design should be walkable and pedestrian friendly and avoid isolating the hospital in the center of a sea of asphalt parking. Hospital buildings should be designed to be transparent and welcoming, with mixed uses and public amenities at street level.

In the U.S., Northwestern Memorial Hospital is an example of a hospital campus fully integrated into its surrounding community. It is situated in the middle of the Streeterville neighborhood in downtown Chicago. The first several floors of hospital buildings are predominantly commercial and civic functions. Street-level sidewalks and elevated public pedestrian pathways that pass through and connect buildings on the campus are lined with dining and retail establishments that serve patients, visitors, staff, and the community at large. The health campus is not simply a place to go when one is sick but an integral part of the local community, and is familiar to the people who work there in addition to the episodic patients and visitors who come onto the campus.

The master plan for the Baton Rouge Health District and proposed plans for St. Anthony's Focal Point Community Campus, introduced earlier in the book, represent two additional contemporary examples in the U.S. of the movement toward the hospital without walls. In each of these cases, traditional healthcare services are planned as part of an integrated urban mixed-use district with a variety of community offerings. Instead of simply being places where people go only to work or receive medical care, they are conceived as vibrant places central to the life of the community and places that serve as models of healthy community planning and design.

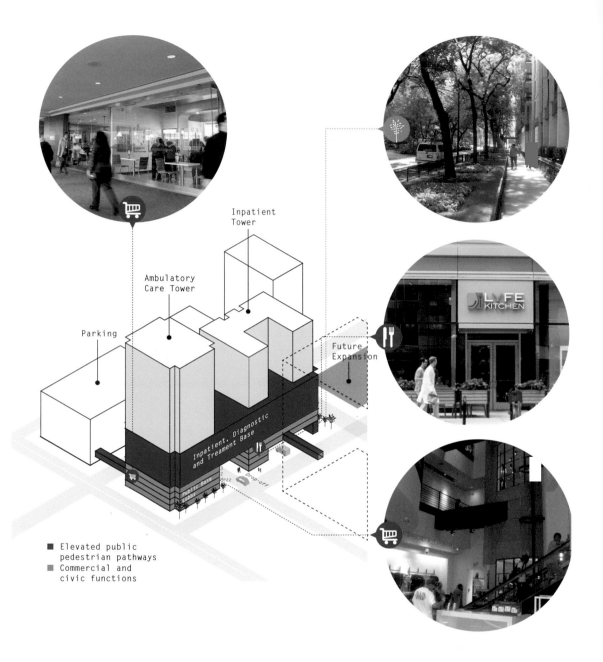

Parking

Ambulatory
Care Tower

Inpatient
Tower

Future
Expansion

Inpatient, Diagnostic
and Treatment Base

Drop-off

■ Elevated public
  pedestrian pathways
■ Commercial and
  civic functions

22.5.3 Resilience and Sustainability

Resilience in general is defined by *Merriam-Webster* as "capable of withstanding shock without permanent deformation or rupture" or "tending to recover from or adjust easily to misfortune or change". In building and urban design, it generally refers to a built environment's ability to withstand and/or recover quickly from man-made and natural disasters. Resilience in the built environment is most commonly considered as a response to sudden, episodic, and catastrophic natural events, such as floods, tornadoes, hurricanes, and earthquakes,

▲ Figure 22.5

Northwestern Memorial
Hospital.
Source: Heinle, Wischer und
Partner

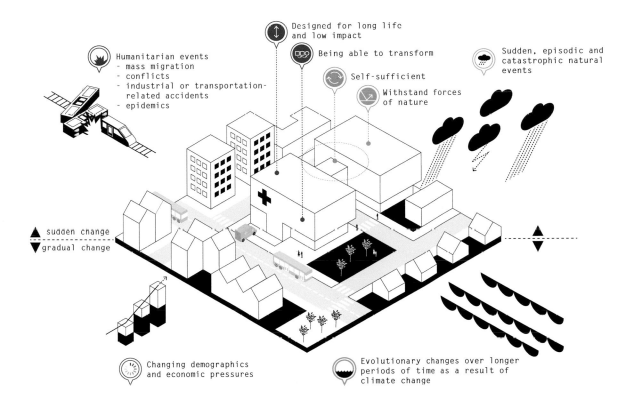

Humanitarian events
- mass migration
- conflicts
- industrial or transportation-
  related accidents
- epidemics

Designed for long life
and low impact

Being able to transform

Self-sufficient

Withstand forces
of nature

Sudden, episodic and
catastrophic natural
events

▲ sudden change
▼ gradual change

Changing demographics
and economic pressures

Evolutionary changes over longer
periods of time as a result of
climate change

▲ Figure 22.6

Resilience and sustainability.
Source: Heinle, Wischer und
Partner

and even man-made disasters, such as refugee crises, wars, and industrial or trans-portation-related accidents.

However, a broader definition of resilience can also include measures of how a built environment adapts to evolutionary change over longer periods of time. This could be the result of climate change, rising sea levels, or even chang-ing demographics and economic pressures. As in the natural world, resilience should be considered a dimension of sustainability. In this sense, it also implies adaptation with the least degree of difficulty, cost, and impact on its surround-ings through the minimized consumption of additional resources. Healthcare environments must be designed to accommodate changes more than most set-tings, changes that occur suddenly as well as over time as healthcare services and technologies evolve.

22.5.3.1 Primary Drivers

The reality is that much of the world's population lives in risk-prone places, and human migration patterns appear to be accelerating this trend. Population den-sity and ongoing migration are occurring increasingly in places subject to severe weather events, flooding and gradual sea-level rise, earthquakes, wildfires, fam-ine, human conflict, and so forth. Healthcare services and facilities inherently need to be close to where people live and need care, and therefore must also tend to be in risk-prone locations. These facilities need to rapidly respond to both normal and exceptional conditions. Since hospitals are considered critical facilities, it is during and immediately following natural and man-made disasters that they are most important to their communities.

At the same time, healthcare organizations, and the settings for the delivery of health and healthcare services, need to accommodate the inevitable evolutionary changes that will occur over the often 50-year or longer life of the buildings or campuses. Changing needs may be driven by a variety of forces, including changing economic and reimbursement contexts, regulations and codes, demographic patterns, scientific/medical/technological innovation, and evolving patient care and treatment patterns. Buildings and places that can adapt and remain valued in their communities ultimately make the most use of the embedded energy and resources that go into building them.

22.5.3.2 Design Considerations

One fundamental attribute of resilience in the built environment is being designed for long life and low impact under both normal and extra-normal conditions. This is also a fundamental characteristic of sustainability and can include both passive and active measures. Passive measures might include being designed to withstand the forces of nature. Active measures might include the ability of the building and its elements to transform in a variety of ways in response to both sudden and evolving conditions and needs. Response to sudden events might include the ability to accommodate a surge in capacity to care for illness and injury in a population impacted by a catastrophic event. In the long term it might include adapting to the impacts of climate change, demographic shifts, or changing technologies.

Self-sufficiency is also important for resilient design, which includes the ability to reduce demand on, or operate independently from, external resources, such as energy, water, and waste systems that can be disrupted at times of natural or man-made disasters. These same design strategies can also be employed to operate more sustainably under normal conditions. A health facility that minimizes its energy footprint, resource consumption, and environmental impact under normal conditions can inherently be more resilient under extraordinary conditions.

One could elevate the idea of resilience further and address the fundamental concepts of restorative and regenerative design. These principles can be manifested in several ways—for example, generating more energy than consumed, having less impact on watersheds after development than before, minimizing or recycling both biological and technological waste, reducing/eliminating toxic loads placed on the environment, and making communities healthier, more vibrant, and desirable.

22.5.4 The Ability to Accommodate Change

As outlined previously, hospitals and large healthcare campuses need to be able to accommodate change. Buildings that cannot change, and especially healthcare buildings, which often remain in operation for 50–100 years or longer, are

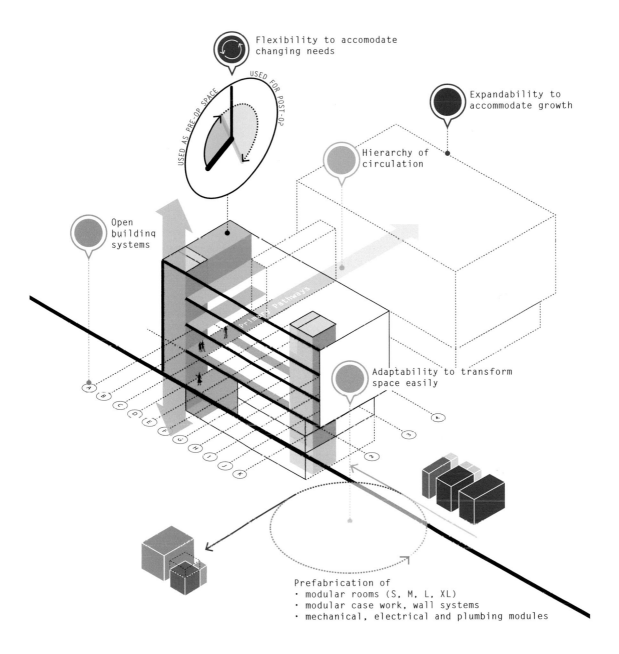

Flexibility to accomodate
changing needs

Expandability to
accommodate growth

Hierarchy of
circulation

USED AS PRE-OP SPACE

USED FOR POST-OP

Open
building
systems

Primary Pathways

Adaptability to transform
space easily

Prefabrication of
· modular rooms (S, M, L, XL)
· modular case work, wall systems
· mechanical, electrical and plumbing modules

▲ Figure 22.7

A change-ready hospital.
Source: Heinle, Wischer und
Partner

at risk of premature obsolescence. There are three ways in which buildings and building complexes can transform and accommodate changing needs: through flexibility, adaptability, and expandability. Flexibility and adaptability have been used interchangeably, but for the purposes of this chapter, flexibility involves the ability of a given space, department, building, or campus to accommodate changing needs with little or no physical reconfiguration. Adaptability involves planning and constructing buildings or building elements with the capability to transform space easily with the least amount of physical, material, and economic impact. Expandability involves planning to accommodate growth and change in a coherent and logical way. It requires planning infrastructure and circulation in a way that anticipates future growth.

22.5.4.1 Primary Drivers

As noted, the healthcare context is incredibly dynamic and influenced by constant changes in medical science and technology, healthcare policy and regulation, demographic transformations in both populations served and caregivers, and evolving clinical practices and approaches. Collectively not only are these forces increasing in their impact but also the rate and pace of change are accelerating. Healthcare as delivered 50 years ago was fundamentally different than today. Facilities that were designed and built then and are still in use were not conceived to easily accommodate changing healthcare needs, practices, and technologies. It was simply impossible then to imagine the scope of changes that have occurred over the life of these facilities, and it will be increasingly impossible to imagine healthcare needs over the next 50 years or how healthcare will be delivered. Therefore, healthcare facilities must be able to accommodate not only changes we can anticipate but also changes we cannot even imagine.

22.5.4.2 Design Considerations

The first principle for accommodating change is to design the overall building for layers of change, as outlined by Stewart Brand (1995) in *How Buildings Learn: What Happens After They're Built*. The fundamental principle is that buildings designed to accommodate layers of change have long lives. These layers consist of site, structure, skin, circulation (added by the authors), services, space plan, and stuff. The key is to design buildings so that more stable elements ("hard spaces"), such as structure and core infrastructure, support frequent changes to the more flexible elements ("soft spaces") around them.

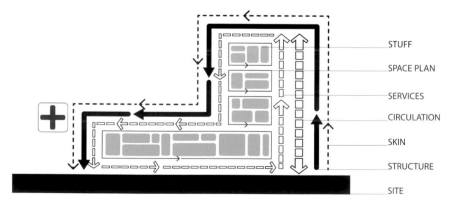

▲ Figure 22.8

Layers of change.
Source: Clemson University Architecture + Health Program

A truly open building system is also designed with a clear hierarchy of circulation where the primary pathways are stable even in the event of changing programmatic use. In cities, we rarely change the location of streets to accommodate the needs of individual development. The most stable elements of the city are its streets and movement systems. Healthcare planners and designers need to employ urban design principles when designing large healthcare facilities and campuses, where movement systems and infrastructure are aligned and stable. Medical planning of a campus, the equivalent of a city block, can then constantly change and transform.

Within an open building framework designed for layers of change, modularity can be employed to accommodate flexibility, adaptability, and expandability. Modularity can occur at multiple scales, from building components and individual rooms to planning strategies that allow departments and larger areas to transform. A key attribute of modularity is that it allows for prefabrication. Standardized and prefabricated modules can also lead to improved construction quality in controlled manufacturing conditions, lower waste, and improve the speed of construction. Finally, modularity enables the delivery of high-quality healthcare settings when and where it may be difficult if not impossible to build on-site with locally available materials, expertise, and labor.

Prefabricated modules are becoming commonly produced at multiple scales:

- Prefabricated and modular casework, headwalls, and wall systems
- Prefabricated mechanical, electrical, and plumbing modules
- Prefabricated and modular rooms (toilets, patient rooms, and other spaces that are repeated multiple times in the design and construction of healthcare facilities)

Finally, modularity should be considered in the overall planning of departments and functional areas within them. Standardized clinical modules not only support the implementation of prefabricated building elements but also can help standardize care practices with replicated and pretested design elements.

22.5.5 Pretest Design

Pretest design involves practices of virtually and physically designing and building mock-ups of significant spaces and design elements and using trials and data to refine their designs prior to final construction. Pretesting is most appropriate in highly repetitive spaces, like bathrooms, patient rooms, exam rooms, and clinical treatment and diagnostic spaces, or elements like patient room headwalls, casework, and mechanical components. These spaces and elements not only are repetitive but also represent those places that impact patient care and significant interactions between patients, families, and caregivers. Pretesting allows broad input from a diverse cross section of design and occupant/user constituencies in a form that enables better understanding than simply the review of traditional design documents, such as floor plans and renderings. This is particularly valuable when new ideas are being explored.

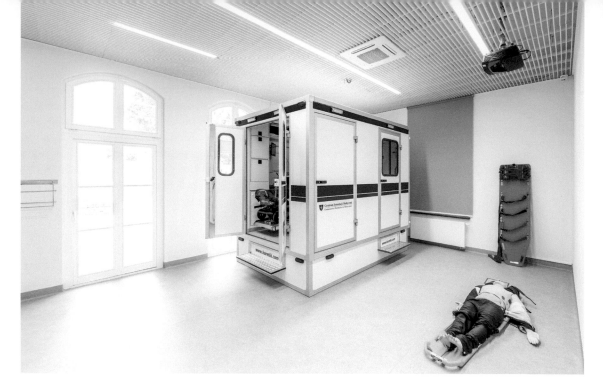

▲ Figure 22.9

Simulation Center, Medical University Breslau, Poland.
Source: Maciej Lulko Photographer

Physical and/or virtual mock-ups or prototypes of these spaces, modules, or elements are then systematically evaluated iteratively through simulations (both computational and physical) and refined based on lessons learned. In an ideal scenario the design, evaluation, and redesign process cycles through multiple iterations with ever increasing fidelity of the mock-up or prototype before finalizing design concepts, fabrication, and construction. Virtual models can allow better visualization of spaces earlier in the testing process, but to date most virtual modeling applications have had limitations. Readily available virtual reality (VR) applications today have not been able to effectively simulate realistic engagement and interaction with moveable equipment, objects, or other people in a virtual space. Studies conducted indicate that while today VR is a better option for allowing non-design constituencies to understand the design of spaces than architecture drawings, physical mock-ups remain the most effective and realistic way to help non-designers visualize a space and simulate care processes.

At a larger scale, simulation modeling applications enable the pretesting of larger functional areas (e.g., departments) to evaluate and predict patient, staff, and material flows, disruptions, and throughput in various functional areas or departmental configurations prior to finalizing design decisions. These tools require significant data on historical and predicted utilization, patient encounters, staffing, and care process. Data can then be implemented into spatial models to test various departmental design configurations against both existing and proposed care processes. This enables the identification of potential choke points in processes and flows and allows for forecasting of flow and throughput for a given design configuration.

22.5.5.1 Primary Drivers

The use of mock-ups, prototypes, simulation models, and virtual reality can improve communication and collaboration between designers, end users, and builders, and allow for more informed design decision making. These strategies help empower all stakeholders to actively take part in the design process. Designs can be evaluated for optimization of workflow, task performance, and safety. They can also enable the identification of conflicting conditions and allow for better conflict resolution earlier in the design and construction process.

22.5.5.2 Design Considerations

As in the work on the Clemson University Patient Room Prototype and "Realizing Improved Patient Care Through Human Centered Design in the Operating Room" (RIPCHD.OR) projects at Clemson University, mock-ups might begin as virtual models and evolve into "tape on the floor mockups". These might later

▼ Figure 22.10

RIPCHD.OR prototype operating room in Charleston, South Carolina. *Source*: Clemson University Architecture + Health Program

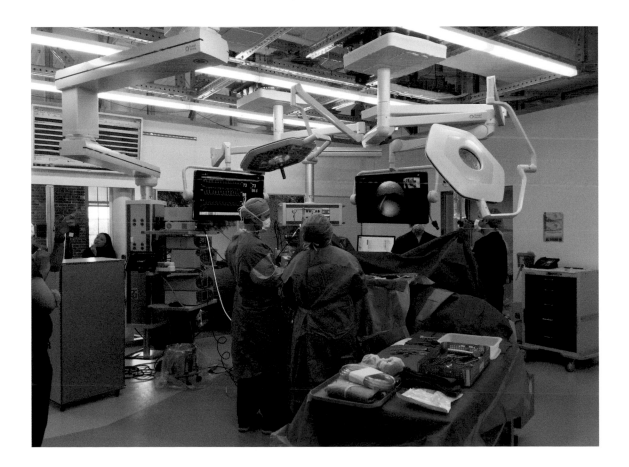

be followed by cardboard mock-ups and ultimately higher-fidelity functioning mock-ups involving actual equipment and design elements. While mock-ups cannot test all design factors that come into play in real patient care settings, they are highly useful in testing care practices and procedures without risk to patients. They enable the testing of fundamental task-related issues and functionality concerns relevant to the physical configuration of the element or space. Working with virtual and physical modeling, the architectural planning process can be shifted to place greater emphasis on the early design phases by allowing the design to fail fast, frequently, and early in the design process (when the impact is minimal on project schedules and cost) and be remedied and optimized. Pretesting also allows the designer to be more experimental, unconventional, and take greater risks in the design process of healthcare environments than is possible when patient care and safety might be impacted.

22.6 Conclusions

Ultimately the design of healthcare environments must be considered beyond traditional building types, like hospitals and clinics. Designers must move beyond providing better settings for the delivery of healthcare to providing a diverse range of health-supporting and -sustaining settings that encompass the home, the workplace, and the community, as well as the clinic or hospital. Healthcare must be considered holistically, respond to the geographic and sociopolitical context, and include principles of healthy community planning and design, sustainability, and resiliency. Healthcare environments should serve as role models for best practices that promote human health and minimize the impact on local and global ecosystems despite ever-changing forces. We need to design in ways that effectively translate and employ the growing body of knowledge on how the built environment impacts health and healthcare. We must avoid designing again and again based on past practices and repeating the same mistakes over and over. Finally, we must realize that what we design and build today will need to accommodate changing needs and changes in healthcare that we cannot begin to imagine.

The cross section of projects presented in this book begin to give some guidance and illustrate the impact of the significant trends outlined and how they are being realized in a variety of ways, contexts, and scales. We are excited about the future of healthcare architecture and think that it will present new challenges and opportunities for demonstrating the potential of the built environment to support improved health and healthcare. Designing with an expanded view toward health has become a much greater focus both within and beyond traditional healthcare settings over the past half-century. Making further advances will require looking beyond convention and the practices of the past and expanding the role of the built environment in human and ecological health. As Robin Guenther articulates in Chapter 17, we must move toward an architecture of and for health as being restorative and regenerative in the broadest terms possible. It must be part of a larger ecosystem of health resources, set within a wholesome and healthful environment, resilient and sustainable, open and accessible, flexible and adaptable. Finally, an architecture for health must be informed by applying the ever-expanding body of knowledge on how and why the built environment impacts health.

David Allison et al.

Bibliography

Allison, David. "Designing Hospitals and Medical Centers as Healthy Livable Urban Districts." Proceedings of the *49th International Making Cities Livable Conference.* Portland Oregon, 2012.

Allison, David. "Going Downtown: Embracing Urban Concepts in Health Care Campus Design." *Health Facilities Management* 26, no. 11 (2013): 27–31.

Allison, David. *Team 2 White Paper: Developing a Flexible Healthcare Infrastructure.* Washington, DC: National Institute of Building Sciences—Academy of Healthcare Infrastructure, 2016.

Bayramzadeh, Sara, Anjali Joseph, David Allison, Jonas Shultz, James Abernathy, and RIPCHD OR Study Group. "Using an Integrative Mock-Up Simulation Approach for Evidence-Based Evaluation of Operating Room Design Prototypes." *Applied Ergonomics* 70 (2018): 288–299.

Brand, Stewart. *How Buildings Learn: What Happens After They're Built.* New York, NY: Penguin, 1995.

Danneberg, Andrew, Howard Frumkin, and Richard Jackson, eds. *Making Healthy Places: Designing and Building for Health, Well-Being, and Sustainability.* Washington, DC: Island Press, 2011.

Guenther, Robin, and Gail Vittori. *Sustainable Healthcare Architecture.* Hoboken, NJ: John Wiley & Sons, 2008.

Joseph, Anjali, Rutali Joshi, and David Allison, eds. "Realizing Improved Patient Care through Human-Centered Design in the Operating Room (RIPCHD.OR)." *Internal CHFDT Publication* 2 (2017).

Joseph, A., D. Wingler, and D. Allison, eds. "Realizing Improved Patient Care through Human-Centered Design in the Operating Room (RIPCHD.OR)." *Internal CHFDT Publication* 1 (2016).

Kendall, Stephen H., ed. *Healthcare Architecture as Infrastructure: Open Building in Practice.* Abingdon, Oxon and New York, NY: Routledge, 2018.

McDonough, William, and Michael Braungart. *Cradle to Cradle: Remaking the Way We Make Things.* New York, NY: North Point Press, 2010.

O'Hara, Susan. "Planning Intensive Care Unit Design Using Computer Simulation Modeling: Optimizing Integration of Clinical, Operational, and Architectural Requirements." *Critical Care Nursing Quarterly* 37, no. 1 (2014): 67–82.

Pentecost III, A. R., Perscield, W. "AI & Architecture, How Will Artificial Intelligence Impact Health Care Design?" *Health Facilities Management* 03 (2019): 40–45.

Schultz, Edzard. "Entwurfsmethodik." In *Krankenhausbau*, edited by H. Stockhorst, L. Hofrichter, and A. Franke, 155–163. Berlin, Germany: Medizinisch Wissenschaftliche Verlagsgesellschaft, 2018.

Topol, Eric. *The Creative Destruction of Medicine: How the Digital Revolution Will Create Better Health Care.* New York, NY: Basic Books, 2012.

About the Editors

Dina Battisto, BArch, MArch, MS, PhD, is an associate professor in the School of Architecture at Clemson University with an emphasis on the Architecture + Health Program. She is also the coordinator of the Built Environment and Health concentration in the Planning, Design and Built Environment PhD Program in the College of Architecture, Arts and Humanities. Her teaching, research, and scholarship activities focus on exploring how environmental design contributes to the health of individuals, communities, and interconnected ecosystems. She is a recognized expert in the area of post-occupancy evaluation and has developed facility evaluation methodologies and modular toolkits for various clients worldwide. She served as chair of the AIA's Academy of Architecture for Health Foundation Grants Committee from 2006 to 2012. In 2008, she was named one of the "Top Twenty People Making a Difference" in Healthcare Design by *Healthcare Design Magazine*. She is passionate about seeking ways to use applied research to advance the design of built environments aimed at improving health and well-being.

Jacob J. Wilhelm holds a Bachelor of Science in design in Architectural Studies from Arizona State University (2016). Currently designing with 359 Design in Denver, Colorado, his work focuses on international ski resort development and solutions to the housing crises in mountain and remote regions. Beyond professional practice, he has published *Adaptive Architecture: Changing Parameters and Practice* (Routledge 2018) and NCARB's monograph series entitled "Indicative, Investigative, and Diagnostic Post-Occupancy Evaluations" (2017). Both as an individual and collaborating with students in the fields of architecture, industrial design, urban planning, and more, he has been awarded in design competitions sponsored by Arizona Residential Architects, the Scottsdale Museum of Art, and Arizona State University, and was the recipient of the Provostal Undergraduate Research Mentorship Grant (2014). He is committed to expanding architectural discourse through interdisciplinary study, research, and theory, specifically around local vernaculars and future trends.

Contributors

David Allison, FAIA, FACHA, is an Alumni Distinguished Professor and has served as the director of graduate studies in Architecture + Health (A+H) at Clemson University since 1990. His teaching, research, and scholarship involve the study of relationships between health, healthcare, and the built environment. The A+H program at Clemson is nationally recognized for its focused curriculum and emphasis on design excellence within the discipline of healthcare architecture. It is committed to the integration of innovative design with academic scholarship and research in healthcare environments and healthy community planning and design, and it has won numerous national and international awards for its work under David's direction. He is a licensed architect in South and North Carolina. He is a board-certified founding member and fellow of the American College of Healthcare Architects (ACHA) and currently serves on the ACHA Board of Regents. He is the founder of the Architecture for Health Educators Summit, held annually as part of the joint AIA/AAH and ACHA Summer Leadership Summit. He is also a cofounder of an annual AIA Academy of Architecture for Health South Atlantic Regional Conference. He was selected in 2007 as one of "Twenty Making a Difference" nationally by *Healthcare Design* magazine and identified again in 2009, 2010, and 2012 by a national poll conducted by the magazine as "one of the most influential people in healthcare design". *Design Intelligence Magazine* named him one of the nation's 30 Most Admired Design Educators in 2013–2014.

Barbara Anderson, RN, MN, is a principal and senior medical planner at ZGF Architects, bringing more than 35 years of expertise to all types of healthcare projects. Her leadership in Lean facility planning translates clinical needs into operationally efficient, patient-centered design solutions. She enjoys collaborating with clients who embrace change to create facilities that support improvements in the healthcare delivery system. Barbara has contributed to the design of several highly integrated and flexible award-winning healthcare environments, including the Everett Clinic at Smokey Point in Marysville, Washington; St. Anthony Hospital in Gig Harbor, Washington, and St. Anthony Hospital in Pendleton, Oregon, both for CHI Franciscan Health; the Marshall and Katherine Cymbaluk Medical Tower at the Providence Regional Medical Center Everett in Everett, Washington; the Playa Vista Physician Office & Urgent Care for Cedars-Sinai in Playa Vista, California; and most recently, two new clinics for Intermountain Healthcare, based in Salt Lake City, Utah. Barbara is a frequent speaker at national conferences, presenting on Lean facility design and the impacts this approach has on patient-centered care. She holds a Master of Nursing from the University of Washington and a Bachelor of Science in Nursing from Sonoma State University.

James J. Atkinson, BS, M.ARCH, AIA, ACHA, EDAC, LEED AP, is Vice President and the Director of Healthcare Planning for HDR Architecture. He is recognized as an expert in the planning and design of complex, state-of-the-art healthcare facilities, bringing transformative ideas to a variety of healthcare planning and design projects. Jim received his highly specialized Master of Architecture degree in Healthcare Design and Planning from the Clemson University Architecture + Health Studio. Throughout his 28-year career, he has become a recognized national expert in designing flexible environments that encourage collaboration, accommodate advanced technology, and support leading research to develop positive outcomes. Jim's projects have received many design awards, which include regional and national awards as well as international design awards. He is a frequent speaker at national and international conferences and has been published in several healthcare architecture publications.

Omniya El Baghdadi is based in industry (Egypt), with a PhD in Economics of Biophilic Urbanism (Queensland University of Technology). She is also an adjunct industry fellow with Griffith University's Cities Research Institute. Her research involves a multidisciplinary context to find rapid and transformational solutions to counteract negative implications for ecosystem health and people's physical and mental health. Coupling sustainability, economics, design, and ecology, her work explores the economics of urban ecology to develop a decision-making framework to inform biophilic urbanism (nature-loving cities). She is interested in emerging concepts, including urban metabolism, biomimicry, green infrastructure, ecosystem services, and holistic approaches to mental health. She is committed to creating a world that sustains our natural environment by embodying a culture that honors our ecosystem.

Mara Baum, AIA, EDAC, WELL AP, LEED Fellow, leads HOK's global health and wellness design practice, with a focus on improving the well-being of the people who occupy the communities, buildings, and workplaces the firm designs. Passionate about bringing healthy building design to those who need it most, Mara also provides strategic leadership to HOK's healthcare practice. Her work focuses on the intersection of ecological and health issues within the built environment. A long-time educator, she is a WELL faculty member and online instructor for the Boston Architectural College Sustainable Design Institute, where she teaches Green Building and Health and Sustainable Design of Healthcare Facilities. She holds a Master of Architecture and Master of City and Regional Planning from the University of California, Berkeley, and a BA in Architecture from Washington University in St. Louis.

Stephen N. Berg, AIA, is an architect and design leader at BWBR based in Saint Paul, Minnesota. Throughout his 18-year professional career, Stephen's passion for design has positively influenced spaces throughout the Midwest. He believes that design has the power to enhance experiences and offers design leadership and insight to a wide range of complex projects, from education to wellness and healthcare. Stephen has worked closely with Mayo Clinic on multiple projects and holds a degree in Architecture and Environmental Design from North Dakota State University.

Allen Buie, BA, M.ARCH, RA, ACHA, NCARB, LEED AP, is an architect and senior health planner with HDR. During his 18-year career he has led both planning and design for projects domestically and internationally, with a focus on award-winning pediatric and inpatient rehabilitation facilities. Motivated by what he considers to be design-focused planning, he seeks holistic design solutions that are beautiful as well as highly functional. The 2013 recipient of the Symposium Distinction Award for contributions to the realm of healthcare architecture, he seeks to elevate the healthcare experience for patients, families, and staff.

Brenna Costello, AIA, ACHA, EDAC, is a Principal at SmithGroup in Denver, Colorado and an architect with extensive experience in healthcare programming, planning, and design. She is a recognized expert in the planning and design of advanced rehabilitation centers, including the National Intrepid Center of Excellence, Bethesda, MD., a world-class facility devoted to military veterans recovering from traumatic brain injuries, and its ten satellite centers across the country. She has also led rehabilitation design projects for the National Rehabilitation Hospital, Washington, DC., Walter Reed National Military Medical Center, Bethesda, Md. Polytrauma Centers at the VA San Antonio Medical Center and VA Palo Alto Medical Center; and the Rancho Los Amigos National Rehabilitation Hospital, Downey, Ca. and Craig Hospital, Englewood, Co., two of the top rehabilitation hospitals for spinal cord and traumatic brain injuries. She holds a Master of Architecture and a Master of Architecture + Health from Clemson University.

Cheryl Desha is an associate professor and Director of Engagement (industry) at Griffith University (Australia), responsible for designing and delivering an unprecedented "twenty-first-century" civil engineering curriculum within a specially equipped new building. She is also part of the university's Cities Research Institute, focused on building capacity for sustaining livable and vibrant cities. For the past decade Cheryl has been working with colleagues in Australia and overseas to foster urban nature for resilient and livable cities, through whole-system thinking, biomimicry, resource productivity, decoupling, and sustainable business practice. Her career goal is to facilitate sustainable development by empowering society with emerging language, knowledge, and skills for sustainable solutions.

Steve Doub, AIA, CSI, has been with The Miller Hull Partnership since 2010, bringing over 20 years of experience in a wide range of project and building types and specializing in high-performance building envelope design. Leveraging his technical expertise, Steve has become a senior technical architect and project manager, as well as leading the firm's specifications effort. As specifier, he is responsible for reviewing all project plans and managing each permitting process. Working on design of the Bullitt Center, Steve served as a project architect.

Robin Guenther, FAIA, LEED Fellow, is a principal of Perkins+Will and senior advisor to Health Care Without Harm. Robin works at the intersection of healthcare architecture, health, and sustainable policy and participates in a wide range of leading-edge advocacy initiatives while continuing to practice. She is a Robert Wood Johnson Foundation Culture of Health Leader 2017–2019 and the co-author of two editions of *Sustainable Healthcare Architecture*. She co-authored the *Green Guide for Health Care* and served on the LEED for Healthcare committee. *Healthcare Design* magazine named her the "#1 Most Influential Designer in Healthcare" in 2010 and 2011. In 2012, *Fast Company* included her as one of the "100 most creative people in business". She co-authored the U.S. Department of Health and Human Services's *Sustainable and Resilient Hospital Infrastructure Toolkit*, and serves on the WELL Building Standard Advisory Board. She led one of the winning teams in the Kaiser Small Hospital Big Idea Competition and was a TEDMED 2014 speaker. Robin served as the project director for the expansion of the award-winning Lucile Packard Children's Hospital Stanford, which opened in 2017.

D. Kirk Hamilton, PhD, FAIA, FACHA, FCCM, EDAC, is the Julie & Craig Beale Endowed Professor of Health Facility Design at Texas A&M University, teaching healthcare design at the graduate level. His research is about the relationship of evidence-based facility design to organizational performance. He has a Bachelor of Architecture and a Master of

Science in Organization Development, and he completed a PhD in Nursing & Healthcare Innovation at Arizona State University, studying nurse movement patterns and interaction with objects in ICU patient rooms. A fellow of the American Institute of Architects, he is board certified by the American College of Healthcare Architects, and a fellow of the American College of Critical Care Medicine. With 30 years of active practice, he is founding principal emeritus of Houston's WHR Architects (now EYP Health). He has received the Lifetime Achievement Award from ACHA and the Center for Health Design's Changemaker Award. Kirk is a founding co-editor of *Health Environments Research & Design* (HERD). He edited *Area Calculation Method for Health Care* with Sarel Lavy (2017), and authored *Rigor and Research Design: A Decade's Advocacy* (2013); *Design for Critical Care: An Evidence-Based Approach* with co-author Mardelle Shepley (2010); and *Evidence-Based Design for Multiple Building Types* with co-author David Watkins (2009).

Jim Hanford, AIA, LEED AP BD+C, has over 25 years of experience in evaluating design strategies and technologies suitable for low-energy buildings. Jim joined The Miller Hull Partnership in 2005 and currently serves as a principal and Miller Hull's lead for sustainable design. He works with each design team to develop project goals, design ideas, and research and analysis tasks related to energy efficiency and building performance. Working on design of the Bullitt Center, Jim served as the building performance lead and specifier.

Chris Hellstern, AIA, LFA, CDT, LEED AP BD+C, is an author, architect, and the Living Building Challenge Services Director with The Miller Hull Partnership. Chris works to integrate sustainability in every project and focuses on occupant health, including materials toxicity, embodied carbon, and biophilia. He co-founded the Seattle 2030 Roundtable and the Healthy Materials Collaborative and also serves as an ambassador for the International Living Future Institute. He has been a speaker at national conferences, publishes articles, volunteers with school groups, and is an affiliate lecturer in the graduate school at the University of Washington, teaching sustainability and advocacy.

Eva Henrich is a healthcare specialist at Heinle, Wischer und Partner in Berlin. She is a registered architect, EDAC and LEED AP certified, and a member of the Association of Architects for Healthcare Architecture (AKG) in Germany. As a Fulbright grantee she received her Master of Architecture at the Clemson University Architecture & Health Program in 2011. Since then, Eva has worked on several hospital projects in Germany and internationally, including the University Hospitals in Berlin, Munich, Tubingen, Ulm, and San Diego. In addition to her project work, she focuses on the study of relationships between health, individuals, and the built environment and regularly shares her experience at conferences and seminars nationally and internationally.

Harm Hollander is a principal with Conrad Gargett (Australia) and has a desire to advance improvements in the healthcare environment. A fellow of the Australian Institute of Architects, Harm has also lectured in construction, professional studies, and design at various universities. He has developed comprehensive skills in leading large projects from commencement to completion, working meticulously through brief, design, and delivery challenges. He seeks to continually be informed by best practice in both strategic and practical health requirements, and this has seen him lead the health planning on major projects, such as the Princess Alexandra Hospital Redevelopment (opened 2001), Great Ormond Street Children's Hospital–Entrance Building (competition top three, 2017),

Zhejiang University Hospital (competition top five, 2013), and the Lady Cilento Children's Hospital (opened 2014), as well as speaking engagements at a number of conferences. As a Doctor of Creative Industries candidate, Harm remains the student in seeking further improvement in collaborations toward better design outcomes.

Keith Holloway is a licensed architect and a vice president at RLF, overseeing operations and architecture. With 30 years of experience at the firm supporting complex military projects worldwide for the Navy, Army Corps of Engineers, and Department of Veterans Affairs, he has extensive knowledge on delivering phased projects in operational mission-critical environments. Keith has been a driving force in the development of RLF's technology practices, successfully transitioning the firm to a fully integrated BIM platform. He is a well-recognized leader in the realm of technology and a past speaker at PDC, SAME JETC, AHCA, AutoDesk University, EcoBuild, AIA NTAP, COAA, and other organizations as an advocate for the advancement of technological practices. Keith holds a Bachelor of Architecture and a Bachelor of Science in Building Construction from Auburn University.

Klavs Hyttel, Chairman of the Board of Directors, Partner, and Architect m.a.a. at C.F. Møller, has been with his firm since 1986, interrupted by a two-year period from 1994 to 1996, in which he worked as an associate professor at the Aarhus School of Architecture, from where he also graduated. Klavs became a partner at C.F. Møller in 1997, and has since been responsible for a wide range of projects, including educational and cultural institutions, and commercial as well as residential buildings. However, the healthcare sector is one of his primary architectural fields, with the planning and design of many large and complex hospital projects in both Denmark and abroad. The healthcare projects have been awarded both nationally and internationally—for example, Architectural Review MIPIM Future Projects Award, Old & New category 2016; Design & Health International Academy Award 2015; Building Better Healthcare Awards 2009/2012; Civic Trust Award 2012/2014; and the AADAIH-IFHE award for Architectural Quality in Healthcare Buildings 2014. He has also received the Københavns Murerlaugs (Copenhagen Masons' Guild) Architecture Prize in 1999 and the Nykredit Architecture Prize in 2006. Klavs serves as adjudicator in numerous architectural competitions and has held a number of honorary positions, most recently as board member of the Danish Association of Architectural Firms.

Brett Jacobs holds a Bachelor of Science in Biomedical Engineering from the University of Rochester (2013). After working in numerous hospitals related to bioengineering he decided to study architecture, with special emphasis on healthcare environments. He enrolled in the Master of Architecture program at Clemson University in 2016 and received his degree in 2019. Immediately following, he became the inaugural Perkins+Will E. Todd Wheeler Fellow for emerging healthcare design and planning leaders.

Christopher W. Kiss, AIA, NCARB, EDAC, is a PhD candidate in the Planning, Design, and the Built Environment (PDBE) program at Clemson University, and a lieutenant colonel in the United States Army. Chris has most recently served as a medical program manager at a Military Medical Center Replacement project office in El Paso, Texas. He has experience with numerous healthcare projects in various states of design through construction and outfitting. Chris has a Master of Architecture from Norwich University and a Master of Science in Construction Management from Texas A&M University.

Shannon Kraus, FAIA, Executive Vice President, HKS Architects, has over 20 years of experience in planning and design at all scales. His work has been honored with design awards from both the AIA and *Modern Healthcare* as well as published in *World Architecture News* and *Healthcare Design* magazines. A provocative thought leader, in 2005 he served as national vice president at the American Institute of Architects, where he helped organize and lead the organization's knowledge and research agenda. In 2007 he launched and founded the HKS design fellowship, focused on bringing together designers across the globe for the purposes of providing design thinking to a community-based need. Most recently he served as a resource member for the National Endowment for the Arts–funded National Session of the Mayors Institute for City Design. His passion for how design impacts the health of communities was the focus of his TEDx Talk in 2017. In recognition of his contributions, in 2013 he was named a fellow by both the AIA and the ACHA. He has a Master of Business Administration and Architecture from the University of Illinois, as well as a Bachelor of Science in Architecture from Southern Illinois University.

Julia Leitman is a senior public relations coordinator at ZGF Architects, with a passion for writing, editing, and content creation. She enjoys crafting the ZGF story through a lens of high-performance design, sustainability, and stewardship of the built environment. Prior to ZGF, she worked at a global communications firm, supporting a diverse portfolio of corporate and sustainability clients, spanning design and construction, higher education, financial services, and footwear and apparel. She holds a Bachelor's degree in Strategic Communications from Seattle University.

Jeffrey Mansfield is a design director at MASS Design Group, whose work explores the mediated space between architecture, landscape, and systems. He received a Graham Foundation grant and was a John W. Kluge Fellow at the Library of Congress for his research on the topic "The Architecture of Deafness", and his work has been published in *The Economist*, *Cooper Hewitt Design Journal*, AD, and Tacet and presented at MoMA PS1, Bergen Assembly, Sao Paulo Biennale, and the Sharjah Biennial. Jeffrey holds a Master of Architecture from the Harvard Graduate School of Design and an AB in Architecture from Princeton University.

Katherine Misel is the communications specialist with The Miller Hull Partnership. Katherine works closely with firm leadership to develop, coordinate, and execute the firm's strategic communications plan, which includes writing and editing, media and publications, social media, research, information management, speaking opportunities, and other marketing needs. She received a Bachelor's degree in Journalism/Public Relations from Western Washington University, where she worked as a writer and editor for *The Western Front* and *Klipsun Magazine* before being hired as editor-in-chief of *Klipsun*.

Jamie Mitchell is the publications manager at Maggie's Centres. Before that, he worked as a journalist writing about architecture, interior design, and art for prominent magazines and websites, including *FX* and *Blueprint*. He holds a Bachelor of Arts in Multimedia Arts from Liverpool John Moores University, a Bachelor of Arts in English Literature and Creative Writing from The Open University, and a Postgraduate Diploma in Online Journalism from Goldsmiths College at the University of London. He lives in London and, alongside architecture and design, his main interests are literature, politics, and cooking.

Michael Murphy is the founding principal and executive director of MASS Design Group, an architecture and design collective that leverages buildings, as well as the design and construction process, to become catalysts for economic growth, social change, and justice. As a designer, writer, and teacher, his work investigates the social and political consequences of the built world. Michael's research and writing advocate for a new empowerment that calls on architects to consider the power relationships of their design decisions, while simultaneously searching for beauty and meaning. Michael's 2016 TED Talk invites viewers to question how architecture can be a tool for healing and the construction of dignity. He is an adjunct associate professor at the Columbia Graduate School of Architecture, Planning, and Preservation, has taught at the University of Michigan, Boston Architectural College, and the Harvard Graduate School of Design. Michael sits on the Clinton Global Initiative Advisory Committee, the Harvard Graduate School of Design Alumni Board, the board of the Center for Healthcare Design, and is an expert in residence of the Harvard Innovation Lab. Michael is from Poughkeepsie, New York, and earned a Master of Architecture from the Harvard Graduate School of Design and a Bachelor of Arts in English Literature from the University of Chicago.

Katharina Nieberler-Walker is a principal and head of landscape architecture at Conrad Gargett (Australia). She is an industry-recognized leader in landscape architecture, responsible for significant projects as designer and project leader in Australia and overseas. Katharina has a passion for biophilic urbanism and the development of nature-related design and the pedestrian-/people-oriented public realm. She has extensive experience in collaborating in large multidisciplinary teams to deliver client objectives. Her focus on place, the importance of nature in design, and the social context drives her when combining the natural and built environments in design. She is a keen proponent of sustainability, integrating cultural context and evidence-based design toward resilient landscapes. This includes using green infrastructure as an important climate change mitigation tool toward a thriving built environment.

Terri Peters is an assistant professor in the Department of Architectural Science at Ryerson University in Toronto, Canada. She is a registered architect in the UK and holds a PhD in Sustainable Housing from Aarhus Architecture School in Denmark. Her research explores the social and human dimensions of green architecture. Previously, she was a researcher at the University of Toronto, where she held a postdoctoral fellowship funded by the Social Sciences and Humanities Research Council of Canada. Her expertise is in sustainable design, digital design tools for environmental building simulation, and the adaptive reuse and renovation of modern housing. She has published 20 peer-reviewed journal articles and conference papers and is co-author of the book *Computing the Environment: Digital Design Tools for Simulation and Visualisation of Sustainable Architecture*, published by John Wiley and Sons in 2018. Terri guest-edited two issues of *Architectural Design* journal, one on mapping workflows/tools among leading sustainability research teams in design practice (2011), and "Design for Health: Therapeutic Approaches to Sustainable Architecture" (2017).

Birgit Prack was born in 1982 in Graz, where she studied art history, philosophy, and European ethnology, earning her degree with a thesis about the French photographer Henri Cartier-Bresson and "the decisive moment" in 2006. In the following years she focused on modern and contemporary art, working as a scientific and curatorial assistant in the Neue Galerie Graz am Universalmuseum Joanneum in Graz. Since 2016 she has worked with Dietger Wissounig Architekten, where she supports the architect's office as a project assistant and is responsible for press and public relations.

Angela Reeve is a senior policy manager in the Sunshine Coast Council (Australia). She has a PhD in Mainstreaming Biophilic Urbanism (Queensland University of Technology), and is an adjunct research fellow with Griffith University's Cities Research Institute. She is an environmental engineer passionate about fostering sustainable cities and systems through a whole-systems perspective and community-based initiatives. Over the last decade Angela has worked on a range of projects relating to behavior change, energy efficiency, climate adaptation, policy change, and resource efficiency.

Kate Renner, AIA, EDAC, Lean-Six Sigma CE, LEED AP BD+C, WELL AP, Associate, HKS Architects, specializes in healthcare and design research, with experience working with several top healthcare systems worldwide. She has worked to develop solutions to the many complex challenges encountered in the healthcare environment to create a healing space for patients, care teams, and the community. Passionate about continually improving projects, processes, and outcomes, Kate has worked extensively with the HKS research team, developing post-occupancy evaluation methodologies focused on overall impact. Most recently, Kate has developed a research fellowship program to expand research beyond the boundaries of the HKS research team to all project teams. Outside of work, she is active in the local and national design community, serving on a number of committees with the American Institute of Architects (AIA) and the U.S. Green Building Council. In 2016, Kate received the President's Volunteer Service Award for her work on the 2015 USGBC Greenbuild Host Committee and the Greenbuild Legacy Project, and she is a member of the Building Design and Construction's 40 Under 40 Class of 2016. Kate is a graduate of the University of Kansas with a Master of Art and a Master of Architecture.

Dr. Naomi A. Sachs, PhD, MLA, EDAC, is an assistant professor in the Department of Plant Sciences and Landscape Architecture at the University of Maryland. After earning a PhD in Architecture, she worked for two years as a postdoctoral associate with Professor Mardelle Shepley at Cornell University in the Department of Design and Environmental Analysis. Naomi is the founding director of the Therapeutic Landscapes Network and co-editor of the peer-reviewed *Health Environments Research & Design Journal*. She has published and spoken nationally and internationally on evidence-based design and the health benefits of access to nature. She is co-author with Clare Cooper Marcus of the book *Therapeutic Landscapes: An Evidence-Based Approach to Healing Gardens and Restorative Outdoor Spaces* (2014) and wrote the chapter on psychiatric hospitals for Cooper Marcus and Marni Barnes's *Healing Gardens: Therapeutic Benefits and Design Recommendations* (1999).

Bart van der Salm is an architect and interior architect. He holds a Bachelor of Design (Interior Architecture) from the ArtEZ Institute of the Arts, Zwolle (the Netherlands) and a Master of Architecture from the Academy of Architecture, Amsterdam, graduating with honors in 2014. His work on a proposal for an in-between home (Tussenthuis) for the last phase of a person's life, located within the medieval fortified city center of Zwolle, was nominated for the Dutch Archiprix Award 2015 for its integrated approach to landscape design and architecture for hospice facilities. He has also received recognition for his work via the Hedy d'Ancona Prize 2016 for excellence in healthcare architecture and presence on the shortlist for the Abe Bonnemaprijs 2018. Directly after graduating, Bart founded VANDERSALM-aim (architecture—interior architecture—model workshop) in Zwolle. The office recognizes an important role for the architect as a master builder and pursues a strong belief in sensitive architecture based on craftsmanship, well-being, and self-evidence. Landscape plays an important role in the studio's work, and assignments are often located in the area between towns and the countryside. Besides his work as an architect, Bart teaches at various architecture academies in the Netherlands (Amsterdam, Arnhem, Groningen).

Edzard Schultz is a principal architect and partner of Heinle, Wischer und Partner in Berlin. He is also the representative of the partnership. Edzard studied architecture at the Technical University in Berlin and is engaged in teaching and research at various institutions, such as the TU Berlin, Institute of Public Health, and Clemson University. He is member of the Association of Architects for Healthcare Architecture (AKG) and was appointed for the DIN 13080 (German Institute for Standardization) committee, which updates and revises the regulations and codes for hospitals and healthcare facilities in Germany. His work encompasses a wide range of complex projects, focusing on healthcare architecture with a holistic approach, including masterplanning, competition, construction, and evaluation. He is especially interested in the structural and communicative synthesis of the work of architects. Among his projects are designs and built projects as well as masterplans for several hospitals in Germany, including Charité University Berlin, University Hospital Munich, University Hospital Essen, University Hospital Tubingen, University Hospital Ulm, and community hospitals across Germany—for example, in Berlin, Brandenburg on Havel, Dortmund, and Munich—as well as projects worldwide—for example, in Italy, Poland, Israel, India, and Venezuela.

Amie Shao is a principal with MASS Design Group, a global nonprofit architecture studio. Amie directs MASS's research initiatives with a focus on health infrastructure planning, design, and evaluation. Her work is aimed at engaging and empowering stakeholders in the design process; supporting and substantiating the impact of design on health, social, and environmental outcomes; and translating research into guidelines that can be used to advocate for policy change. She coordinated the production of National Health Infrastructure Standards for the Liberian Ministry of Health and has been involved in the design and evaluation of healthcare facilities in Haiti, Africa, and the United States. Amie has also managed a range of research initiatives aimed at understanding the impact of the built environment on individual and community health, including a collaboration with Cincinnati Children's Hospital, studying the spatial needs of children with cerebral palsy, and more recently with Ariadne Labs on the impact of design on clinical care in childbirth. Prior to joining MASS, Amie worked for the Office for Metropolitan Architecture in Beijing, WORK Architecture Company in New York City, and EnSitu, S.A., in Panama. Amie received her Master of Architecture and a Certificate in Urban Policy & Planning from Princeton University.

Dr. Mardelle McCuskey Shepley, BA, MArch, MA, DArch, is the chair and an endowed professor in the Department of Design and Environmental Analysis and associate director of the Institute for Healthy Futures at Cornell University. She serves on the graduate faculty in the Cornell University Department of Architecture. Mardelle is a fellow in the American Institute of Architects and the American College of Healthcare Architects. She is LEED and EDAC certified. She has authored/co-authored more than 100 peer-reviewed works and six books, *Design for Mental and Behavioral Health* (2017), *Design for Pediatric and Neonatal Critical Care* (2014), *Health Facility Evaluation for Design Practitioners* (2010), *Design for Critical Care* (2009), *A Practitioner's Guide to Evidence-based Design* (2008), and *Healthcare Environments for Children and Their Families* (1998). To enhance the link between research and practice, Mardelle has worked full- and part-time in professional practice for 25 years and is founder of ART+Science design research consultants. She has led more than 50 design and research projects providing pro bono services to community partners. In 2017 she received the Changemaker Award from the Center for Health Design.

Peter G. Smith, FAIA, is the President and CEO of BWBR, one of the Upper Midwest's largest and oldest design firms, offering services in architecture, interior design, and planning. A licensed architect with more than 30 years in the profession, Peter has spent a major portion of his career in healthcare design and has overseen the firm's development of a knowledge management program that leverages evidence-based research to enhance healing and workplace environments. He is a member of AIA's College of Fellows and a graduate of the University of Minnesota.

Margaret Sprug, AIA, has been with The Miller Hull Partnership for nearly 20 years, bringing a passion for design and sustainability. Margaret is committed to continual improvement of the design process, believing that a better process will further design excellence. She has driven sustainable performance through seamless team integration, resulting in numerous award-winning projects and proving disciplinary integration leads to excellence in design that positively impacts our communities. Working on design of the Bullitt Center, Margaret served as project manager.

Megan Stone, founder and owner of The High Road Design Studio, is a pioneer of cannabis retail design, and has provided interior design and branding services to discerning cannabis retailers across the country since 2013. She has an Associate of Arts from the Interior Designers Institute in California and a Bachelor of Science in Marketing from the University of Minnesota's Carlson School of Management. She has won numerous awards for her work, including two 2018 Shop! Design Awards for Gnome Grown as well as recognition from Retail Design Institute as a 2017 Store of the Year Finalist. She also received the 2017 Shop! Design Award for Level Up dispensary and a 2016 Shop! Design Award for the TruMed Concentrate Bar. She has been honored with *design:retail* magazine's 40 Under 40 Award in 2016, and *VMSD* magazine's Designer Dozen Award in 2015. She is a contributing editor on design for *MG Magazine* and has been featured in *Forbes*, *Entrepreneur*, and *Cosmopolitan Online*. She has presented on her work at international conferences and trade shows in both the design and cannabis realms, including GlobalShop in 2017, the 2014, 2015, and 2016 International Retail Design Conferences, and the National Marijuana Business Conferences in 2015 and 2016.

Matthew Suarez, B.ARCH, AIA, ACHA, EDAC, is a health planning principal with HDR, and has been instrumental in the design and planning of numerous high-profile, large-scale replacement hospitals. He has a Bachelor of Architecture from the University of North Carolina at Charlotte, where he studied the impacts of the built environment on human behavior. He has focused his 17-year professional career exclusively on the understanding of world-class facilities, and he uses this professional knowledge to enhance the complete patient experience. The broad spectrum of domestic and international projects he has completed has won numerous national and international awards. Matthew received the 2016 Symposium Distinction Award for his contributions to the healthcare architecture profession; he has led multiple evidence-based design research initiatives; and his efforts have been featured in national publications.

Stephen Verderber, ArchD, NCARB, DP-ACSA, is a professor of architecture at the University of Toronto, where he has served as associate dean for research (2014–2018), is the founding director of the Centre for Architecture, Design + Health Innovation at the Daniels Faculty of Architecture, Landscape and Design, and is an adjunct professor at the Dalla Lana School of Public Health. He is a registered architect in the United States and founding co-principal of R-2ARCH. He previously taught at Tulane University and Clemson University, and holds a doctorate from the University of Michigan. He has received numerous awards, taught and lectured widely at universities in North America, Asia, and Europe, and published extensively in scholarly journals and conference proceedings. His nine books include *Healthcare Architecture in an Era of Radical Transformation* (2000), *Innovations in Hospice Architecture* (2006), *Innovations in Hospital Architecture* (2010), *Innovations in Transportable Healthcare Architecture* (2016), and *Innovations in Behavioural Health Architecture* (2018). His research-based design scholarship and critical practice activities explore the frontiers of history, theory, and design therapeutics for human and ecological health.

Dietger Wissounig, director of Dietger Wissounig Architekten, is an architect and certified civil engineer born in 1969. After graduating from the higher technical college for structural engineering in Villach in 1989, he went on to study architecture at Graz University of Technology, where he earned his degree with a thesis project in Klang Valley, Malaysia. In the following years he worked as a project architect for several offices in the fields of health service, residential building, and transportation. In 2003 he opened his own architecture office, Dietger Wissounig Architekten. In 2015 the office became a limited liability company (GmbH). Since 2005, Wissounig has earned several Austrian timber and state awards and international prizes. Furthermore, he has participated as a member of various boards, including having served on the board of directors for the Haus der Architektur (HAD), the architectural advisory boards of Naturpark Südsteirisches Weinland, Wels, Bad Klainkirchheim, and the society of Baukultur Steiermark, and the editorial board for the magazine *Zuschnitt*. He has also served as a lecturer on design at Graz University of Technology, and remains involved in architectural discourse through publication and practice.

Melanie Yaris is a marketing manager at ZGF Architects. As a passionate writer, she is interested in exploring design from every angle, examining how the built environment can influence human performance and well-being, and how environments uniquely respond to their programs, climates, and places. She is also a photographer and her work has appeared in the *Seattle Times*. She holds a Bachelor's degree from Washington University in St. Louis, with dual majors in Art History and English Literature.

Index

Note: Page numbers in *italic* indicate a figure and page numbers in **bold** indicate a table on the corresponding page.

Aarhus University Hospital *142*, 145–150, *145*, *147–148*, *150*
accessibility: and community health 160–161, 186–187, 219–220; and individual health 46–47, 51, 54, 85–86, 109–110
adaptability 143–144, 222, 297–299, 304–305, 361–362, 373–375; for program evolution and future expansion 41–42
aesthetics **78**, 79, **79**, 185, 209–211
affordable elegance concept 209–211
African Center for Excellence in Infectious Diseases (ACEGID) 353–357, *353–355*
age-specific spaces 36–37
Akershus University Hospital 143, *143*
alternative therapies 230; *see also* cannabis
ambulatory clinics *29*, *33*, 42
ancient civilizations 8–9
anti-prototype 351–358
arcades *147*
architecture *see* architecture for health; healing architecture; landscape architecture; preventative architecture; regenerative architecture
architecture for health: driving forces of 360–361, *360*; framework for *14*; scalar domains of consideration for 362; three domains of 12–18, *13*; trends moving forward 364–366; *see also* healing architecture
arrival 146–148, 160–163, 302–303, 305
art program 337–338, *338*
atriums 48, 88, *162*, 306, *306*; and pre-design planning 178–179, *178*; and residential care *50*, *53*
autonomy 43, 55; and designing for dementia 43–46; and the Erika Horn Residential Care Home 48–55; and the nursing home typology 46–47

Baton Rouge Health District 132–137, *133–135*, 369
beach chair 253–254, *254*
beauty 276–277
behavioral health 201, 300, 304; *see also* mental and behavioral health (MBH)
behavioral outcomes 78–73, **79**, *81–82*
biophilia **18**, 80, 251, 329–331, 339; and living buildings 273; and outdoor oncology 247; *see also* biophilic design
biophilic design 16, 311, 314–322, *316*, *321*, 324; the case for 328–331, *329*; case studies 332–339, *331*, **331**, *333*, *336*; and global rating systems 311–313; and inclusive rating system 322–323; and user well-being 313–314
brand 238–240; brand design 231–234
briefs 99–102, 179, 190–191, 288; brief development 170–176, *173*
built environment 16, 274–276, 280–281, 370–372, 378; influence on health 1–2; and regenerative design 283–294; and swarm rules 281–283
Bullitt Center 260–262, *261*, *265*, *267–271*, *273–275*, *277*, *277–278*; and beauty 275–277; and the Bullitt Foundation 260–261; design process 263; and energy 267–270; and equity 274–275; and health and happiness 270–272; and the Living Building Challenge 262–263; and materials 272–274; and outcomes 263–264; and place 264–265; and water 266–267
Bullitt Foundation 260–261, 264, 275, 277–278

calm 69–71, 211
cannabis 243; and brand design 232–234; and history and evolution 229–232; and interior design 235–237; and retail

design 238–240; and security-led design 240–242
carbon-neutral 267, 308–310
care delivery 73, 155–157, 162–163, 196
caregivers 25–31; efficient and effective workplace for 40–41; *see also* caregiver teams; employee wellness; staff spaces; workplace
caregiver teams: co-located *208*; multidisciplinary 28
Center for the Intrepid (CFI) 65–67, *66*
change: ability to accommodate 364, 372–375, *373–374*; over the life span of the hospital **156**, 166; transformative change 276–277
chapels *37*, 48, 84, 91, 92, 159–161
check-in 203–204, *204*, 210–211, 241
chemotherapy 108; *see also* Chemotuin
Chemotuin (Chemo-Garden) 247–248, *248*, 253–257, *254–256*
child-life 28, 36–37
circulation pathways *see* flows
civic wellness 8–9, *12*
client expectations 155, **156**, 159
client vision 155
climate change 280–281, 339, 371–372
clinical experience 29, 31, 33, 215
cohesiveness 220
collaboration 128–129, 206–208, *208*
co-locating **156**, 162, 167, 186–187, *187*, 354; and Lean Design 208, *208*
comfort 34, 172–173, 233–235, 238–240, 312–314, 355–357; environmental strategies for 353, **356–357**
communication 27–28, 62–64, 198–199, 208
community health 15–16, 127–128, 136–137; community health spectrum *118*; creating a healthy community 119–120; defining a healthy community 116–118; guidelines for creation of **117**; overview of **17**; planning typologies for *119*
comorbidities 58, 73, 76
conference room 71, *277*
continuous improvement 199–200, *199*, 203, 216, 282
corridors 32–33, 86, 87, 209, *211*, 347–348 courtyards 49, *53*, 108, 110, *126*; and biophilic design 320, 337; and employee wellness 217, *223*, 224; and local solutions in community health 348, 352–355, *353*, **356–357**; and mental and behavioral health

84–89, *86, 89*, 92; and outdoor oncology 248; and regenerative architecture 287; and superhospitals 146–147, *147*, 149
Craig Hospital 62–64, *63–64*
culture 335–337
curiosity 104–106, 221
current solar income 267–270, *268*

Dan Abraham Healthy Living Center (DAHLC) 227; design goals and solutions 218–226, *219–226*; evidence of successful design 226–227; goals and objectives 216; and Mayo Clinic's journey to wellness 214–216, *215*; programmatic elements 216–218, *217*; programs across levels *218*
dance therapy *61*
daylight: and community health 140–146, 222–224; and global health 271–274, 306–307, 312–314, 335–337; and individual health 35–36
decentralization 152, 154, 155, 163, 167, 269
dementia 43–48, 51–55, 81
democratic process 144
demonstration kitchen 136, 217, 225–226, *225*
design: brand design 231–234; design concepts 57, 62, 263, 306, 376; design goals 76, 100–110, **117**, 155, **156**, 159–166, 203, 218–226; design objectives 59, 191, 298–308; design principles 49–55, 146–150, 183–184, 286–287; design responses 1, 264–277; design strategies 31–42, 305–307; emergent 191–193, *191–192*; evidence-based 78–80, 140–144, 150–151, 323; evidence of successful design 226–227; green design 285, **291**; healing design principles 146–150; holistic approach to 203, 209–212, 229, 243; interior design 103, 232, 235–237; nature-inclusive 250–251, 253, 256; passive design strategies 286, 296, 305, 307, 310; patient-focused 30–31; pretest 364, 375–378, *376–377*; retail design 232, 238–241; security-led 232, 240–243; *see also* biophilic design; healthcare design; integrated design events; Lean Design; regenerative architecture
disabilities 75, 184, 288; *see also* rehabilitation care

Discovery Health Center 288–291, *289–290*

dispensaries 231–232, 243; and brand design 232–234, *234*; and interior design 235–237, *237*; and retail design 238–240, *239–240*; and security-led design 240–242, *242*

distractions 36–38, **90**, 169–170, 206–207

Dordtse Buitenschool *249*

durability 211; environmental strategies for 353, 355–357, **356–357**

dynamic blinds 269–270, *270*

eating habits 122, 225–226; *see also* nutrition

Ebola 350–351, 354, 357; treatment unit *347*

ecological health 13, 16–19, 260, 362, 378

ecosystems 16–19, **18**, **117**, 333–335

educational activities 36–37, *92*

efficiency 40–42, 203–209

employee wellness 213–214; *see also* Dan Abraham Healthy Living Center

empowerment 61, 106–108, 165

energy 260–263, 267–270, 272–278, 291–293, *293*; and biophilic design 311–312; and local solutions in community health 356–357; *see also* renewable energies

environmental press model 44–46

environmental qualities and features 78–83, **79–80**, *81–82*, **90–91**

equity 116–117, 274–275

Erika Horn Residential Care Home 43–44, *44*, 47–55, *47*, *49–50*, *53–54*

Eskenazi Health *329*, 330–339, *331*, **331**, *333*, *338*

Everett Clinic, The (TEC) 196, *197*, *205–208*, *210–212*, *212*; and circulation paths 206–207; and collaborative teaming areas 208; and a holistic approach to design 209–212; and Integrated Design Events 197–200, *202*; Lean planning and design process 201–202; and Lean thinking 196–197; and a one-stop shop concept 209; overview of 200–201; and a standardized clinical module 204–206, *204*; vision, guiding principles, and goals 203; and wayfinding 203–204

evidence-based design mental and behavioral health (EBD MBH) 78–80, 83, 90

exam rooms 28–31, 157–159, 201–209, *207*, 210, *212*

exercise 108–110, 185–186, 224–227

expansion 41–42, 62–63, *63*; and employee wellness 215, *215*, 220, *220*

exteriors: Aarhus Kommunehospital *142*; African Center for Excellence in Infectious Diseases *355*; Bullitt Center *261*, *265*, *267*, *270*; The Craig Hospital *63*; Erika Horn *44*; Everett Clinic *197*, *210*; Focal Point *127*; Maggie's Centres *100*, *102*, *104–106*, National Intrepid Center of Excellence *67*; Nemours *39*; The Next Door *92*; Parkland Hospital *153*, *160–161*; Queensland Children's Hospital *170*; Rancho Los Amigos *72*; Weed Army Community Hospital *303*, *309*

exterior spaces: balconies 48, *307*, 332–333; outdoor café *223*; Queensland Children's Hospital *183–186*; resiliency area *223*, *226*; roof garden *35–36*; trellis roof superstructure 354–355, *354*; *see also* courtyards; gardens; healing gardens; parks; plazas

facility size 320, 322

facility type *319*, 320–322, **321**

farms 289, *333*

Fibonacci *211*

fitness 127–128, 214–219, 222–227; fitness centers 127, *222*, 224

flexibility 41–42, 83–88, 203–206, 210–212, 222, 236–238; and the future of an architecture for health 360, 373–375; and remote locations 304–305

flows 40–41, 45, 174, 178, 241; and the consolidated health campus 163–164; and Lean Design 202–204, 206–209; and superhospitals 149–150, *150*

Focal Point Community Campus 123–127, *125–127*, 137, 369

galleries 77, *145*, 146, 354

gardens 29–37, *35*, 46–53, 71–72, 88–89, *89*, *90*, 91; and biophilic design 332–337; and Maggie's Centres 101–104, 107–108; *see also* Chemotuin; healing gardens

Gehry, Frank 105, *105*, 111
germ theory 9–11
global health 13, 16–19, **18**
green space 122, 182–183, 187–188, *188,*
   211, 268–269
guiding principles 198, 201, 203

happiness 115, 260, 263, 270–272; world
   happiness rankings 5, *8*
healing 169–176, 229–233, 247–253,
   256–258, 285–286; implementing
   healing design principles 146–151;
   and interior design 235–237
healing architecture 140–143
Healing Center, The 241–242, *242*
healing gardens 65, 71, 181–182, 193,
   328; and normalcy 182–190, *183,*
   185–190; and the role of landscape
   architecture in healthcare design
   190–192, *191–192*
health: determinants of 2–6, *3–5,* 12,
   118–120, 137; models of 6–11, *11,*
   369; recognizing health needs 57–58;
   see also behavioral health; community
   health; ecological health; global health;
   individual health; mental health; mental
   and behavioral health (MBH)
health campuses 16–17, **17,** 152–153,
   369; and the decentralization of care
   154; and health improvement goals
   155; and healthy community 115–120,
   117, *118–120,* 136–137; and the
   immersive planning process 155–157;
   integrated 120–127, *121–122,*
   124–127; overview of case studies
   for *121*; patient- and family-centered
   154–155; and wellness districts
   128–136, *129–135*; *see also* New
   Parkland Hospital
healthcare design 140–145, 190–192,
   196–197
healthcare spending 2–6; as a percentage
   of GDP *7*; in relation to health
   determinants *5*
health improvement goals 155
health intensity *366*
health outcomes 2, 116–117, 313–314,
   358, 359–360, *360*
holistic approach 140, 183, 203, 209–212,
   229, 243
hope 101–104
hospitals *see* hospitals without walls; rural
   hospitals; superhospitals

hospitals without walls 264, 367–370, *368*
human experience 31, 312, 259–261, *360*
human spirit 98, 110–111; and curiosity
   and imagination 104–106; and design
   for a diverse array of programs
   108–109; design goals and strategies
   for 100–101; and the first Maggie's
   Centre 99–100; hopeful and healing
   environment for 101–104; and
   inclusion and accessibility 109–110;
   and the philosophy and approach of
   Maggie's Centre 98–99; and self-
   reliance and empowerment 106–108

ideas 98–99, 116–118, 174–175,
   198–202, 222
imagination 104–106, 169, 187
inclusion 109–110
independence 46, 53, 58, 60–62,
   258, 308
individual health 13–15, 339; overview
   of **15**
inefficiencies 206–207, 298, 310, 346, 351
infrastructure 116–120, 346–353,
   362–364, 374–375
inpatient rooms 31, *39,* 300, 303–304,
   304; *see also* patient rooms
inspiration 62
Integrated Design Events (IDEs) 197–202,
   202, 212
Irresistible Stair 267–269, *267, 269,* 272

Jacobs, Jane 116
Jencks, Maggie Keswick 98; *see also*
   Maggie's Centres
John F. Kennedy Medical Center
   345–348, *345*
John Kane Hospital *345,* 346

landmark building 221, *221*
landscape architecture 62, 105, 176;
   African Center for Excellence in
   Infectious Diseases *355*; and biophilic
   design 311; and living buildings 266;
   and outdoor oncology 250, 253; *see*
   also gardens; healing gardens
Las Vegas Medical District (LVMD)
   128–132, *128–132,* 137
layouts 144, 347–348; universal 42; urban
   146; *see also* modular layout
Leadership in Energy and Environmental
   Design (LEED) 16, 29, 287–288,
   288, 311, 324; and biophilic design

patterns 314–319, *315*, *318–319*, **321**; and facility size 320; and facility type 320–322; and global rating systems 312–313; and inclusive rating system 322–323; and user well-being 313–314; and Weed Army Community Hospital 305, 309–310

Lean Design 196, 201; and integrated design events 197–200; *see also* Everett Clinic, The

Lean planning 201–202

Lean thinking 196–197, 199–200, *199*, 212

Level Up Dispensary 236–237, *237*

life-cycle cost analysis (LCCA) 305, 310

light 35–38, 62–71, **78**, 79, **79–80**, 81, 85–87, 89, 177–178, *271*; and biophilic design 337–338; and employee wellness 222–224; *see also* daylight

Living Building Challenge (LBC) 16, 260–263, *262*, 274, 278, 312; and beauty 276–277; and energy 267–270; and equity 274–275; and health and happiness 270–272; and materials 272–274; and place 264–265; and water 266–267

living buildings 16, *287*; *see also* Bullitt Center

living wall *223*, *224*

lobbies 69, *70*, *92*, 132, 161, 178; and biophilic design 339; and designing for distinct age groups 32–33, *32*, 35, 38, 41; and employee wellness 222, *223*, *224*; and healthcare retail design 233–234, *234*; and Lean Design 210; and living buildings *275*; and renewable energies in remote locations 306, *306*

Maggie's Centres 98, 110–111; design goals and strategies 100–110; first Maggie's Centre 99–100; Maggie's Aberdeen *106*; Maggie's Dundee 104–106, *105*; Maggie's Edinburgh 100, *100*, 104; Maggie's Glasgow 101–102, *101*; Maggie's Lanarkshire 108, *108*; Maggie's Manchester 102–103, *102–103*; Maggie's Newcastle 109–110, *110*; Maggie's Oldham 103, *103*; Maggie's Oxford *107*; Maggie's West London 104–105, *104–105*, 109; philosophy and approach 98–99

Maison Tropicale 343–349, *344*, 357

material choices 65–71, 85–86, 163–164, 233–235; and biophilic design 311–312, 320–321, 329–331, 338–339; building material transparency 282–283; and the Bullitt Center 272–274; and the future of an architecture for health 373–376; and local solutions in community health 343–344; material health in the workplace *283*; and regenerative architecture 289–293; therapeutic and sustainable material choices 211–212

Mayo Clinic 58, 213–216, *223*; campus *219*; demonstration kitchen *225*; fitness studio *222*; landmark building *221*; natatorium *224*; pillars of wellness *217*; project timeline *215*; resiliency area *226*; teaching studio *225*; vertical expansion *220*; *see also* Dan Abraham Healthy Living Center

Medical University Breslau *376*

mental and behavioral health (MBH) 76, 81, 93; environmental qualities and features for **78**, **79–80**, **90–91**; framework **79**; *see also* evidence-based design mental and behavioral health (EBD MBH)

mental health *see* mental and behavioral health (MBH)

MetroHealth 122–123, *122*, *124–125*

miasma theory 9–10

Military Health System (MHS) **18**, 296–297, 310; design objectives of 298–309

models of care *45*, 196, *360*

modern medicine 1, 9–11, 238, 260

modular layout 42, 204–207, *204*

multidisciplinary care 31, 59–60, 73

multidisciplinary teams *see under* caregiver teams

natatorium 217, *221*, *224*

National Intrepid Center of Excellence (NICoE) 67–71, *67–70*

nature 42–43, 77–82, **78**, **79–80**, 88–92, 177–179; and biophilic design 313–314, 329–333, 337–339; coexistence with 264–265; and employee wellness 222–226; innate connection to 328–329; and Lean Design 211–212; and living buildings 274–276; and outdoor oncology *250–251*; and regenerative architecture 284–288, 290–291; and superhospitals 140–141, 144–146; *see also* biophilia; Chemotuin

neighborhoods 115–119, **117**, 122–123, 128–129, 263–264, 272–274; inpatient 40, 42

Nemours Children's Hospital 28–30, *28*, 42; and an efficient and effective workplace 40–41; exterior at night *39*; and a flexible and adaptable environment 41–42; functional stacking *30*; inpatient room *39*; and patient-focused design 30–31; and a positive experience for patients and families 32–36; and a safe and secure environment 36–40; tower-level plan *33*

Net-Zero (NZE) 261, 266–268, 277–278, 308–310

New Parkland Hospital (NPH) 152–155, *153*, 166; design goals and strategies 159–166, *160–166*; master plan and program 157–159, *158*

Next Door, The 91–93, *92–93*

Ng Teng Fong General Hospital and Jurong Community Hospital (NTFGH-JCH) 18, 330–339, *331, 334, 336*

normalcy 182–184, 191, 193

Northwestern Memorial Hospital 369–370, *370*

nursing home *see* residential care

nursing units 78, *163*, 361

nutrition 108–109, 214–219, 225–227

office space 148; Bullitt Center 272–275, *273–275*

offstage flow *see* flows

oncology *see* outdoor oncology

one-stop shop concept 126, 154, 161, 209

onstage flow *see* flows

open space 187–188, *188*

outdoor oncology 256–259; and the Chemotuin 253–256, *248, 254–256, 258*; and grounding 251–253, *251*; and nature and healing 247–249; and nature-inclusive design 250–251, *250*

outpatient services 40–41, 57–58, **60**, 76–78, *175*; and biophilic design 338–339; and remote locations 298–300, 304–306

parks 2, 9–10; and community health 116–118, **117**, 123, 126–127, 136, 146; and global health 275–277, 369; and individual health 37, 49, 51, 65, 71–72; and New Parkland Hospital 159–161, 164–165, *165*

pathogenesis 9–12, *12*, 247

patient population 25–28, 41–42, 154, 212, 331

patient rooms: and biophilic design *336*; and the consolidated health campus 157, 163, 165–166, *166*; and designing for distinct age groups 28, 31, 36, 38, 40; and the future of an architecture for health 361, 375, 377; and mental and behavioral health **79**, 83, 86, 88–89, **91**, 93, *93*; and rehabilitation 60, 62–64; and remote locations 304; and superhospitals 141, 146, 148, *148*

physical activity 117–118, 217–218, 224–227; *see also* exercise; fitness

Pictou Landing Health Centre 285–286, *285–286*

plans: Bullitt Center *274*; The Everett Clinic *205*; Focal Point Community Campus *125*; MetroHealth *124–125*; and models of care *45*; Nemours typical tower-level plan *33*; New Parkland Hospital 157–159, *158*; Sahlgrenska University Hospital *88*; Tergooi Hospital *255*; Vermont Psychiatric Care Hospital *85*; Weed Army Community Hospital *300–302*

play 37–39, 42

plazas 47, 63, 72, 116, 134, 369; and biophilic design 333, 335; and healing gardens 183–185, *185*

point of care 28, 40, 366

pre-design planning 169, 179; brief development 174; building a project team 172–173; establishing a vision 174–179; and project-specific principles 170–172

pre-modern medicine 9–10

preventative architecture 351

preventative healthcare 351

program evolution 41–42

programming 48–49, 108–109, 157–159, *158*

prospect 188–189, *189*, 330, 339

prototypes 376–377, *377*; colonial 343–345, *344–345*; emergency

prototype 350, *350*; postcolonial development 346–349, *347*; prototype clinics 349; *see also* anti-prototype
psychological health 67, 270–272
public space 38, 61, 86, *161*, 352, 369; and living buildings 275; and pre-design planning *175*

Queensland Children's Hospital (QCH) 169–170, *170*, *175*, *177–178*, 179; brief development 174, *173*; building a project team 172–173; establishing a vision 174–179; and healing gardens 182–190, *182–183*, *186–190*; project-specific principles 170–172, *171*

Rancho Los Amigos National Rehabilitation Hospital *61*, 71–72, *72*
rating systems: global 312–313; inclusive 322–324; *see also* Leadership in Energy and Environmental Design (LEED)
Redemption Hospital 350–354, *350–352*, **356**
refuge 188–189, *189*, 256, 330, 369
regeneration 174, 226, 288
regenerative architecture 16, 280–281, *284–286*, 291; future of 291–293, **291**, *293*; in practice 286–291, *287–290*; and sustainability 283–284; and swarm rules 281–283; theory of 284–286
rehabilitation care 57, 73, 186–187, 258–259; case studies 62–72; and design objectives 59; and evolution of care 58–59; history of 58; key concepts 59–62; overview of needs for **60**; recognizing health needs 57–58
renewable energies **117**, 261, 291, 296, 310, 322, 324; *see also* Weed Army Community Hospital residential care 43, 55; and designing for dementia 43–46; and models of care *45*; nursing home typology 46–47; *see also* Erika Horn
resilience 226, 370–372, *371*
resiliency area *223*, *226*
responsibility 281–283
retail 120–122, 127–128, 229, 243; and brand design 232–234; and interior design 235–237; retail design 238–240; retail dispensaries 231–232; and security-led design 240–242
River Beech Tower 292–293, *293*

rural hospitals 296–297; *see also* Weed Army Community Hospital (WACH)

Sachs, Jeffrey 5–6
safety 36–40, 183–185, 235–237, 272–274, 361–362, 367–369
Sahlgrenska University Hospital 87–91, *87–89*
salutogenesis 8–9, 11–12, *11*, 247, 313, 323
Scandinavia 150–151; implementing healing design principles in 146–150; Scandinavian healthcare design 140–145
security 36–39, 53–55, 88–89, *89*, 128–129, 238–239; security-led design 240–243, *242*
self-reliance 106–108
senses 187, 189–190, *190*, 259
Smokey Point Medical Center *see* Everett Clinic, The (TEC)
staff spaces 40, 337
stairs *see* Irresistible Stairs
superhospitals 140, 150–151, 367; and building for the future 144; and democratic process 144; and healing architecture 141–143; and transformation of the healthcare sector 140–141; and urban layouts 146; and wayfinding 149–150; and zoning 146–149; *see also* Aarhus University Hospital
superstructure 354–355, *354*
supplies 40, 47–48, 164
sustainability 54–55, 260–264, 287–288, 291–299, 310, *371*; and biophilic design 311–312, 323–324; and regenerative design 283–284; and resilience 370–372; sustainable material choices 211–212
swarm rules 281–283

Tappita Regional Referral Hospital 348–349
teaching studio: Mayo Clinic 224–225, *225*
teams *see* caregiver teams; project team
Tergooi Hospital *248*, 253, *255*; *see also* Chemotuin
Texas Original Cannabis Company/Texas Original Compassionate Cultivation (TOCC) 233–234, *234*
therapeutic experiences **156**, 164–165

timber 292–293, *293*
treadmill workstations 224–225, *225*
Triple Aim objectives 155–157, **156**, 159, 196, 212
Tru|Med Dispensary 239–240, *239*
trunk and branches 177–179, *177–178*
typologies 119–121, *119, 121*, 254, 257–259, *262*

ubiquitous healthcare 364–367, *365*
Unilever Marketplace 287–288, *288*
unintended consequences 281–283
user experience 128, 141, 203, 209–212

value 197–203, 209–211, 277–278
VanDusen botanical Garden 287, *287*
ventilation 271–274, 335–337, 347–348, *352*, 353, **356–357**
Vermont Psychiatric Care Hospital 83–87, *84–86*
vertical reveals 209, *211*
views 35–36, 141–149, 164–165, 186–190, 274–276, 328–337
vision 154–155, 174–179, 203

waiting areas 101, *164*, 204, 233, 306; and designing for distinct age groups 34–35, *34–35, 38*; and rehabilitation 69–70, *70*
water **117**, 248–249, 260–263, 274–281, 287–289, 309–310; and biophilic design 311–312, 332–335; and

local solutions in community health 355–356; water independent 266–267
wayfinding 51–53, 69–72, 144–146, 149–151, *150*; and Lean Design 203–204, 206–207, *207, 211*
Weed Army Community Hospital (WACH) 296–298, *297, 299–304, 306–307, 309*, 310; and design objectives of the MHS 298–308; and net-zero and carbon-neutral 308–309
well-being 5–6, 91–93, 181–183, 191–193, 256–257; and biophilic design 311–314, 329–330, 337–339; and living buildings 270–272, 274–277
wellness districts 16–17, **17**, 136–137, 158, 369; and healthy communities 115–120, **117**, *118–120*; overview of case studies for *121*; the rise of 128–136
wetlands **117**; constructed 266–267, *267*, 276; restored 351–352, *351*, **356**
windows 46–48, 69–71, 88–89, 92, 100–102; and biophilic design 335–337, *336*; and Lean Design 210–211, *210–211*; and living buildings 268–277, *270, 277*
workplace 40, *283, 288*; *see also* staff spaces

zoning 128–129, *135*, 146–149, 264, 272, 275